1988

MEDICAL DIRECTION IN LONG TERM CARE

A Clinical and Administrative Guide

MEDICAL DIRECTION IN LONG TERM CARE

A Clinical and Administrative Guide

Edited by Steven A. Levenson, MD

(NHP) National Health Publishing

Printed in the
United States of America
First Printing
ISBN: 0–932500–61–7
LC: 87–62905

To the memory and the spirit of three grand old men:
S.R., R.V.W., and J.S.

Contents

        Steven A. Levenson, M.D.

Contributors

Kay E. Jewell, M.D.
Assistant Medical Director of The Wisconsin Peer Review Organization, Chair of the State Medical Society Committee on Aging and Extended Care, Consultant, Bureau of Quality Compliance, Wisconsin Department of Health and Social Services, Madison, Wisconsin.

Angelo J. Lucco, M.D.
Assistant Medical Director, Levindale Hebrew Geriatric Center and Hospital, Baltimore, Maryland.

Jane F. Potter, M.D.
Chief, Geriatrics Section, Department of Internal Medicine, University of Nebraska Medical Center, Omaha, Nebraska.

Elizabeth L. Rogers, M.D.
Director, Geriatric Faculty Training Program; Associate Professor and Associate Dean, University of Maryland School of Medicine; Chief of Staff, Baltimore Veterans Administration Medical Center, Baltimore, Maryland.

Susan G. Scholer, M.D.
Assistant Professor, Geriatrics Section, Department of Internal Medicine, University of Nebraska Medical Center, Omaha, Nebraska.

Debra S. Wertheimer, M.D.
Assistant Professor, Director of Geriatric Programs of the Division of General Internal Medicine, Department of Medicine, University of Maryland School of Medicine, Baltimore, Maryland.

Editor

Steven A. Levenson, M.D.
Medical Director, Levindale Hebrew Geriatric Center and Hospital, Baltimore, Maryland.

Foreword

As physicians become more involved with all aspects of aging and long-term care, greater attention must be paid to the many accompanying organizational and administrative concerns. Yet, medical literature is truly lacking in these areas. With this in mind, Dr. Levenson has written a comprehensive, scholarly book, describing models of physician participation in long-term care; the role of the nursing home medical director; and practical administrative aspects involving the physician's role, including quality assurance, infection control, utilization review, information systems, legal and regulatory issues, as well as ethical issues.

The medical director concept came about in 1974, following a series of seminars on medical directorship sponsored by the American Medical Association. In 1973, the AMA published *Guidelines for a Medical Directory in the Long-Term Care Facility* "to help ensure the adequacy and appropriateness of the medical care provided to patients." In May, 1974, the Department of Health, Education and Welfare (HEW) published regulations for participation in Medicare and Medicaid, requiring each skilled nursing facility to retain a physician to serve as medical director on a part-time basis. In 1977, the American Medical Association published the handbook, *The Medical Director in the Long-Term Care Facility.*

Topics related to long-term care have been the subject of increased continuing medical education of the American Geriatrics Society, the American Medical Directors Association, and specialty physician organizations, particularly within family medicine and internal medicine. In the last ten years, there has been greater interest in the concept of the teaching nursing home. Nevertheless, physicians serving in such capacities need more guidance and additional resources, with thorough analyses of their varied roles in the rapidly changing field of long-term care.

Dr. Levenson's book, *Medical Direction in Long-Term Care*, accordingly offers a comprehensive guide for any physician involved in any aspect of long-term care. He stresses the need to understand the complex problems involved in caring for the elderly from a physician's standpoint. Despite the increasing number of textbooks on clinical geriatrics, Dr. Levenson's book provides equally invaluable and practical information for the physician, describing the many components of long-term care. These include: models of physician participation, quality assurance, the long-term care team, economic and financial issues, and many other important issues. The book also examines information systems and computers in medical care, an area in which Steven Levenson has played a leadership role. Clearly, information systems and computers will be vital to the successful operation of long-term care facilities in the future. Dr. Levenson likewise provides significant information on legal, policy, and regulatory issues, as well as on managing ethical issues. The book also examines the teaching nursing home, and provides a look at the future of long-term care.

Dr. Levenson is a pioneer in a field which is still being neglected 14 years after the promulgation of regulations regarding the medical director concept. The book demonstrates his firsthand experience as a medical director of an outstanding long-term care facility. Of the existing publications in this field, *Medical Direction in Long-Term Care* will be a unique and thorough resource physicians will turn to for guidance and information pertaining to the organizational and administrative aspects of long-term care.

William Reichel, M.D.
Chairman, Department of Family Practice
Franklin Square Hospital Center
Baltimore, MD
Clinical Professor, Department of
Community and Family Medicine
Georgetown University School of Medicine
Washington, D.C.
July, 1987

Preface

While many editors may explain their books by describing what they are about, I will attempt to explain this book by first describing what it is *not* about. This is not a book about how to diagnose diseases in the elderly, nor is it about the biology of aging or the clinical aspects of aging. It is not simply about Medicare, hospitals, or nursing homes. Rather, it is a book about long-term care (LTC), about physicians and other health professionals, and about roles, attitudes, and goals.

The emergence of LTC has surprised everyone except, perhaps, for those who have worked in it over the past decade. Acute care, once the primary focus of mainstream medicine, has been de-emphasized, as expanded LTC services respond to greater demand. This is not so much because of relative merit, but because of the realities of demographics, society, and economics.

The acute general hospital of the past is not likely to ever again perform all of its traditional roles. Although many hospitals have begun offering LTC services, the hospital itself moves inexorably toward serving as a center for the treatment of severe acute and emergency illness. Meanwhile, many other facets of patient care have shifted into community-based and LTC operations.

Although it consists of both acute and non-acute care, geriatric medicine—medical practice concerned with the specific problems and needs of the elderly—is much more involved with the long-term, than with the shorter-term, acute care system. As one observer notes:

> Geriatric medicine is not a duplication of acute hospital rhythm, style, technology, and goals. It is an approach to health care that is based on realistic and attainable goals appropriate to the elderly, especially the frail elderly and the institutionalized elderly. Its rhythm fits the patient, not the health profession. Its major specialized instrument is the team concept. It is not only cost effective, but human effective (Libow 1982, 135).

Nevertheless, geriatric medicine is *not* the same as long-term care. Therefore, any assumption that the only important physician contributions to improving the LTC system are discovering more facts about gerontology, practicing good geriatric medicine, and teaching others to practice good geriatric medicine, is erroneous. All knowledge remains of mainly academic value unless it can be applied at some level. The discovery of new knowledge is not an end in itself, but a means to an end – in this case, the successful achievement of the goals of care for the geriatric patient. If the system in which that knowledge is to be applied does not facilitate the timely and consistent accomplishment of those goals, the knowledge is wasted.

The operation and management of the LTC system demands as much attention as the quest for scientific and clinical knowledge. How, for instance, is the physician even to know if the LTC patient requires his intervention in a system where observation and reporting of changes in patient condition is notoriously incomplete and inaccurate? One thesis of this book is that good medical practice is not enough and will be lost on this system without substantial thoughtful physician input into improving the system itself.

Therefore, admonishments about the failings of the LTC system and lectures to physicians about needing to learn more principles of geriatrics and attend more to other nonmedical aspects of their older patients' care are wasted, without equal concern for finding practical, cost-effective, efficient ways of delivering the care within the system and supporting those physicians and other professionals who often struggle to do the best they can, given the system's realities and limitations.

In fact, both geriatrics and long-term care are still evolving within a changing environment. We have yet, for example, to establish conclusively the details of what actually constitutes quality medical care in the NH and how best to achieve it. Public policy has greatly affected the practice of medicine at all levels – office, community, and institution. Accustomed to dictating the course of treatment and institutional policy, doctors must now consult other professionals, often sharing responsibility for more complex problems.

Physicians are still trying to ascertain their role in the LTC system and its institutions. With increasing medical involvement, numerous administrative and clinical questions arise. Not all the answers to the problems of LTC are known at this time. But often the first step in solving any problem is to know the right questions to ask. This book attempts to pose and clarify the questions that are being, and should be, asked, and to suggest some helpful answers. At the back of this book, a section entitled *Strategy Worksheets* offers the reader specific guidelines to achieve various tasks (e.g., establishing a geriatrics service).

Although some background information and theory is presented, this is mainly a "how to" book; that is, how does the physician in geriatrics and LTC go about selecting standards, establishing and managing programs, monitoring medical care delivery, and practicing medicine in the LTC system of the present and future? Some of it is grounded in information already in the literature, while much of it is new, simply because the literature on such topics is relatively sparse. Therefore, I ask the reader's understanding in those areas where information is somewhat thin and invite comments from those with programs and ideas they have also found successful, in the hope that any deficiencies of this initial effort can be subsequently alleviated.

Long-term care in the future means far more than its previous definition within the nursing home setting. It is a *continuum*, ranging from the bedbound nursing home patient to the ambulatory older person needing occasional medical assessment or intervention. This book will therefore cover not just the nursing home (NH), but the broader spectrum of LTC; everything, in fact, *except* the acute hospital setting.

Nevertheless, the NH is the centerpiece of LTC, and the main domain of the medical director. References to the "LTC facility" (or "LTCF") are sometimes used interchangeably with the "nursing home" (or "NH") because the associated principles are applicable, with some modification, in any LTC setting. In other cases, the term "NH" is specifically used where the idea is most pertinent to that setting.

In addition, while this book focuses on the medical director and medical direction in LTC, it is intended for *both* medical directors and the physicians practicing under their direction. After all, as a physician, the medical director must be aware of those facts which his medical staff needs to know, so that he can help them provide the necessary care. On the other hand, attending physicians need to understand the role and responsibilities of the medical director, so that they can understand what he does, what he expects of them, and why. Here again is an interchange of terms, as "LTC physician" may be used where ideas apply to both medical directors and practicing physicians.

Finally, women clearly constitute the vast majority of LTC patients, and more women are needed as medical directors. Therefore, all uses throughout the book of the pronouns "he" and "his" should be considered as merely a generic, more readable representation of "he/she" and "his/her."

In this book, we have tried to present the most information possible about a broad range of subjects. Clearly, not all LTC physicians, facilities, or programs will care to implement all the ideas and recommendations to the same degree. In fact, it may help to view these concepts on three levels: those necessary to provide *basic* quality care while complying with laws and regulations; those useful to achieve an *intermediate* level of care or to support more extended programs; and those that might facilitate *optimal* levels of care within an even broader spectrum of LTC-related programs. Ultimately, the appropriate level will be chosen based on the needs of patients, facilities, or programs. More importantly, perhaps, it will depend on the understanding, interest, and initiative of the involved physicians.

This book is intended to serve as both a sourcebook for all physicians involved in LTC and as an educational reference for those physicians who may become involved in the future. In addition, it is hoped that these suggestions and guidelines will help physicians provide quality care at reasonable cost and time investment, to dispel long-standing criticisms of inadequate and indifferent participation.

Reference

Libow, L. 1982. Geriatric medicine and the nursing home: A mechanism for mutual excellence. *The Gerontologist* 22:134-141.

Chapter One

A Brief History of Medical Participation in Long-Term Care

Steven A. Levenson, M.D.

Introduction

Like atomic energy, long-term care (LTC) is an issue with roots in the past, but whose problems are mainly unique to the 20th century. Until recently, the care of the elderly did not require a system, because there were not enough old people to utilize that system. Even now, it is mainly relevant to the industrialized nations of the West. The LTC concept is therefore relatively new, even though some pieces of the system (like the nursing home) have operated for many decades. In addition, significant physician involvement has been severely limited, if for no other reason than the lack of a medical foundation to adequately evaluate and treat the problems of the sick and disabled elderly.

The British medical community has a somewhat longer history of involvement in geriatrics, probably because of the inauguration of the National Health Service, and the subsequent recognition of geriatrics as a specialty. Since the British experience to some extent parallels our own, it is instructive to describe it, as well.

In both the U.S. and Great Britain, the care of the elderly has traditionally been linked with the care of the poor (Libow 1984). American nursing homes originated in the late 19th and early 20th centuries, in five types of facilities: county poorhouses, state mental hospitals, voluntary homes for the aged, proprietary boarding houses, and hospital-affiliated nursing homes. Prior to the Depression, U.S. state governments supported almshouses and other "poorhouses." Specialized institutions gradually evolved to care for those who were previously confined to these poorhouses. The poorhouses themselves were gradually closed by reformers in the 1930s and 1940s.

Meanwhile, the British in the 19th and early 20th centuries often handled the needs of the elderly in workhouse infirmaries. Unfortunately, these institutions attracted only the desperate. Such facilities were unable to address the needs of the growing elderly population. As a result, many patients were improperly assessed, treatable illness was not diagnosed, and numerous patients who should have been placed elsewhere lived in these institutions permanently (Coakley 1982).

In addition, since medicine has until fairly recently lacked the means to understand and treat cognitive, emotional, and behavioral disturbances, many impaired elderly have routinely been confined to mental hospitals, and have been given only custodial care. Today, as mental institutions increasingly are being (not always appropriately) cleared of their residents, LTC facilities have taken over the care of many of these persons.

Today's LTC system includes a voluntary, proprietary, and governmental sector. Forerunners of this system included homes for the aged, established in the late 19th and early 20th centuries by various immigrant groups and voluntary and religious organizations. As additional services were added, these evolved from voluntary homes for the aged into the voluntary, nonprofit portion of the nursing home (NH) industry. Such facilities have traditionally been among the first to provide skilled nursing, medical, and social services, and to serve as more sophisticated models of geriatric care.

The proprietary sector, by far the largest portion of the NH industry today, began in the late 19th and early 20th centuries as boarding home accommodations for those needing room, board, and limited personal care. It has evolved into today's multibillion dollar industry, striving to find a comfortable accommodation of the changing patient population and growing expectations for care and services, while still being mainly a business operation. The principal physician, traditionally the primary physician in the proprietary NH, is also attempting to find his place as the demands of more regulations, greater expectations, and sicker patients force proprietary NH owners and administrators to seek more medical input and support.

In the middle 20th century, some hospitals established nursing home affiliates as adjuncts, which have evolved into today's hospital-affiliated institutions, most of which are either governmental or voluntary (nonprofit). The Veteran's Administration NH-hospital network is probably the most extensive.

Government Support and Legislation

The Social Security legislation of 1935 marked a major turning point for LTC in the U.S. (Libow 1982). By providing income maintenance for the aged and disabled, residents could afford alternative arrangements to poverty-stricken old age. In 1950, additional legislation provided for means-tested aid to the disabled, similar to the Old Age Assistance (OAA) of Social Security. The 1965 Medicare amendments established a government funded payment program for hospital and physician services for the elderly.

The Moss amendments of 1967 offered the first federal authorization for establishing standards for nursing homes participating in federal funding. These included 24-hour nursing coverage, the services of a registered nurse (RN), and qualified charge nurses, as well as other regulations on such things as safety and drugs (Reichel 1983).

Amendments in 1972 replaced OAA and other previous legislation with the Supplemental Security Income (SSI) program, providing monthly payments to the aged and disabled, as part of a federally financed and administered program.

In Great Britain, at much the same time, similar reports and investigations to those in the U.S. led to the conclusion that hospitals should establish special geriatric services to handle the multiple complex needs of the elderly—which was done.

Physicians and Long-Term Care

Physicians have become involved in LTC in different ways. In the past, the physician role was limited by the near absence of genuine medical advances in geriatrics, leaving little more to offer than hand-holding and vague reassurances. Today, however, social imperatives, demographic changes, political involvement, and medical progress have all contributed to an expanded medical role in LTC.

L. I. Nascher (1914) is credited with having coined the term "geriatrics," as well as with having published, in 1914, the first American textbook on the subject. In 1942, the American Geriatrics Society was founded, to serve the interests of physicians caring for the elderly, followed in 1945 by the Gerontological Society of America, to facilitate a broader group of professionals.

Meanwhile, in Great Britain in the 1940s, Dr. Marjorie Warren was among the first to establish a geriatrics service. This hospital-based program included assessment, treatment, and rehabilitation. Around the same time, Bluestone at Montefiore Hospital in New York was establishing a home care program, which demonstrated the benefits of noninstitutional services for many of the elderly, and which was adapted by the English for some of their medical and social service needs (Coakley 1982).

Besides building up the institution-based geriatrics services, British primary care physicians also became attuned earlier than their American counterparts to the importance of the team approach to the care of these patients, and the need for close cooperation with and among many community-based agencies and resources. The British reimbursement system has also made such community-based alternative services as day hospitals and home health services more generally available than the American Medicare system, which has so far mainly paid only for some home health services to supplement institutional care (Coakley 1982).

Today, despite considerably more medical attention to the needs of the elderly, there are still probably only about 1,000 physicians in the United States whose primary specialty or practice emphasis is *geriatrics*, although the age 65 and older population clearly comprise a major portion of the practices of thousands of primary care physicians.

Most medical care for the elderly is provided by primary care physicians in private practice or in clinics, increasingly supplemented by physicians in HMOs or other prepaid programs. Given the small number of geriatricians, these primary care providers will continue to offer the bulk of medical services to the elderly for many years to come. Unfortunately, only a small minority of primary care physicians will even enter a NH to provide care for institutionalized elderly (Mitchell and Hewes 1986). There is thus still a disparity between care for the ambulatory, basically well elderly (the vast majority) and that for the minority with multiple complex medical and psychosocial problems and functional deficits.

Academically, geriatrics is emerging in the United States not as a specialty, but as an area of special competence – almost considered a subspecialty – in the fields of family medicine, internal medicine, and psychiatry. The rapid spread of fellowship training programs throughout the United States in the 1980s promises an unprecedented number of physicians with the interest, enthusiasm, and knowledge for the medical care of the elderly at a time of growing need (Beck and Vivell 1984). As yet, however, most of the graduates of such programs are filling academic manpower needs, while relatively few have dedicated themselves primarily to providing long-term care.

In the past, LTC has been equated with the NH, and physician involvement has meant little more than NH visits. The newer, far broader, concepts of LTC place the NH in its proper context, as one very important part of an overall spectrum of programs and services to the elderly. Physician involvement in LTC therefore encompasses a broad spectrum of activities and services.

The Medical Director Concept

As described in more detail by Reichel (1983), the medical director concept is less than two decades old, having evolved out of government investigations and subsequent regulations in the early 1970s. In collaboration with the American Geriatrics Society (AGS), the American Medical Association (AMA) proposed to the U.S. Department of Health, Education, and Welfare (HEW, now known as the Department of Health and Human Services, or HHS) that the position of medical director be required in all skilled Medicare and Medicaid NHs.

In 1973, the American Medical Association published "Guidelines for a Medical Director in a Long-Term Care Facility," setting forth a basic list of job responsibilities for the medical director. In 1974, HEW issued regulations requiring every skilled nursing facility retain a full- or part-time medical director, either directly by the facility, or through arrangements with local physician groups, medical societies, or hospital medical staffs.

Today's medical director certainly owes much to the tireless efforts of Herman Gruber (1977), whose efforts and influence with the American Medical Association's Committee on Aging in the early 1970s were largely responsible for the acceptance of the concept, and the establishment of the basic roles and responsibilities of medical direction (Reichel 1983).

As the position evolved, the medical director's role has at times been considered uncertain and unnecessary. Currently, medical directors are still required only in skilled nursing facilities (SNFs). Medical directors have often been expected to provide backup and minimal intervention, maintaining the status quo. It should be noted that many physicians and administrators still feel that formal medical staffs and vigorous medical administration are not practical in the vast majority of NHs (Blumberg 1984).

Unfortunately, minimal involvement has often been viewed as reflecting disinterest and deficiencies of care. Several reports—most recently, that of the Institute of Medicine (1986)—have suggested that while most of the medical community's energies have gone into treating the acutely ill in high-technology hospitals, physicians have largely shunned their responsibilities for caring for nursing home patients, and for monitoring that care. Patient care in long-term-care facilities is hampered by poor physician motivation, low payments for services, and a shortage of capable and well-motivated support personnel and equipment.

Today, the roles, job descriptions, interest, and participation of medical directors still differ considerably throughout the country. Expectations are often vague and nonspecific, or mainly reflect what a facility or nursing director needs, rather than an understanding of what a medical director *could* do. Because medical care in LTC has often been separate from other aspects of care, medical directors have often been distant from the needs and problems of other staff, and the institution as a whole. Unfortunately, in most American NHs, while the principal physician or medical director has reported to the administrator, owner, or board, he has not had any real authority because no one has reported directly to him. This is an untenable situation, lacking real incentives to improve without appropriate feedback or without consequences for inadequate performance.

But this may change for several reasons. First, there are many degrees of organization, and even the least organized setting can have *some* basic order. Second, already, shifts to older, sicker, and more functionally impaired patients are sure to require more frequent medical attention, and will inevitably require some adjustments in medical input and organization. Efforts are now underway to try to produce a more standardized basic list of medical director responsibilities and objectives.

Today, given the importance of LTC in care of the elderly, and increasing expectations for a positive outcome of such care, the medical role looms ever larger. Advocates of greater medical involvement suggest that physicians can help correct a broad spectrum of deficiencies, not just in medical care, but in physical environment, infection control, and employee health, among other things.

The following chapters will, among other things, focus on the prospects for merging the past and the present into a coherent whole for physicians who will be caring for the elderly *and* managing, or helping manage, the services and programs for such care in the future.

References

Beck, J. C. and S. Vivell. 1984. Development of geriatrics in the United States. Volume 2, Chapter 5 in ed. by Cassel, C. K., and J. R. Walsh, *Geriatric Medicine* (2 volumes). New York: Springer-Verlag.

Blumberg, H. 1984. The role of the nursing home medical director. *Minnesota Medicine*, Feb. 1984, 109.

Coakley, D. 1982. *Establishing a Geriatric Service*. London: Croom Helm.

Gruber, H. W. 1977. The medical director in the nursing home—a catalyst for quality care. *Journal of the American Geriatrics Society* 25:497-499.

Institute of Medicine. 1986. *Improving the quality of care in nursing homes*. Washington, D.C.: National Academy Press.

Libow, L. 1982. Geriatric medicine and the nursing home: A mechanism for mutual excellence. *The Gerontologist* 22:134-141.

Libow, L. 1984. The teaching nursing home: Past, present, and future. *Journal of the American Geriatrics Society* 32:598-603.

Mitchell, J. B. and H. T. Hewes. 1986. Why won't physicians make nursing home visits? *The Gerontologist* 26:650-654.

Nascher, L. I. 1914. *Geriatrics: The diseases of old age and their treatment*. Philadelphia: Blakiston & Sons & Co.

Reichel, W. 1983. Role of the medical director in the skilled nursing facility: historical perspectives. In ed. by W. Reichel. *Clinical aspects of aging (2nd ed.)*, Baltimore: Williams and Wilkins, 570-579.

For Further Reading

American Medical Association Committee on Aging, Council on Medical Service. 1973. *Guidelines for a medical director in a long-term care facility.* Chicago: American Medical Association.

Gladue, J. R. 1974. Evolution of the medical director concept. *Journal of the American Geriatrics Society* 22:43.

Shaughnessy, M. E. 1973. The role of the medical director in the nursing home. *Journal of the American Geriatrics Society* 21:569.

Chapter Two

Long-Term Care: Components and Goals

Steven A. Levenson, M.D.

Chapter Objectives

This chapter will:

- Discuss the sudden growth of long-term care
- Describe the general components of the LTC system
- Explain the major goals of LTC and how they differ from those of acute care
- Illustrate the need for more physician involvement in long-term care
- Discuss alternatives to institutionalization
- Review alternatives for the arrangement, management, and control of services for the elderly
- Offer some suggestions to help physicians recommend appropriate LTC plans to their patients.

The Growth of Long-Term Care

As the number of elderly—especially those over age 85—grows rapidly there is a remarkable increase in chronic, disabling, and degenerative conditions. In addition, many older people suffer acute illnesses and injuries either associated with, or which worsen, those chronic problems.

In the past, older persons admitted to acute hospitals were treated for their acute illnesses, and then discharged home or to a nursing home, left to fend for themselves. Attention to functional status, mental changes, or community and family support systems was not generally considered the proper realm of the physician.

Today, we recognize that the treatment of acute or chronic illness alone is insufficient for adequate care of the older patient. Function is often more important than illness, and the maintenance and restoration of function often become central to this care.

Unlike acute care, LTC is not provided almost exclusively by trained medical and nursing specialists, but may be rendered by the elderly individual, the individual's family, neighbors, formal or informal community supports, institutions, private providers, or government.

For the health care professional, delivering LTC services is often time-intensive and costly, requiring extensive evaluation, multidisciplinary collaboration, extended treatment periods, and long-term follow-up. This is in marked contrast to the acute care setting, in which immediate treatment of an acute illness may be the beginning and the end of medical attention for years at a time, except for occasional office or clinic visits.

Though the NH remains the centerpiece of LTC, and will continue to command the most medical attention, LTC medicine is neither solely the practice of clinical geriatrics nor merely the provision of NH care. Rather, it is the application of knowledge and skills about the problems of the elderly, *coupled with* knowledge and skills about choosing and applying the many possible people, services, therapies, programs, options, and plans that might help deal with those problems.

Even now, for instance, physician involvement in the research and clinical (diagnostic and treatment) aspects of geriatric medicine is far greater than in these ancillary areas. This unbalanced perspective is probably the result of trying to apply old perspectives to a field emerging in a wholly new era of medical care and practice. A new balance will have to be struck before long.

Goals of the LTC System

Increasingly, physicians are being asked to help set standards for LTC – not just for physician performance, but for the entire system. As with everything else, however, we must first establish our goals before we try to establish standards which tell us how best to meet those goals.

A systematic approach to analyzing the medical role, needs, or performance standards for LTC is still widely lacking. Ultimately, greater physician participation in each of these areas will encourage further clarification of goals for system design and outcomes of care.

In acute care, the major medical goal for the individual is resolution of an acute illness and return to his previous setting. In LTC planning, however, additional factors beyond illness affect subsequent care or placement.

Categories of desired outcome in LTC may include:

- maximum functional independence

- humane care (including terminal care)

- prolonged longevity

- prevention of avoidable medical and social problems (Vogel and Palmer 1982, 11).

Each one of these categories demands a somewhat different approach.

For example, fostering maximum functional independence for one patient may require a plan centered around a rehabilitation program, with little medical intervention, while prolonging life for another patient may emphasize direct medical intervention to treat one or more acute illnesses or complications.

Another prominent feature of LTC is that the goals for the elderly are not monolithic. They vary among individuals, and they change at different times for the same person. Depending on the current medical problem, the underlying chronic condition, the prognosis, and the persons's wishes, the same person may be a candidate at various times for a program designed to cure an acute illness, maintain function and prevent further deterioration, restore full function, die comfortably, or control difficult behavior.

Medical training and expertise to care for the elderly center on correctly diagnosing, and on choosing and implementing selected treatments and prescriptions. Reversal of treatable mental status changes, for example, requires physician expertise in diagnosis, testing, and prescribing. Setting the *goals* for that treatment or care, however, is not solely a medical prerogative, and may sometimes hardly involve the physician. Nevertheless, choosing the goals and implementing the measures to achieve them are tightly intertwined.

Even as the prescriber of final authority, the physician practicing LTC medicine cannot act properly without considering and including patient, family, and other health professionals in the decision-making processes. This is an unfamiliar situation for the traditionally trained doctor, and still makes many feel uncomfortable. Part of the requisite physician reorientation is to accept and adapt to this different position.

In addition, LTC decisions are increasingly influenced by broader social and political objectives, such as conforming with regulations, meeting the needs of constituents, or controlling costs.

The Expanded Physician Role

The LTC system also has certain major administrative and organizational functions, including:

- reference and referral
- assessment and reassessment
- monitoring of use
- client advocacy
- maximizing available financial resources
- coordination of the timing of services
- reporting gaps in services
- creating cooperative agreements
- purchasing services
- case finding (Vogel and Palmer 1982, 17).

Inevitably, many physicians will become involved in at least some of these administrative and organizational activities, perhaps by:

- receiving a patient referred from a social service or nursing agency
- referring a patient to such agencies
- evaluating a longstanding patient for new mental or physical problems
- following up on prior treatment or referral
- consulting on a patient referred by a colleague
- treating a patient in a nursing home
- completing forms for placement, evaluation, or legal or financial matters
- becoming involved in administration, management, or planning for a LTC system, program, or agency.

Thus, in considering their role and participation, physicians should keep the following general guidelines for good LTC management in mind:

- Facilitate the easiest possible access to the LTC system for the dependent person and his family.
- Try to help maintain individuals in their "natural" setting for as long as possible.
- Coordinate medical services with other LTC professionals and services.
- Consider overall individual goals and objectives to be as important as diagnoses and treatment in care planning.
- Recognize that any such care plans may need to be recast from time to time, as a person's needs and condition change.

The System's Constituency

The LTC system does not just serve the elderly. For example, chronic rehabilitation facilities serve large numbers of younger trauma victims for extended periods, and psychiatric facilities treat persons of all ages over many years. Though the focus of this book is on LTC for the elderly, many of the same principles apply to any LTC system.

The number of elderly in the community needing supportive care is not precisely known. Kane (1984, 383) estimates that there are three similarly disabled persons living in the community for each person living in an institution. If we equate the need for assistance with the presence of some disability limiting a person's ability to perform an activity of daily living (ADL) or instrumental activity of daily living (IADL), then 19% of those 65 and older have some limitation, with disability rates increasing with age from 12.6% of those 65 to 74, to 45.8% of those 85 and older (Senate Special Committee 1986, 87). For the most part, people in need of assistance require services that can be provided only by another person (National Center for Health Statistics 1986, 2). The number of dependent elderly in need of assistance living in the community in 1985 was approximately 5.2 million, with that number expected to double between 1985 and 2020 (Day 1985, 6).

Thus, the elderly constituency for LTC spans a wide spectrum, including the institutionalized, the homebound, the partially functional, the mentally impaired, the chronically ill, and the mostly well. But the NH population as a rule consists of those with:

- multiple concurrent chronic illnesses
- some cognitive, emotional, or behavior impairments
- reduced functional capacity
- a need for daily nursing care and some periodic medical care
- a higher risk for injury and acute illness
- advanced age (average 80-83 in many studies)
- high mortality
- a female:male ratio of 2:1 or more

- prescriptions for an average of 6-10 medications daily
- extensive previous medical histories
- considerable, often incomplete, medical records.

The number of elderly in NHs has increased both in absolute numbers and as a percentage of the elderly. In 1970, 0.8 million elderly were in homes for the aged or disabled (4% of the elderly population), while 1.2 million were in NHs in 1980 (4.8% of the elderly), representing an annual increase of 4.5% (Waldo and Lazenby 1984, 13). By 1985, this increased to an estimated 1.5 million elderly (about 5% of the elderly population) in NHs. The NH population is expected to more than double again between 1985 and 2020 (Day 1985, 6). The rate of NH use by the elderly has almost doubled since the introduction of Medicare and Medicaid.

The proportion of the elderly in NHs varies with age, currently 2% of those age 65 to 74, 7% of those 75 to 84, and 16% of those 85 and older (Senate Special Committee 1986, 97). The portion of NH residents requiring assistance in one or more ADLs also varies with age, from 86% of residents age 65 to 74, to 96% of those 85 and older (Waldo and Lazenby 1984, 13).

About two-thirds of NH residents stay for one year or more, while 1 in 4 stays less than 6 months. Most NH residents require assistance with activities of daily living, especially bathing, walking, dressing, and toileting. Only a minority (1/5 to 1/3) have significant sensory impairments. Most have adequate vision and hearing for reading, watching television, or carrying on conversations.

A growing number of NH residents have enough cognitive, emotional, or behavioral dysfunctions, such as agitation, aggression, wandering, depression, or withdrawal, to cause some management or treatment problems.

Components of the LTC System

In the past, LTC and nursing home care were often considered synonymous. But the newer concept of LTC is as a *system*, not as an institution or a single program (see Fig. 2-1). In addition, LTC is care delivered over time, rather than at one time.

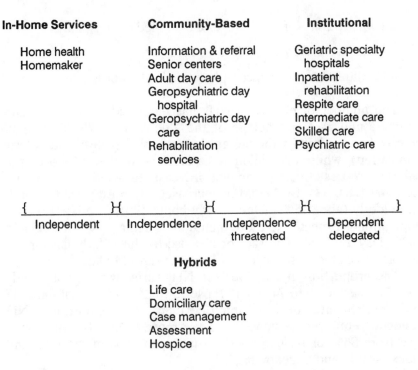

Figure 2-1 The continuum of long-term care services.

One way to categorize the components of this system is according to site, which may be *home-based, community-based, institutional, or some hybrid* of these. Since dysfunction, rather than illness, is usually the most important determinant of need, it also helps to divide the LTC system components according to individual functional levels. Four major dependency categories range from independent, to independence threatened, to independence delegated, to dependent.

Thus, a person who has been medically stable for years, for example, with mild osteoarthritis or asymptomatic coronary artery disease, may be considered independent until he starts to have trouble sleeping, shopping, or keeping house, because of progressive congestive heart failure or dementia, at which time he would be considered in the "independence threatened" category. Later, if he became chairbound or too confused or weak to care for his basic personal needs, he would be considered dependent.

Home-Based Services

In-home services include home health services, meals on wheels, homemaker assistance, and supervised living.

Home health services include the following provisions: part-time or intermittent nursing care provided under the supervision of a registered nurse; physical, occupational, or speech therapy; medical social services under a physician's direction; part-time or intermittent services of a home health aide; and medical supplies other than drugs. Such services are usually provided by a public or private agency, such as the Visiting Nurses Association.

The home health nurse, or visiting nurse, is a licensed nurse who goes into the home, and may assist with activities of daily living (ADL), dispense medicines, monitor blood pressure or other vital signs, evaluate changes in condition, and issue periodic telephone or written reports to the treating physician.

The home health aide is an unlicensed person who assists an older person, under the supervision of a registered nurse, in personal care, ambulation and exercise, household services essential to health care at home, and in the taking of self-administered medications; who observes and reports changes in condition and needs; and who completes appropriate records.

The *homemaker* is an unlicensed person—often another elderly individual—who goes into the home to assist in various chores, such as cleaning or cooking.

Community-Based Services

Community-based services include information and referral, senior centers, day care, day hospitals, mental health services, and rehabilitation.

Information and referral is a community-based nonmedical program serving one or several functions, including: providing lists of aging-related agencies, programs, and practitioners; providing information on self-care, prevention, illnesses, or medications; and channeling individuals both into and within the system.

Senior centers are community-based programs, often owned and operated by local governments, which function as recreational and social sites that generally provide one meal, but no licensed or supervised medical, nursing, or social services. They may offer educational programs on health-related topics, and they can serve as a source of referral to local health agencies, programs, and practitioners.

Adult day care offers programs that provide adults with various health and social services in a supervised ambulatory group setting. There are currently over 1,000 adult day care centers in the U.S. They may be sponsored by government, hospital, religious, or other agencies.

Adult day care generally exists as either a freestanding facility or as part of another institution, such as a NH. Participants are transported to and from home, usually three to five days per week. The programs are supervised by a licensed nurse, and must comply with many federal and state regulations.

Adult day care services may be categorized as *restorative* (moderately intensive health care focus including active therapy); *maintenance* (longer duration emphasizing individual care plans with less intense monitoring and treatment); or *social* (mostly activity-oriented). They may include some nursing care and medication administration, nutrition, meals, activities, social services, and various evaluations, such as hearing, speech, and podiatry.

Since most adult day care patients are functionally disabled to some degree and require some assistance with ADL, rehabilitation services, including physical, occupational, and speech therapy, and psychological testing and treatment are often included.

Adult day care is helpful for those individuals who need partial assistance with their ADL, monitoring or observation, or good nutrition; or who are socially isolated or confused, unable to manage personal care and hygiene, or who are physically or functionally impaired. Adult day care often complements other services, such as domiciliary care, home health, and homemaker services. While any of these alone might not suffice, the combination is often enough to help keep the older person in the community, especially by allowing family members some respite from responsibilities.

The physician's duties include referral, patient management and follow-up, completion of necessary forms, and communication with adult day care staff regarding patient problems or needs.

The *day hospital* is not a hospital at all, but a program of intensive goal-directed medical, rehabilitation, or psychiatric services which would otherwise be provided in a hospital setting. The goal is to provide the services without the hotel costs, and other attendant problems of hospitalization.

Geropsychiatric day hospitals (GDH) provide intensive psychiatric treatment to older persons whose problems are severe enough to otherwise require an inpatient stay. Active psychotherapeutic and psychopharmacologic management for a limited time is emphasized, with the goal of stabilizing or improving the individual as quickly as possible. Experienced multidisciplinary professionals treat patients directly, rather than merely supervising nonprofessionals. These are usually located in the acute general or psychiatric hospital setting.

Geropsychiatric day treatment programs (GDTP) offer psychiatric supervision, and drug and psychotherapy treatments with limited rehabilitation and social services for persons with problems not severe enough to otherwise require inpatient treatment. Emphasis is on maintenance of current function and independent living. Though time limited, treatment is usually longer than in the GDH. These services are often offered as part of an adult day care program, rather than as a separate program.

Rehabilitation programs offer supervised physical, occupational, and speech therapy programs to which patients are transported on a regular basis as needed. These are usually based in hospital rehabilitation or outpatient centers, or in freestanding facilities.

Institutional Services

Institutional services include geriatric specialty hospitals, inpatient rehabilitation, respite care, and skilled and intermediate nursing care.

Geriatric specialty hospitals, sometimes referred to as subacute or chronic hospitals, are licensed in some states as nonacute hospitals, which in fact provide acute, postacute, and chronic medical and nursing services, plus patient assessments and such specialty services as care for incontinence and severe decubitus ulcers. Elderly individuals in these settings require much more extensive medical or nursing attention than in the NH, but less high-powered medical and technological intervention than in the acute hospital. Such programs are also likely to provide an important foundation for the geriatric medical center of the future, which could offer many of the same diagnostic and treatment programs that were once part of an acute hospital stay, but at much less cost.

Inpatient rehabilitation units, licensed at either the acute, specialty hospital, or skilled levels, offer intensive, short-term, goal-oriented rehabilitation services, including physical, occupational, and speech therapies, plus medical intervention, and often the services of a rehabilitation medical specialist (physiatrist).

Respite care is a program of supervised short-term institutional placement of individuals usually cared for at home or in the community, often to allow caretakers to take vacations, enjoy a break from responsibilities, or deal with emergencies.

The *nursing home* (NH) is the centerpiece of LTC. While residential care facilities emphasize protected living arrangements and minimal assistance with psychosocial, activity, and personal care needs, NHs provide around-the-clock medical and nursing care, as well as other social services.

The 1982 National Master Facility Inventory of Nursing and Related Homes noted 17,819 NHs in the United States excluding residential facilities, hospital-based facilities, and 238 nonresponding facilities. These homes account for about 1.5 million beds. Three-quarters of all homes and 71% of all beds are under *proprietary* (for-profit) ownership. Five percent are government operated and 20% are nonprofit institutions, with 7% and 22% of the beds, respectively (National Center for Health Statistics 1985, 3).

Of all NHs, fully 40% have under 50 beds, 3 of 10 have 50 to 99 beds, 1 in 5 have 100-199 beds, and only about 5% have over 200 beds.

The staffing ratio per 100 beds in the NH is only about 1/6 that of the community hospital. With lower levels of care, there are fewer of both general staff and skilled nursing staff.

NH levels of care have frequently been classified as either *Intermediate care facilities (ICFs)* or *skilled nursing facilities (SNFs)*. The ICFs provide health care to those who require less than hospital or skilled NH, but more than domiciliary care. This would include homes for the aged and the institutionalized mentally retarded, and some homes classified previously as Medicaid SNFs. *Skilled nursing facilities (SNFs)* provide more intensive nursing care than ICFs. The distinctions between ICF and SNF are often representative of a particular state's definition rather than of any clear differences in needs, and many facilities now house ICF and SNF patients on the same units.

For payment purposes, however, Medicare has explicit criteria for the skilled level, and will not presently reimburse for ICF services, while Medicaid will generally pay for both, for those who meet the eligibility criteria (See Chapter 8).

Hybrid Services

Hybrid services include life care, domiciliary care, hospice, case management, and assessment.

Life care is a hybrid of inpatient, home, and community-based services and benefits, ranging from housing to medical care, usually arranged as a package for an initial entry fee plus additional monthly fees. Typically, the housing choices may include apartments, condominiums, or a room in a nursing home. Medical care includes prescription medicines, professional counseling, preventive and screening programs, and various physician and nursing services.

Domiciliary care, another hybrid of institutional and community-based care, refers to arrangements for providing food, shelter, and limited supervision in a home-like setting. Definitions and applications vary widely, and may include foster homes, private homes, family home care, and community residences. One proposed definition is:

> ... any facility, operated for profit or otherwise, which accommodates or is designed to accommodate two or more adults unrelated to the owner or operator and which provides room and board on a 24 hour basis to primarily non-transient aged or handicapped (physically or mentally) persons who require some personal care, supervision, or assistance in daily activities such as bathing, dressing, or the taking of medicine prescribed for self-administration (Vogel and Palmer 1982, 438).

Increasingly, the domiciliary care facility is viewed as another option for those elderly and mentally ill/retarded who do not need institutionalization or medical care.

Hospice programs are formal multidisciplinary services which provide comfort and care to both a terminally ill individual and to family. They may be hospital-based, LTC-based, or home-based, or a mixture. Services include medicine, nursing, social, clergy, and psychological counseling. Major goals are comfort and relief of pain, plus assisting the dying individual in dealing with death and helping the family to cope afterwards.

Case management services incorporate assessment, referral, and treatment planning to help coordinate the care and payment for an individual. A *case manager* supports and advocates for the older person as he moves through the health care system, following up on appointments and problems. These are often sponsored by social service agencies and local governments.

Assessment programs may be social, medical, psychiatric, or multidisciplinary, either outpatient- or inpatient-based, providing a variety of evaluations, testing, and referrals for elderly with multiple complex problems, changes in condition or mental status, or in need of placement or management beyond the capacity of current family or professionals (see Chapter 5).

Clearly, much of the LTC spectrum is nonmedically oriented. But since physicians frequently order, authorize, arrange for, or support the services, they should know something about which programs, agencies, tests, treatments, orders, and care plans may be most likely to accomplish desirable goals at the least cost to a given patient.

Looking for Institutionalization Alternatives

In LTC, alternatives to institutionalization are preferable wherever possible, for two reasons. First, the cost of institutional care is usually, though not always, greater than that of noninstitutional care. Secondly, helping a person remain in a more familiar and private surrounding is preferable to providing those same services in a nursing home, all other things being more or less equal.

Use of alternatives is hampered by financial factors, including limits on payment from third-party payors, like Medicare and Medicaid (see Chapter 8). The multiple services provided in LTC facilities are often covered as part of the institutionalization, while community-based services providing the same support are often not. Sometimes, the cost of NH care may actually be less when all other factors (such as transportation, supervision, physical resources and meals) are considered. In addition, many people simply will not or cannot use alternatives to nursing home care.

Thus, in assisting with the search for alternatives to institutionalization, the physician may very well have to deal with social, financial, psychological, and political factors.

Creating A Geriatrics Service

Chapter 13 discusses in some depth the elements of a teaching nursing home program. This is one kind of geriatrics *service*, which we may define as an organized, coordinated collection of programs for the assessment, treatment, and care of the elderly. The principles of formulating and managing such a service are similar, regardless of who establishes or controls the individual programs or the overall service.

Creating a true geriatrics service requires that we:

- assess the needs of an area or patient population
- evaluate the available resources and patterns and levels of medical care and other professional services
- project likely needs at certain future points
- select the elements to include in the particular geriatric service
- decide on participants for managerial, clinical, evaluative, and other functions
- define overall operational policies and goals (See Chapter 4)
- establish procedures and roles (see Chapter 4)
- refine or establish the elements of the service, such as assessment programs or a day hospital
- encourage certain attitudes, teamwork, communication, and coordination (see Chapter 7)
- establish programs for the monitoring and follow-up of care and services (see Chapter 6).

With so many possible programs, and an ever-growing constituency, each situation presents issues of administration, planning, management and control. We must decide who will manage and coordinate the services, and how those services will be arranged and offered.

Important participants in this area may include: acute hospitals, long-term care facilities, private corporations, physicians' groups, community agencies, and government agencies.

Common arrangements for the management and coordination of such services include:

- for-profit or nonprofit hospitals with vertically integrated multilevel geriatric programs or centers
- multilevel nursing home/geriatric centers with or without affiliations with acute hospitals
- community or government programs, such as day care and senior centers, with or without coverage arrangements with local hospitals or universities.

Options for arrangement of the services include:

- integration in one physical setting
- availability in several settings, but managed by one organization or agency
- coordination among several independent agencies or sites
- separate independent programs, which may or may not collaborate.

Planning for such projects may occur at the *institutional*, *governmental*, *corporate*, or *community* levels. Physicians may be involved as consultants, advisers, or direct participants at any of these levels.

Day-to-day operations of these projects or programs may be handled by:

- existing administrative staff of a hospital, nursing home, or community or government agency

- new staff, either within its own department or division, or within an existing department or division in a parent organization

- a person designated by a board of directors

- a government official or his designate.

Collaboration among agencies or programs may include sharing of management, caregivers, consultants, resources, funds, information, planning, and sites.

Coakley's book (1982) is recommended as a more detailed review of the many considerations in establishing a geriatrics service.

Governments and LTC Services

The Older Americans Act of 1965 was an important stimulus to state and local governments to create a coordinated system of services for the elderly. Today, there are 10 regional offices of the national aging network, and over 50 state and 660 area agencies on aging, along with 15,000 community organizations offering supportive social and nutritional services. State and area governments do not usually provide direct services, but instead subcontract with others. Extent and number of services vary with state and local area.

Several states employ a channeling concept as a starting point for state-sponsored geriatric services. This establishes a single point of entry for clients in need of health and social services. It may include screening, assessment, case management, and a mix of cost-saving services to meet needs, with the ultimate goal of providing more efficient, effective, coordinated, and less costly delivery of needed services. Such programs have had varied success.

Realizing future fiscal and social constraints, state and local governments have made unprecedented efforts to plan and coordinate needed services for the elderly. Statewide plans are then presented as guidelines for the development of private or academic interests or programs.

Many states have established committees or task forces to study the needs and service utilization of their elderly population, and to make recommendations based on projections of future trends.

In Maryland, for example, the Maryland Health Resources Planning Commission proposed a long-range plan for LTC programs after finding that a disproportionate amount of public funds had been spent on institutional versus community-based services. From 1970 to 1981, the average annual growth rate of expenditures for institutional services had increased almost twice as rapidly as that for noninstitutional LTC expenditures. A 1983 estimate of disability by level of the community-based elderly showed 20.4% mildly, 7.2% moderately, and 7.8% severely disabled (Maryland Health Resources Planning Commission 1985).

This 1985 study therefore recommended the following goals and objectives:

- Develop a system for identifying high-risk disabled persons as priority recipients of LTC services, including an instrument to measure the physical, psychological, and social needs of disabled individuals requesting publicly funded LTC services.

- Develop and expand services identified for priority, focusing on home health care, home-delivered meals, specialized transportation, homemaker services, heavy chore services, and respite care.

- Establish a state-level management strategy for implementing the LTC plan and addressing future LTC issues.

- Integrate a system for delivering LTC services throughout the state, including a channeling agency, a comprehensive needs assessment, case management, a services audit, and central data collection and planning.

- Provide support for informal support systems such as counseling, training case managers, and volunteers and voluntary organizations in the care of the disabled elderly.

In Miami the LTC experience represents one positive community-wide approach to these issues. "In 1984, about 98,000 of Greater Miami's elderly population—one-third of those over age 65—were hospitalized for an average of 9.5 days each. Medicare covered 35 percent of hospital admissions, compared with 37 percent paid for by Blue Cross and other non-government insurers (*Hospitals* 1986, 58)." Though there are more than enough hospital beds for Miami's elderly, NH beds are in demand. The state funds such alternative services as home health care, homemaker services, meals on wheels, and activity programs. The issue was how to reduce costs while still providing acceptable levels of essential services.

Among the programs available for the elderly in the greater Miami area are: medical day care, where patients are picked up at home and spend three days a week in rehabilitation and socialization programs; caregiver, which teach spouses and others how to cope with those with such chronic disabling conditions as Alzheimer's disease or Parkinsonism; home health services; mobile labs, providing senior citizen testing and prehospital screening, or offering education programs; transportation, free or for nominal charges, to local hospitals and doctors' offices; rehabilitation and preventive services; HMOs and other primary care; and education and instruction regarding the illnesses and chronic problems affecting the elderly.

These are typical government concerns and planning efforts to be expected in the future. Emphasis will be on coordinated planning of services to avoid duplication of cost and effort.

Advising on Programs and Placement

Again, the LTC physician in this LTC system may serve as either planner, administrator, or clinical patient manager. In this third area, he will invariably be called upon by family, colleagues, or other health care professionals to assist in making decisions about placement or services. Although patients or families, rather than physicians, usually determine NH preference, physicians still make or influence most decisions concerning utilization of health care facilities and resources. On what basis should we make these recommendations?

One guiding principle is that the *level of function*, not the diagnosis, is key to the recommendation. For example, some patients with Alzheimer's disease are quite active and minimally impaired intellectually, while others are severely impaired, and still others are bedbound and completely dependent. The same is true for people with strokes, heart disease, musculoskeletal disturbances, or any other ailments.

Keeping this point in mind, the following are recommended steps for the LTC physician to follow:

Assure that accurate diagnosis has been made. In addition, be sure that potentially reversible problems are treated. For example, mental dysfunction from toxic side-effects of medications can be improved or reversed by change or discontinuation of medications. Possible misdiagnosis as organic brain disease in this case, could force unnecessary institutionalization.

Ascertain patient function. For example, use psychological, rehabilitative, or in-home evaluations.

Determine patient goals. Some people will want to do everything possible to stay in their homes. For them, the physician can help by prescribing and certifying home care services or special equipment. Others will have no desire, or will be unable, to stay in their homes, and must be sent to day care centers, live with relatives, or be admitted to a NH.

Ascertain family goals and expectations. Many elderly persons are cared for by their families. Therefore, it helps to understand family resources, their limits in handling a disabled person, and what they want or expect from a NH, day care programs, or other services.

Determine realistic objectives. Base these on condition and prognosis. Do we want to improve functional ability, psychological well-being, and independence, or simply make it easier for others to care for someone?

Ascertain available resources and options. Review what the community offers in the way of in-home, community-based, institutional, or hybrid services. Consider referrals to case management, channeling, assessment, or other such broad programs that can assist in handling a difficult case and with referrals and follow-ups.

Match patient needs with available services. Combine the evaluation of patient needs and goals with the understanding of available services, to present a recommendation likely to meet those needs and accomplish the goals. Where possible, several different options should be offered to patient or family, giving them the opportunity to choose.

Many of the aforementioned steps can be performed or assisted by such nonmedical professionals as social workers and nurses. But even when not directly involved, the physician should at least be aware of what various programs and services exist, what they can offer their patients, how a solution might be reached by matching needs to available services, and what the likely results are for the patient's management and care.

References

Coakley, D., ed. 1982. *Establishing a geriatric service*. London: Croom Helm.

Day, A. T. 1985. Who cares? Demographic trends challenge family care for the elderly. In *Population Trends and Public Policy*, No. 9, edited by P. M. Scommegna. Washington, D.C.: Population Reference Bureau.

Kane, R. L. 1984. Long-term care: Policy and reimbursement. In *Geriatric Medicine, Vol. 1: Medical, Psychiatric, and Pharmacologic Topics*. Edited by C. K. Cassel and J. R. Walsh, 380-396. New York: Springer-Verlag.

Maryland Health Resources Planning Commission. 1985. *Report to the Maryland General Assembly: Long Term Care Services*. Baltimore: Maryland Health Resources Planning Commission.

Miami's elderly: the future of health care. 1986. *Hospitals* 60(6):58-63.

National Center for Health Statistics, B. A. Feller. 1986. *Americans Needing Home Care, United States*, Pub. no. PHS 86-1581. Washington, D.C.: Government Printing Office.

Senate Special Committee on Aging. 1986. *Aging America: trends and projections*, 1985-86 ed. Washington, D.C.: Department of Health and Human Services.

Sirrocco, A. 1985. *An overview of the 1982 National Master Facility Inventory Survey of Nursing and Related Care Homes*. Advance data from vital and health statistics, No. 111, Pub. no. PHS 85-1250, National Center for Health Statistics. Washington, D.C.: Government Printing Office.

Vogel, R. J., and H. C. Palmer. 1982. *Long-term care: Perspectives from Research and Demonstrations*. Washington, D.C.: Health Care Financing Administration.

Waldo, D. R., and H. C. Lazenby. 1984. Demographic characteristics and health care use and expenditures by the aged in the United States: 1977-1984. *Health Care Financing Review* 6(1):1-29.

For Further Reading

American Hospital Association. *Guide to the Health Care Field*. Chicago: AHA. An annual directory of hospitals, accredited long-term care facilities, multihospital systems, and international, national, regional, and state organizations and agencies involved in the administration, planning, review, monitoring, and provision of health care services, including LTC.

Campion, E. W., A. Mahoney, and A. Bang. 1984. Acute care hospitals providing elderly and long-term care services: A survey of the Massachusetts experience. *Journal of the American Geriatrics Society* 32:727-733.

Furukawa, C., and D. Shomaker. 1982. *Community Health Services for the Aged*. Rockville, Md.: Aspen. A detailed overview of the development, management, and delivery of community-based health promotion and maintenance services for the elderly.

Gillick, M. and K. Steel. 1983. Referral of patients from long-term to acute-care facilities. *Journal of the American Geriatrics Society* 31:74-78.

Hughes, S. 1986. *Long-Term Care: Options in an Expanding Market*. Homewood, IL: Dow-Jones-Irwin.

Kane, R. L., and R. A. Kane. 1980. Alternatives to institutional care of the elderly: beyond the dichotomy. *Gerontologist* 20:249-259.

Kayser-Jones, J. S. 1984. Physicians and the care of nursing home residents. In *Geriatric Medicine*, Vol. 2, Edited by C. K. Cassell and J. R. Walsh, pp. 397-412. New York: Springer-Verlag.

Rocheleau, B. 1983. *Hospital and Community Oriented Programs for the Elderly*. Ann Arbor: AUPHA Press. A book which documents and advocates hospital participation in community-based programs for the elderly, with a number of examples of existing efforts.

Shapiro, E. et al. 1980. Long term patients in acute care beds: Is there a cure? *Gerontologist* 20:342-349.

Also, many geriatric textbooks and periodicals (see Chapter 10) have sections on programs and services for the elderly, from the physician's viewpoint.

Chapter Three

Models of Physician Participation

Steven A. Levenson, M.D.

Chapter Objectives

This chapter will:

- Review the broad areas of medical involvement in LTC, and some options for provision of physician services
- Review the advantages and disadvantages of these service options
- Consider the place of bylaws to accommodate different options
- Propose some guidelines to help choose appropriate options for specific settings
- Detail the role and responsibilities of the attending physician in LTC.

Areas of Physician Involvement in LTC

Not all physicians associated with geriatrics are involved in LTC (some may only teach or do research, for example). But most physicians' activities in LTC fall into one of three categories (see Fig. 3-1):

- system management
- operational management
- patient management.

System Management	Operational Management	Patient Management
Planning	Integration of service	Delivery of care
Financing	at community,	Referral
Development	program, or	Assessment
System control	institutional level	Placement
System evaluation	Quality monitoring	Case management
	Performance	Advocacy
	evaluation	Quality control

Figure 3-1 Categories of medical involvement in LTC.

Many LTC physicians have responsibilities in more than one area, and activities (e.g., quality monitoring) in different categories may overlap.

System management refers to planning, financing, system development, system control, and evaluation. The physician may be involved with state, federal, private, or local governments, department, or agencies (such as the Health Care Financing Administration (HCFA) or state health departments), and focuses on comprehensive coordination and the integration of money, personnel, and agencies.

Operational management refers to integration of services at a community, program, or institutional level, including delivery of care and the monitoring of the quality of that care. This encompasses the level of activity of the medical director as administrator.

Patient management refers to the delivery of care and services, and other associated activities, including referral, assessment, placement, case management, patient information, quality control, and advocacy. This is the level of both attending physicians and medical directors as patient care providers.

The extent of medical involvement in each area varies with the needs of the institution or program, the needs of patients, and the interest of the physician. The current and future need is for physicians willing to become actively and extensively involved, to design and improve individual programs and facilities, to serve as role models, and to actually deliver the care. An active, vigorous physician role is believed by many to have a far-reaching effect, improving the interest and understanding of nursing and other professional services, and encouraging facilities to provide a better environment and level of response to patient and professional needs.

Options for Physician Coverage

There are four major models of clinical physician coverage in LTC:

1. Full- or part-time employment

2. Arrangements for routine physician coverage at regular intervals

3. Arrangements for physician on-call coverage, as needed

4. Medical coverage in the community, such as in private physicians' offices.

Each of these has an important place in the LTC continuum.

Sources of such medical care may include: community practitioners; acute hospital medical staff; university faculty; group practitioners (including HMOs and PPOs); medical residents or fellows under faculty supervision; and nurse practitioners or physician assistants, under physician supervision.

Typical Arrangements

Most community-based and home-based programs continue a person's preexisting community-based medical arrangements. Group homes or life-care facilities may provide some full- or part-time salaried medical coverage (models 1 or 2), while giving individuals the option to retain their own physicians (model 4), often at their own expense.

Day hospitals are most often staffed according to model 1. Day care medical backup is most often provided to each individual patient by a community attending physician (model 4). Some programs, however, retain a physician consultant to evaluate acute problems, sign forms, renew orders, and review continuing eligibility for the program (model 1), though these are truly the responsibilities of attending physicians. Outpatient assessment programs are generally staffed according to model 1, frequently by trainees or attending physicians who are already in the geriatrics department of medical school faculty.

Medical coverage for LTC institutions has been drawn from many sources, including private practitioners, hospital medical staff, medical school faculty, and shared staff from other LTC facilities.

Nursing homes are most often staffed according to models 2 or 3, and sometimes model 1. About a third of NHs have arrangements for regularly scheduled visits, and about half have physicians with on-call arrangements. Usually, only larger facilities or teaching nursing homes have a structured arrangement for full-time and regularly scheduled physicians (Solon 1983). NH physicians are increasingly using nurse practitioners and physician assistants to provide many NH medical services under their supervision.

Medical coverage in the NH should be likened more closely to the community-based or home-based model than to the hospital-based model. Although NH residents are indeed institutionalized, and often bedbound or dependent, the NH is really a home setting. Unlike in the hospital, medical care is not the primary reason for the stay, but is instead one part of an overall care plan. Even while the care is rendered, the patient remains a NH resident. The medical record is episodic and long-term, and follow-up care is often as important as, if not more important than, the initial medical action. Therefore, physician coverage for the NH should be a hybrid of both the community-based and the institutional models, but certainly not modeled exactly after the hospital situation. Nursing home residents needing intensive medical care should be transferred to either a geriatric specialty hospital, or to an acute facility.

Medical Staff Structures in the Nursing Home

Whereas medical staff arrangements in acute hospitals have evolved towards formal, often complex, organizations with a governing structure, bylaws, and a full array of committees, medical staffs in NHs have remained loose and unstructured, often without authoritative leadership or specific requirements. Traditionally, a physician's hospital privileges have also covered his NH practice.

While given certain responsibilities for compliance, medical directors have often lacked the authority for adequate enforcement. Without the granting of formal clinical privileges or mechanisms to review quality of care, it is extremely difficult to establish criteria and standards against which to compare physician performance, or to take action when performance is lacking.

More accrediting agencies, medical directors and LTC administrators are considering a more formally organized medical staff as one means for improving quality of care. The question is whether, and to what degree, these arrangements should imitate those of acute hospitals, and to what extent they should differ.

Open and Closed Staffs

Medical staffs may be classified as either *open* or *closed*. Membership on an open staff is available to any practitioners who meet specified requirements, and who wish to admit and attend to the NH residents. Closed staff membership, on the other hand, is available to a restricted group of physicians; for example, only to those who are in a particular group, those who are salaried by a facility, or those faculty in the geriatric division of a hospital department of medicine. When residents are admitted to a facility with closed staffing, they are frequently assigned to, or select, a physician who will remain as their attending as long as they live in the facility. Most NHs have open staffs.

Each has its advantages and disadvantages. Open staffing allows for broader participation by the practicing community, and may help enhance physician interest and involvement in LTC. It may improve continuity of care by allowing the individual to keep the same attending physician no matter where he may receive treatment within the LTC system.

On the other hand, the open staff makes medical administrative supervision and control more difficult. Each individual practitioner has his unique personal ways of practicing, and incentives for coming or not coming to the NH. Consensus may be very hard to reach, and performance monitoring difficult to achieve. There is little incentive for such nonreimbursable tasks as completing necessary forms, meeting with families, or reviewing medications with the nursing staff. A closed staff allows for closer control, supervision, and enforcement of policies and procedures. Also, with a closed staff, the community-based attending physician can still act in a consultant role, although the financial and professional incentives to do so are limited.

The "Organized" Staff

Medical staffs may also be seen as organized or nonorganized. The organized staff has bylaws, officers, committees, rules and regulations, and regular meetings. The nonorganized, or informal, staff is simply a group of individuals with privileges to practice. Of course, there are varying degrees of organization (and some "organized" staffs may be rather *dis*organized), and many settings may find it advantageous to be somewhere in the middle.

Yet whatever the arrangement, some degree of organization is always possible and desirable. In addition, the right to practice in the NH, like that in the acute hospital, is increasingly viewed as a privilege with commensurate responsibilities, not as an unconditional right.

Bylaws Options

The broad rights and responsibilities of medical staffs are customarily defined by medical bylaws.

Bylaws are a formal, legally enforceable set of policies, instructions, and guidelines which define an organization and its relationships with those within and outside that organization. Medical bylaws are documented with definitions of the responsibilities, prerogatives, criteria for membership, leadership, and circumstances of monitoring and discipline, for all those providing medical care in an institution. They are, in effect, a contract between individual practitioners and the facility, in that the individual must agree to abide by them as a condition of membership or privileges, and failure to keep that agreement has enforceable consequences.

Basic Elements of Nursing Home Bylaws

Federal regulations require a NH medical director, with appropriate medical staff input, to develop written bylaws, rules, and regulations for the medical staffs of Medicare and Medicaid facilities. These must be approved by the board (where such exists), and must define attending physician responsibilities. Today, there are still few guidelines to help those medical directors who are trying to comply.

Appropriate bylaws may range from a few pages of simple definitions and descriptions, to a fairly lengthy and detailed production. This will vary with the institution and physician needs. We can, nevertheless, describe both essential and optional components.

The following elements of NH medical bylaws are *essential*:

- Purpose of the medical staff organization
- Definition of the organization
- Description of a governing structure, or lines of authority
- Qualifications for staff membership
- Conditions and duration of appointment and reappointment
- Basic expectations for service to patient and facility
- Structure for corrective action, due process, suspension of privileges, and appeal
- Provision for immunity from liability for providing information in good faith
- Provision for amendments and adoption of the bylaws.

Optional parts of such bylaws include:

- Definitions of staff categories (active, associate, etc.), and criteria for each
- Arrangements for, and notification of, regular and special meetings of the staff
- Procedures for requesting and granting privileges
- Definitions of specific privileges (such as temporary or emergency)
- Description of allowable privileges (such as surgical procedures)
- Arrangement of staff into services or divisions
- Definitions and descriptions of committees.

It should be noted that in Joint Commission on Accreditation of Hospitals (JCAH)-accredited facilities, these "optional" portions are required by JCAH standards.

Some of these elements deserve additional discussion.

Governing structure. The hospital medical staff typically has officers, and is ruled by a medical executive committee (MEC), with a chairman and both elected and appointed members. The NH medical staff may or may not benefit from officers (president, vice-president, secretary-treasurer), and may or may not need the formal structure of the MEC. In many instances – especially, small staffs in small facilities – the medical director can assume the roles of chief of staff and MEC chairman, even if not actually having the titles. Critical medical executive functions (quality of care review, privileges, etc.) may be accomplished by the medical staff meeting as a committee of the whole. If this is done, minutes of the staff meetings should reflect these specific functions by recording them separately from other medical staff discussions and activities. In addition, a utilization review or quality assurance committee, consisting in part of attending physicians, can perform some governing functions, by conducting medical care evaluation studies and handling basic medical administrative problems of inadequate patient care.

In short, the structures can be flexible, as long as the essential tasks are accomplished. In addition, the lines of authority and responsibility – whatever they might be – must be defined clearly and understood.

Qualifications for membership. The chronic care in the NH is not the same kind of medicine as that practiced in the acute hospital. Therefore, having privileges at one or more acute hospitals should not be assumed to qualify a person to provide geriatric medical care, and should not substitute for a credential review process for the NH medical staff. Certain paperwork (letters of recommendation, state license) could be copied and shared, but a separate file ought to be kept within the NH for each persons with privileges. This assures consistent information and standards for every practitioner, regardless of their practice locale, specialty, or acute hospital privileges.

Duration of appointment and reappointment. Nursing home privileges, like hospital privileges, should be granted for a limited time period, and renewed periodically, to assure compliance with standards and responsibility. Indefinite privileges, like a long-term contract for an athlete, often depend too much on uncertain personal motivation, and lack incentives for continued adequate performance.

Expectations for service. The bylaws should describe in general what the practitioner is expected to do to meet regulations, laws, and standards, to comply with institutional and medical staff policy and procedures, and to provide quality medical care. More specific performance standards (timely completion of records, proper prescribing of medications, advance notification of family of discharges) should be delineated in rules and regulations, or departmental policies.

Due process. This does not necessarily require a formal structure and a judicial-type hearing, but it does demand equitable treatment of all individuals. Each practitioner should be judged by the same set of standards as his peers in the same specialty. A physician has the right to answer those charges, to present his own case, and to examine the evidence against him. Charges of poor practice or patient management must be explicit and presented before any disciplinary hearing is held, to allow the accused to prepare a defense. The hearing body should be as impartial as possible, and there should be some option for appeal.

Immunity from liability. As with hospital bylaws, this is essential to permit acquisition of information about a person's clinical competence and patient care, as long as such information is offered in good faith.

Staff categories. The majority of NHs have 10 or fewer practitioners, while others have a larger number of doctors, each caring for only a few patients. Those physicians with many patients may want more involvement in staff matters, but they should also have additional responsibilities, such as attendance at meetings and service on committees. It may therefore be appropriate in the NH, as in the hospital, to designate active, associate, courtesy, and consulting staff — each with certain prerogatives and responsibilities to the patients and to the medical staff.

For example, active staff privileges could be granted to those who admit or attend at least a dozen persons per year, while those who only occasionally admit or attend patients could be given courtesy privileges, or even just temporary privileges as needed.

Allowable practices. Many services performed in acute hospitals (diagnostic radiology, surgery under general anesthesia) are not and cannot be done in the NH. Neither are all practitioners equally qualified to provide all the services that could be offered to NH patients (such as minor surgery, biopsy of lesions, or sigmoidoscopy). Therefore, it is appropriate to delineate specific privileges for each physician, in addition to the general prerogatives of his specialty.

See the appendices of this chapter for examples of model bylaws, definitions of staff categories, and a description of clinical privileges.

Selecting A Model

Since NHs, like hospitals, are not all homogeneous, the same arrangements cannot be recommended for all. In trying to select a model for a particular setting, one should consider:

- facility and community goals
- costs
- academic interests
- politics
- program goals

Facility and Community Goals

Ostensibly, every NH wants to give quality service to its residents, but not all have the same ideas about what that means. In addition, some have more resources than others to commit to the effort. Proprietary (for-profit) facilities are typically investor-owned, and may emphasize return on investment more than other factors.

However, just as well-run, for-profit hospitals have been shown to offer comparable service at less cost than some "nonprofits," so too it may be quite possible to combine quality care with a good investment return. Physicians providing service to LTC facility must be prepared to reach some understanding with ownership and management about their relative commitment to quality, as well as to cost control.

Communities or owners may wish to commit to some additional programs or services beyond basic care, such as academic teaching programs or special dementia or assessment centers. Physicians should encourage such commitments where appropriate, and help that community or those owners identify their expectations and firm commitments. (See Chapter 13, on "The Teaching Nursing Home," for additional discussion.)

Thus, the extent of medical involvement and the appropriate staffing arrangements vary with the wishes of the community and the facility. At a minimum, physicians are expected to provide adequate medical coverage. How much they offer in addition, from advice to the administration to education of the staff to participation in patient care planning, depends substantially on such commitments.

Costs

A partially or fully salaried medical staff costs more up front. To the basic salary of employed staff must be added 15 to 20% or more for such fringe benefits as liability and health insurance and vacations. Less than half-time salaried staff do not generally qualify for most fringe benefits.

On the other hand, salaried physician employees may be less costly than apparent at first glance, if enough of the following factors are true:

1. Patient visits and services are reimbursable to the facility

2. Significantly less nursing staff time is spent tracking down physicians to manage patient problems, or to obtain or clarify orders

3. The physicians contribute to a teaching program that benefits both trainees and institution staff

4. Better control of practices within the facility results in fewer medication orders and errors, and better compliance with licensure and other regulations

5. There is greater accountability for actions, resulting in more rapid response to correcting deficiencies or violations

6. Doctors are more available to evaluate and manage changes in patient condition, reducing the frequency of patient transfers to emergency rooms or acute hospitals for assessment.

Academic interests

A university or medical school interested in using a facility for teaching will want some control of staffing and program planning. Obviously, such an arrangement will affect costs, not just for medical care, but for other professional service time, as well. Some salaried physician time is necessary in teaching NH programs for rounding and educational activities (see Chapter 13).

Politics

Local or state politics and regulatory agencies can affect level of expectations, reimbursement, staffing, and licensure review. Some states have more stringent requirements for NH care than do others. These requirements can likewise affect costs and may require greater physician input.

Program Goals

As discussed in Chapter 2, the nature of the elderly population as a whole, and that of many NHs, is changing. What is to be accomplished within the program or facility? Is the primary goal custodial care, or is it aggressive, rehabilitation-oriented, or somewhere in between? Are there many patients with psychiatric problems, requiring additional consultations and posing difficult management and ethical issues? An institution's financial and administrative support and staffing needs vary with the degree of interest in such issues.

The Role of the Attending Physician

Realistically, the majority of medical care in LTC, including NHs, will continue to be rendered by primary care physicians, as one part of their overall practice. The attending physician in LTC has a critical role, especially in the NH. In 70% of NHs, care is provided by fewer than 10 different physicians (Rabin 1981).

Whether or not a NH has an open or closed staff, bylaws, rules, regulations, and committees, the attending physician can nevertheless have an impact by his interest in the many small details that together meet the needs of an older patient. Many of these are discussed in other chapters, including: knowledge of available services; understanding of basic principles of geriatric medicine; collaboration with other professionals; maintaining good documentation; accepting and using the team approach; and responding to deficiencies and quality assurance notices.

The following are some suggested guidelines for the responsibilities of attending physicians in LTC:

- Recognize that the ultimate responsibility for care in any setting rests with the governing body.

- Be aware of the role and responsibilities of a medical director, to facilitate a working relationship.

- Observe a facility's patient care policies.

- Perform an appropriate and adequate preadmission evaluation, and provide all necessary information to facilitate the best possible admission and placement decision.

- Provide for alternate medical coverage, in the event of emergency or absence.

- Collaborate with the medical director or chief of staff in designing and implementing appropriate medical policies and procedures.

- Attend necessary staff or committee meetings, and contribute appropriately.

- Bring to the medical director's attention concerns about quality of patient care, or opinions about additional equipment, personnel, or services to adequately meet the needs of patients admitted to a facility.

- Be aware of the services available for patients and families, and make referrals where necessary to facilitate provision of such services.

- Be aware of medical consultative support for primary medical care in LTC, and request such support whenever indicated.

- Be aware of the special wishes and needs of a patient or family, and consider these in medical decision making.

- Help devise, and periodically review, a multidisciplinary care plan for each patient.

- Comply with federal and state requirements for patient visits and documentation.

- Attempt, when writing orders, to minimize possibilities for error, misinterpretation, drug incompatibilities, and therapeutic duplication.

- Renew medication orders in a timely fashion, and periodically reconsider the need for continuing each drug.

- Be aware of the many sources of iatrogenic illness among the elderly, and try wherever possible to minimize the possibilities.

- Provide legible, timely, and accurate documentation, which adequately reflects a patient's condition, prognosis, and need for services.

Appendix 3-A Example of medical bylaws, rules, and regulations for a NH (Reproduced with permission, courtesy Paul Spilseth, M.D.; Stillwater, Minnesota)

Medical Practice Agreement for Attending Physicians
A Model for Nursing Homes

Compiled by Paul Spilseth, M.D., Stillwater, Minn. as a project of the Minnesota Association of Medical Directors of Nursing Homes and the American Medical Directors Association, 1987.

Introduction:

_____ Care Center is a ____ bed skilled/intermediate care facility located in _____ and operated by _____.

Purpose:
The purpose of this agreement is to achieve a high level of quality health care for each patient. This agreement defines the relationship of the attending physicians, the medical director, and the nursing home.

Organization:

_____ Care Center has an open medical staff. This means any licensed physician who agrees to these rules and has an established primary care practice within the service area may make application to admit and care for patients in the home by signing this agreement. The physician will then be accepted as an attending physician after approval by the Medical Director and the Administration.

The Medical Director will function in a manner similar to the Chief of Staff of a hospital where there is an organized medical staff. He is responsible for the overall coordination of the medical care in the facility. He is to ensure the adequacy and appropriateness of the medical services provided to the residents. He will maintain surveillance of the health status of employees. The Medical Director is responsible for advising the Director of Nurses in the daily execution of patient care policies. He will also serve as a liaison to other physicians, and he will represent the facility in the hospitals and the community.

The Utilization Review Committee functions as the governing body of the open medical staff. It is composed of the Medical Director, ___ additional physician members. The Director of Nurses, the Administrator, and other staff will attend the meetings but have no vote. The Utilization Review Committee will meet every ___ months. They will conduct medical care evaluation studies on a regular basis. This committee will provide a means whereby problems of a medical or administrative nature may be considered.

Attending Physicians Qualifications:

I am a physician licensed in the state of _____ and I have a license to prescribe narcotics. I have an established primary care practice within the service community and seek to admit patients to _____ Care Center. I have an adequate amount of professional liability insurance. I will promptly notify the Medical Director if the status of these qualifications change.

Admission Requirements:

When my patient is admitted, I will provide the facility with pertinent information regarding the patients past medical history, an admitting diagnosis, level of care, rehabilitation potential, medication and treatment orders, and a diet order. I will do a history and physical within five days prior to admission or within two days after admission. If the patient comes from the hospital, a discharge summary will be sent. I will provide medical supervision of rehabilitation services as needed, including physical therapy, occupational therapy, speech therapy, and mental health programs.

Expectations from the Nursing Home:

I expect trained nursing home personnel to provide a clean and safe environment for my patients. I expect to have adequate equipment, supplies and nutrition for my patients. I expect dietitians, pharmacists, social workers, and therapists to complement my services. I will treat the staff with courtesy, and I will expect mutual courtesy from them.

Visits:

I will visit my patients in the nursing home as frequently as is consistent with good medical practice. I will also satisfy the government regulations, and I will visit skilled patients at least once every 30 days for the first three months following admission. Subsequently, an alternative schedule for physician visits may be requested, and if approved by the Utilization Review Committee, the patient may be seen every ___ days. Patients with unstable conditions or those receiving rehabilitative services will be seen every ___ days.

I will write a meaningful progress note and sign it after each patient visit. These notes will contain an evaluation of changes in the health status of the patient. They will also contain a rationale for starting, continuing, and discontinuing drugs and other treatments.

I will provide a yearly physical examination or health appraisal that addresses the overall plan of care.

I will designate an alternate physician who can be reached in my absence. If neither I nor my alternate can be reached, the Medical Director or an emergency physician will have the authority to treat my patient.

When a physician assistant assists me in providing care, I will furnish a protocol to the facility establishing the physician assistant's role, tasks, and responsibilities.

Upon discharge of a resident I will provide a written discharge order, discharge diagnosis, and discharge summary.

Disciplinary Action:
My privileges as an attending physician at _____ Care Center may be suspended if there are allegations that I have engaged in substantial misconduct or wrongdoing, or if it is determined that my practice is below reasonable professional standards. Violations of this Medical Practice Agreement, violations of state and federal regulations, or professional conduct unbecoming of the profession or _____ Care Center shall constitute reason for withdrawal of privileges.

In any case of disciplinary action the procedures established in the appendix attached to this agreement shall be followed.

Acknowledgement:
I have read and understand this agreement, and I agree to abide by its provisions. I understand that _____ Care Center may revise this agreement as appropriate and will advise me of such changes.

Signed_____ **License number** _____ **Date** _____
        Attending Physician

Signed _____   Date _____
        Medical Director

Appendix to the Medical Practice Agreement: Hearing and Appeal Procedure

If an Attending Physician is accused of substantial misconduct or wrongdoing, or if it is determined that the physician's practice at _____ Care Center is below reasonable professional standards, or if the physician fails to follow the Medical Practice Agreement for Attending Physicians, the following procedures apply:

Investigation by the Medical Director:

Prior to any action, the problem will be investigated by the Medical Director and the physician under investigation shall have an opportunity for an interview with the Medical Director. If the Medical Director decides there is a need for further investigation and/or corrective action, he shall notify the Utilization Review Committee and the involved physician of this decision in writing within 30 days. The Medical Director will have the authority to temporarily suspend the physician pending a determination by the Utilization Review Committee.

Action by the Utilization Review Committee:

The Utilization Review Committee will investigate and determine the appropriate action within a period of 90 days. They may interview the physician and receive other information as they deem appropriate. The committee's decision will then be transmitted to the Administrator in writing. Within 48 hours after receiving the committee's decision, the Administrator shall notify the physician in question of the action by certified mail. He shall receive written notice of the specific problems, issues, or charges to be considered, as well as the disciplinary action which may be taken. He shall also be notified that he has a right to a hearing of a committee of peers if he disagrees with the Utilization Review Committee's decision.

Appeal to a Hearing Committee:

The physician must notify the Utilization Review Committee within 7 days of receipt of the administrator's notification that he desires a hearing; if he fails to provide this notice, he shall waive his right to a hearing, and the decision of the Utilization Review Committee will be final. If he requests a hearing, it shall be held not less than 7 days nor more than 30 days after the physician requests a hearing.

The Hearing Committee shall consist of 2 physician members appointed by the Medical Director in consultation with the Utilization Review Committee, and 1 physician appointed by the physician under investigation. The administrator shall be a non-voting member of the Hearing Committee.

The Hearing Committee will choose its own chairman. The physician shall have the right to present evidence and arguments on his own behalf, and he may be accompanied by legal counsel. _____ Care Center shall have the right to present evidence on its behalf and may have legal counsel. All information necessary for the committee to make a fair determination will be freely received and formal rules of evidence shall not apply.

The Hearing Committee shall prepare a written report of its findings and recommendations within 7 days and the physician will be notified by certified mail. The decision of the Hearing Committee shall be final.

Appendix 3-B Example of definitions appropriate
to nursing home privileges

Definition of Specialties and Subspecialties

Allergy

Evaluate and advise regarding treatment of those with problems of immune
system dysfunction, atopic diseases, and related syndromes.

Cardiology

Evaluate and advise regarding treatment of those with problems of the cardiovascular system, such as ischemic heart disease, infective endocarditis, val-
vular heart disease, cardiomyopathies, pericardial disease, hypertension, and
diseases of the central and peripheral arteries and veins.

Dentistry

Evaluate, treat, and advise regarding treatment of, conditions and disorders
of the teeth and oral cavities. Perform uncomplicated tooth extractions and
fittings of dentures.

Dermatology

Evaluate and advise regarding treatment of those with problems of the skin,
such as skin lesions, pruritis, and photosensitivity.

Endocrinology

Evaluate and advise regarding treatment of those with problems of the endocrine glands, disorders of calcium and bone, and metabolic disorders.

Gastroenterology

Evaluate and advise regarding treatment of those with problems of the
gastrointestinal system, such as bleeding, pain, nausea, vomiting, anorexia,
peptic ulcer disease, tumors, diarrhea, constipation, disorders of intestinal ab-
sorption, inflammatory bowel disease, obstruction, jaundice, liver disease and
diseases of the pancreas.

Gynecology

Evaluate and advise regarding treatment of those with problems of the female genitourinary tract, such as incontinence, vaginal bleeding, or breast diseases.

Hematology

Evaluate and advise regarding the treatment of those with problems of the hematopoetic system, such as anemia, polycythemia, bone marrow failure, thrombocytopenia and disorders of platelet function, disorders of blood coagulation, lymphoma, and leukemia.

Infectious Diseases

Evaluate and advise regarding the treatment of those with problems of immune system deficiency and infections involving any of the organ systems.

Internal Medicine, General

Evaluate, treat, and advise regarding treatment of those with problems of the organ systems, including nervous system, cardiovascular system, skin, endocrine system, gastrointestinal system, hematologic system, immune system (including infectious diseases), renal system, pulmonary system, muscles, bones and joints, and cancer.

Nephrology

Evaluate and advise regarding the treatment of those with problems of the genitourinary system, such as hematuria, proteinuria, dysuria, acute nephritic syndrome, nephrotic syndrome, acute and chronic renal failure, nephrolithiasis, and disorders of electrolyte and acid-base balance.

Neurology

Evaluate and advise regarding treatment of those with problems of the central and peripheral nervous system, such as cerebrovascular disease, tumors, trauma, myelopathies, neuropathies, and degenerative and demyelinating diseases.

Neurosurgery

Evaluate and advise regarding treatment of those with problems of the central and peripheral nervous system which might require surgical intervention, such as head injuries and tumors.

Oncology

Evaluate and advise regarding the treatment of those with cancer of any of the organ systems.

Ophthalmology

Evaluate and advise regarding treatment of conditions and problems of eyesight, such as cataracts, glaucoma, and macular degeneration.

Orthopedics

Evaluate and advise regarding treatment of disorders of the musculoskeletal system, such as chronic musculoskeletal pain, fractures, and mobility disorders. Perform closed reduction and casting of uncomplicated acute fractures.

Otolaryngology

Evaluate and advise regarding treatment of conditions and problems of the ear, nose and throat, such as hearing loss, tinnitus, and swallowing difficulties.

Podiatry

Evaluate, treat, and advise regarding treatment of conditions and disorders of the feet and nails.

Psychiatry

Evaluate, treat, and advise regarding treatment of disturbances or disorders of behavior, emotions, personality, and thinking, consistent with commonly accepted psychiatric principles.

Pulmonary Diseases

Evaluate and advise regarding treatment of those with problems of the lungs, such as chronic obstructive disease, aspiration, fibrosis, vascular diseases, sarcoidosis, mediastinal diseases, pleural diseases, cancer, and disorders of respiratory control.

Rehabilitation Medicine

Evaluate, treat, and advise regarding treatment of functional disturbances and disorders which might respond to physical, occupational, or speech therapy, or other physical and mechanical treatments within the domain of the specialty.

Rheumatology

Evaluate and advise regarding treatment of those with problems of the immune system, rheumatic disorders, and joint diseases related to metabolic and biochemical disorders, such as rheumatoid arthritis, systemic lupus erythematosis, vasculitis, polymyalgia rheumatica and temporal arteritis, septic joints, osteoarthritis, gout, and pseudogout.

Surgery, General

Evaluate and advise regarding treatment of those with medical problems which might require surgical intervention.

Urology

Evaluate and advise regarding treatment of conditions and disorders of the kidneys, ureters, and bladder, such as incontinence, urinary tract infections, and kidney stones.

(Reprinted courtesy of Levindale Hebrew Geriatric Center and Hospital, Baltimore, Maryland)

Appendix 3-C Examples of clinical privileges for a geriatric specialty hospital

Clinical Privileges Request

Please check desired privileges:

Dentistry

_____ General dentistry
_____ Minor dental surgery (1)

Dermatology

_____ Skin testing
_____ Skin biopsy

General Surgery

_____ Sigmoidoscopy
_____ Proctoscopy
_____ Colonoscopy
_____ Minor surgery (2)
_____ Anoscopy

Gynecology

_____ Minor GYN surgery (3)

Internal Medicine

_____ Gastric analysis
_____ Thoracentesis
_____ Lumber puncture
_____ Paracentesis
_____ Peritoneal dialysis
     (nephrology)
_____ Minor surgery (4)
_____ Arthrocentesis
_____ Joint injection
_____ Bone marrow
_____ Soft tissue injection
_____ Liver biopsy (GI)
_____ Proctosigmoidoscopy

Ophthalmology

_____ Medical ophthalmology
_____ Minor ophthalmologic
     surgery (5)

Orthopedics

_____ Minor surgery (6)

Podiatry

_____ General podiatry

Psychiatry

_____ General adult psychiatry,
     excluding hypnosis, amytal
     interview, E.C.T.
_____ Hypnosis

Rehabilitation Medicine

_____ Medical rehabilitation
_____ Joint aspiration
_____ Joint injection
_____ Soft tissue injections
_____ Phenol nerve blocks
_____ Acupuncture

Urology

_____ Urethral dilatation
_____ Urethral catheterization
_____ Minor urologic surgery (7)
_____ Irrigation of bladder

Notes

1. Uncomplicated tooth extractions, fittings of dentures, biopsy and repair of lesions of the oral cavity

2. Biopsies under local anesthesia, repair of lacerations, debridement of wounds

3. Biopsies or curettage under local anesthesia

4. Repair of lacerations and debridement of wounds

5. Foreign body removal, biopsies, repairs under local anesthesia

6. Closed reduction and casting of uncomplicated fractures

7. Removal or replacement of complicated suprapubic catheters, emergency cystoscopy, biopsies under local anesthesia

(Reprinted courtesy of Levindale Hebrew Geriatric Center and Hospital; Baltimore, Md.)

References

Rabin, D. L. 1981. Physician care in nursing homes. *Annals of Internal Medicine* 94(1):126-128.

Solon, J. A. 1983. Alternative models of physician engagement with nursing homes. In *Clinical Aspects of Aging*, edited by W. Reichel. Baltimore: Williams & Wilkins.

For Further Reading

Joint Commission on Accreditation of Hospitals. *Long Term Care Standards Manual*. Updated annually.

Joint Commission on Accreditation of Hospitals. *Accreditation Manual for Hospitals*. Updated annually. Both this manual and the aforementioned one contain sections outlining the JCAH requirements for medical bylaws.

Joint Commission on Accreditation of Hospitals. *Medical Staff By-Laws*. A monograph available from the JCAH, discussing bylaws in more detail.

Vogel, A., and T. Henderson. 1984. Attending physician by-laws for nursing homes. *Minnesota Medicine*. April, pp. 225-226.

Chapter Four

The Medical Director As Physician Administrator

Steven A. Levenson, M.D.

Chapter Objectives

This chapter will:

- Consider how physicians relate to LTC administrators and boards
- Review general concepts of medical administration
- Discuss the forms of physician administration in LTC
- Discuss the specific role of the medical director in LTC
- Review the elements of a medical director's contractual agreement
- Analyze the medical director's role as policymaker, educator, and advocate
- Discuss the critical fundamentals of medical policies and procedures, and department organization, for which the medical director is responsible
- Consider how committees can be used effectively in LTC.

The Physician Administrator

The role of physician administrator is relatively new. In the past, some physicians became chief executives of hospitals and NHs, but most have considered the work unsuitable for those with medical training and patient orientation. In addition, the administrator generally had less power than the collective medical staff.

Many of those called upon to run geriatrics programs, including newly trained fellows, will have had extensive training in clinical medicine, research, and teaching. But few of them will have had any significant training or experience in administration.

Today, medical administration by trial and error is unworkable. Changes in health care have made the role of the physician administrator much more significant. Physicians collectively have less power than in the past, and administrators—who control the budget, policies, personnel, and allocation of money for resource usage— have considerably more. Physicians now recognize that the way to share power in health care facilities is to have representation in the management hierarchy.

But with the physician administrator's multifaceted role comes a divided constituency. As an employee of a health care facility, he is expected to carry out the policies and procedures and conform to the goals and objectives of the institution. As the administrative representative of the physicians, he is expected to advocate their position. As a physician, he is expected to advocate for the individual patient and for quality patient care. This is not always an easy balance to strike.

The terms variously used for physicians with administrative responsibilities in nursing homes have included "principal physician," "house physician," and "medical director." In general, the medical director has most often been the primary physician in nonprofit facilities, and the principal physician has been the primary physician in proprietary facilities, called upon by the administrator or owner for advice on medical affairs.

The physician administrator's role may range from directing a single activity or program, such as day care or geriatric assessment, to coordinating an entire medical service while serving as part of an institution's management team. The physician administrator is almost always either an independent contractor paid a certain sum for services, or a full- or part-time employee.

Most, if not all, physician administrators in the acute hospital setting are active managers, rather than mere advisors. But in most NHs, the medical director or principal physician has had much less authority than responsibility, and the role has traditionally been custodial rather than managerial. The question for LTC physician advisors is becoming: When, if at all, do they shift to a true administrator's role?

The answer depends in part on those factors discussed in Chapter 3: patient characteristics, community, ownership, or board interests and goals, and costs. But the key overriding principle is accountability. When the medical care in any setting is–or should be–held to certain standards, and a specific physician is–or should be–held accountable for his efforts, or for supervising the performance of others in meeting those standards, then the physician is no longer just an advisor, but a physician administrator.

While the extent of such a role is certainly not the same in all settings, the same principles of medical management are broadly applicable. This chapter focuses on the physician who is more than a mere advisor.

The Physician Administrator's Broad Responsibilities

Any physician administrator has responsibilities in four major areas:

- policymaking (setting goals and objectives)
- ongoing operational review and evaluation
- assuring adequate provision of medical services
- individual performance review and evaluation.

Many principles applicable to clinical problem solving or patient management are just as relevant for staff or departmental management and problem solving, including:

- setting performance standards
- designing a system for measuring performance against those standards
- collecting sufficient data to permit evaluation
- ensuring continuous review to see if measures are effective and problems are resolved or controlled

- allowing feedback about performance, problems, and achievement of goals to department members and within the institution.

In short, the physician administrator in LTC may have considerable influence, but cannot be too effective without some reasonable authority and systematic approaches.

The Management of Health Care

There are three major power groups within health care facilities: ownership or board, administration, and medical staff. In owner-operated facilities, policymaking and management roles often coincide. Ultimate responsibility for and control of any health care facility does not lie with the professional staff, but rather with the owners or board, who are also empowered to make the overall policy for the institution, and to choose its operating officers for day-to-day management (see Fig. 4-1).

The chief executive officer (CEO), a key person in any corporate structure, is known by many names. In many corporations, and in the executive branch of the federal government, this person is called the president. Other synonyms in different settings include superintendent, warden, director, manager, and executive director.

He is appointed by and works intimately with the owner or board to help formulate policy and to ensure that it is carried out. The CEO's preoccupation with his relationships with the owner or board may in turn influence his relationships with staff.

The CEO is empowered, with rare exception, to hire and fire all of the professional staff serving administrative functions, who in turn hire and fire their own personnel to carry out their departmental responsibilities. This obviously gives that person considerable power in the organization.

The physician administrator must work within these boundaries, since physician power and authority in medicine are not by themselves adequate to support medical input in decision-making. As one observer notes: "The 'old' administration used to be bypassed by the doctors and trustees, who used the administrator as just a secretary . . . . The doctors are holding to this system, while the trustees are

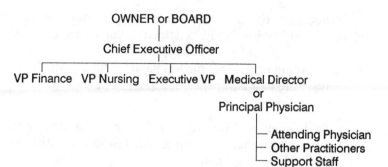

OWNER or BOARD
|
Chief Executive Officer
|
VP Finance   VP Nursing   Executive VP   Medical Director
or
Principal Physician

— Attending Physician
— Other Practitioners
— Support Staff

OPTION 1: Physician Reports to Administration

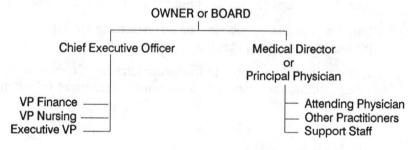

OWNER or BOARD
|

Chief Executive Officer   Medical Director
or
Principal Physician

VP Finance ——
VP Nursing ——
Executive VP ——

— Attending Physician
— Other Practitioners
— Support Staff

OPTION 2: Physician Reports to Board or Owner

Figure 4-1 Typical lines of authority in long-term care facilities.

coming around to the fact that the administrator should not be left out." (Bennett 1978, 28).

While each individual has a different style, certain approaches are essential. First, the physician administrator should be accessible to, and collaborate with, the CEO. Secondly, the physician administrator should develop and foster a good working relationship with other key clinical personnel. In LTC this especially involves working well with the nursing and social service departments.

Third, the physician administrator should view other clinical personnel as equals, rather than as professionals who exist mainly to carry out doctors' orders. Nevertheless, the physician administrator should feel obliged to bring unsound patient care practices to the attention of any pertinent department.

In addition, the physician administrator may enhance his working relationship with the administration and board by:

- attending board meetings regularly, during which he is available to answer questions and contribute to policy discussions

- establishing and serving on a liaison committee to consider, discuss, and make recommendations to the entire board on medically related matters

- contributing his expertise to board members or committees on clinically related issues or debates

- providing evidence that the medical staff delivers quality care

- handling disputes, problems, or infractions related to physician practice or medical staff promptly

- issuing a periodic report to the administrator of concerns and observations, and helping to assure some consistent follow-up.

The Medical Director

General

The most important physician administrator in LTC is the medical director.

Background and Qualifications. Most medical directors have been either family practitioners or internists by training. Both of these specialties have recently established fellowships and other special training in geriatrics. As Figure 4-2 suggests, the medical director has divergent responsibilities for the patient, community, public, facility, and medical staff. Therefore, regardless of specialty, medical direction requires broad interests and a holistic approach. The medical director should be someone who at least understands:

- the need for a team approach to patient care

- general principles of aging and the difference between changes of age and disease due to aging

MEDICAL DIRECTOR'S
PERSPECTIVES ON THE NURSING HOME

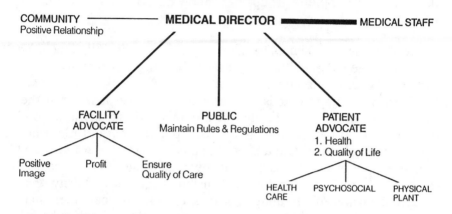

COMMUNITY ————————— MEDICAL DIRECTOR ▬▬▬▬▬▬ MEDICAL STAFF
Positive Relationship

FACILITY ADVOCATE

PUBLIC
Maintain Rules & Regulations

PATIENT ADVOCATE
1. Health
2. Quality of Life

Positive Image   Profit   Ensure Quality of Care

HEALTH CARE   PSYCHOSOCIAL   PHYSICAL PLANT

*Boldness of line indicates degree of strength of the relationship for intensity of contact, frequency and regularity of contact, information gathering and support.

Reprinted with permission by Kay Jewell, MD, Madison, Wisconsin.

Figure 4-2

- the special problems of interviewing, examining, diagnosing, and treating the older patient

- the problems and potentials of drug therapies in the elderly

- the potential for rehabilitation of selected elderly patients

- issues surrounding dying and terminal care

- basic psychological and psychiatric problems involved in caring for the elderly

- general payment and reimbursement issues in LTC

- the specific needs of a particular institution or setting.

In addition, the medical director should be someone willing to keep current in the field; be available for consultation as well as for crises; *and* be able to work well with others within an institutional setting. This last requirement is especially important, because not everyone who shows clinical or research expertise knows how to manage and deal with groups of people. Too often, making managers of bright or accomplished physicians who do not or cannot deal well with people in groups has simply been a costly and painful mistake.

Lines of authority. Figure 4-1 shows that the medical director may be responsible either to the chief executive officer, or directly to the owner or board of directors.

Even more important is the issue of who is responsible *to* the medical director. Theoretically, all attending physicians and non-physician practitioners such as dentists, podiatrists, and physician assistants should be accountable to the medical director, whether acting as a chief of staff or as a department chairman. In practice, the medical director has often had responsibility without authority; that is, he was answerable to administrators, owners, or boards, but had no way to hold the other practitioners accountable for their clinical care. Steps are now being taken to remedy this untenable situation.

Roles. Five major categories of roles for the medical director are as:

- An *advisor* to ownership, administration, and other professional staff
- A *guarantor* of compliance with laws and regulations
- An *overseer* of medical care in a facility
- A *consultant* to attending physicians
- A *provider* of direct patient care.

Some positions involve only one or two of these; others combine them all.

The job description. The following is a comprehensive list of the possible specific responsibilities for a medical director:

- Be responsible for the medical direction and overall coordination of medical care
- Be responsible for the establishment of goals and objectives and an appropriate program development for the medical staff and department

- Assist in the development of written bylaws, rules and regulations applicable to each physician attending patients in the facility

- Help assure the adherence of the medical staff to its bylaws, policies and procedures, rules and regulations

- Assist in arranging for continuous physician coverage for medical emergencies and in developing procedures for emergency treatment of patients

- Participate in developing a system providing a medical care plan for each patient, covering medications, nursing care, restorative services, diet and other services, and if appropriate, a plan for discharge

- Be the facility's medical representative in the community and at appropriate medical meetings and conferences

- Work with the attending medical staff physicians in efforts to ensure effective medical care

- Participate in developing written policies governing the medical, nursing, and related health services provided in the facility;

- Participate in developing patient admission and discharge policies

- Participate in an effective program of long-term care review and quality assurance

- Consult on the development and maintenance of an adequate medical record system

- Advise the Chief Executive Officer (CEO) as to the adequacy of the facility's patient care services and medical equipment, as well as environmental health and safety

- Consult with the directors of nursing and social services, to evaluate the adequacy of the facility's efforts to meet the psychosocial, medical, and physical needs of patients

- Be available for consultation and participation in in-service training programs

- Advise the CEO on employee health policies, and be responsible for the surveillance of the health status of the facility's employees

- Be knowledgeable concerning policies and programs of public health agencies which may affect patient care programs in the facility

- Be a member of appropriate medical staff, institutional, and board committees;

- Coordinate the activities and programs of the medical department with all other departments

- Coordinate transfer and care arrangements for the facility's patients with other institutions

- Take note of and work to resolve medically related problems noted by administration or other departments

- Review and authorize medical clearance and level of care on all admissions

- Prepare and oversee the annual medical budget and an annual departmental report

- Be responsible for the medical education program

- Coordinate physician coverage schedules and responsibilities.

Factors influencing the breadth and extent of medical director involvement in a facility have been discussed earlier in this chapter. At this point, certain aspects of the job description deserve further comment.

Policies and procedures. The institution should make the medical director aware of policies and changes in policies, and his input should be requested for ongoing review and revision of these. The medical director should define clearly the responsibilities of physicians practicing within the facility, and the procedures for dealing with those who do not follow them. Bylaws can set general guidelines, while policies and procedures offer more specifics. As with other responsibilities, these may be done by the medical director alone, or with the input of the attending physicians as a staff or in committees (see below).

Meetings. Both formal and informal meetings are important. Formal meetings include such committees as utilization review (UR), infection control, and pharmacy. Informal ones are those necessary to resolve problems or issues of patient care or physician performance. (See below for further discussion.)

Review of care. A part-time medical director should visit a facility at least twice a month, or more frequently if possible. He should meet with appropriate nursing staff and walk through the facility. He should review various administrative, nursing, dietary, and other concerns, and offer suggestions for resolution. Patient problems can be addressed both as care and as educational issues. At revisits, both full- and part-time medical directors should ensure that patient care issues have been addressed, even in their absence.

Facility representative. The medical director should be the medical representative for both the medical staff and the facility. For example, in the event of an infectious outbreak, the medical director may have to speak to the health department, family members, or the press. He can also help educate the community about the goals of the facility and the various programs for helping residents.

The medical director should also represent the facility in discussions or problem resolution meetings with hospitals, other NHs, or regulatory agencies. As an example of such a problem, hospitals may send medically unstable patients, or not provide adequate medical information. Similarly, health departments sometimes cite deficiencies without understanding what has actually been done to deal with problems.

Education. The medical director should work with the nursing director to create a relevant continuing education program for professional staff. This can include information on new discoveries and practices in geriatrics, drug prescribing and interactions, diet and exercise, or preventive measures in the institutionalized elderly.

The medical director can contribute to the administrator's, owner's, or board's fulfillment of responsibilities by providing occasional reports or in-service programs on issues relevant to medical service and care of the elderly (see Chapter 10).

Admissions. The medical director should assist in devising protocols for the evaluation of prospective admissions, help the facility decide which patients it can accept, and help review the appropriateness and adequacy of individual placement (see Chapter 6).

Quality of care. The medical director should work with other professional staff to establish a quality assurance (QA) program, including standards, measuring tools, and criteria for care (see Chapter 6 for more details). He should review the medical aspects of patient care incidents, or family complaints or disputes. He should follow through to ensure that policies are made and implemented to cover various aspects of care, and to correct and resolve care-related problems.

The medical director should relate to attending physicians to assure their compliance with regulations, including timely visits and adequate documentation. He should be prepared to educate as well as to reprimand.

If the UR or QA committee is used as a medical staff governing committee, the medical director should head the committee, be present at its meetings, and help enforce its decisions.

Provisions for care. Coverage should be available for backup to absent or unavailable doctors, and for emergencies. In many facilities, the attending physicians are responsible for emergencies, and the medical director has no further obligations, unless such coverage fails in individual cases. The medical director should develop a list of available and capable primary care doctors and consultants in all medical and surgical specialties and subspecialties, from which the staff may draw if the resident has no preferences or appropriate physicians.

Advisory role. The medical director should periodically transmit a report summarizing his actions, recommendations, and concerns to the CEO. Besides proving that he is carrying out the contractual and regulatory obligations, the report also serves as an important educational and informational tool.

The Medical Director's Agreement

Every physician serving as a medical director should consider a formal agreement as important as it is in any other business arrangement. It is important for both the facility and the physician to have written specifications of expectations and responsibilities, as well as the support that each will provide the other.

Terms of the arrangement. A service agreement between a medical director and a LTC facility should include at least the following:

- Date of agreement
- Term of agreement
- Job description (as an appendix)
- Privileges, rights, responsibilities, and duties
- Terms of compensation
- Responsibility for professional liability coverage
- Hours per week, and a description of what is included in compensable time
- Rights to retain moneys for patient care services
- Fringe benefits
- Any items or personnel furnished by the facility (e.g., office, secretary, supplies, etc.)
- Terms of the relationship (employee, contractor, etc.)
- Terms of renewal or termination of agreement

Time commitment. This is often difficult to determine, and frequently ends up being more than that for which the physician is actually paid. Much depends on the overall expectations and responsibilities of the position. More time may be needed to start up a program or initiate a position than to subsequently oversee and manage the situation. Suggested minimum weekly hours for medical direction are: 2 to 5 hours/week for facilities of fewer than 100 beds; 4 to 10 hours/week for 100-150 beds; 8 to 15 hours/week for 150-200 beds; and at least half-time (20 hours/week) for over 200 beds. Time spent on administrative responsibilities (including acting in the medical director's consultative role for other physicians' patients) should be considered separately from time allocated to primary patient care responsibilities.

Compensation. As one of the biggest issues regarding physician participation in LTC, many physicians still feel that the compensation is inadequate for the time and responsibility involved. Compensation on an hourly basis for part-time medical directors ranges from $25 to $100 an hour, and annual compensation for a full-time medical director from about $45,000 to $125,000 per annum. These salaries all vary with experience, responsibilities, total time commitment, facility size and location, level of care and medical complexity of patients, and third party reimbursement to the institution for administrative costs. Each individual should consider these factors and his own personal commitment to the job before negotiating compensation.

As always, third-party payors and NH administrations should recognize that they will generally get what they pay for. A competent individual who will devote the necessary time and energy to the task deserves adequate compensation. The failure to provide this can only decrease the likelihood of attracting qualified individuals to do a difficult job, and will perpetuate the problems.

Liability. The facility should be prepared to support the medical director in his efforts to reduce facility and professional liability, and to do what it can to protect the medical director from the liabilities inherent in his role. (See Chapter 11 for a review of liability issues for medical directors.)

Fringe benefits. These might include any or all of: health, life, disability, or liability insurance; paid vacation; paid educational leave; prescription drug payment plan; or participation in a retirement plan.

See Appendix 4-A for a sample service contract between a nursing home and medical director.

The Medical Director As Patient Care Provider

Many principal physicians and medical directors have also provided some, or most, of the patient care in the NH. This raises several additional issues.

First, compensation for medical direction may be separate and distinct from that for patient care. Practice privileges should be considered and reconsidered separately from the administrative position, so that the qualified physician can still care for patients even if he is no longer retained by the facility as its medical director. This clarification should be written into any bylaws and definitions of privileges, and into a service contract.

The medical director who provides patient care must also be just as accountable as the attending staff for the quality of his patient care. He should always be willing to have his patients included in all QA monitoring activities. The absence of such an attitude dissuades other physicians from providing conscientious service and care.

A medical director's failure to provide adequate patient care, or to allow his own work to be subject to the same reviews as is that of other physicians, should be dealt with according to the same procedures as applied to other staff physicians. If necessary, impartial outside reviewers may need to be brought in, since the medical director may not be in a position to adequately judge his own conduct.

Medical Organization, Policies, and Procedures

Since not all LTC programs or facilities will have extensive medical staffing or organization, there is not just one proper approach to organization. However, certain principles of establishing policies and procedures apply in every setting.

While good organization without foresight and imagination does not itself guarantee an innovative, productive program, it is still the solid foundation of every medical system, including physician groups, and essential for long-term success. A poorly organized program may stay together for a while, but the stresses will eventually weaken and possibly destroy it.

Organizational charts. LTC physician services may be either *departmental* or *nondepartmental*. No matter how loose the structure of any organization or department, it never hurts to have an organizational chart. This should allow an insider or outsider to get a quick overview of that group and the working relationships among all the group's divisions. It should also indicate the relationship of the department to the ownership and administration. If there is an organized medical staff with leadership different from the medical director, the lines of responsibility and authority and the interactions among the doctors should be clarified. Such information is invaluable in understanding the relationship between structure, function, and achievement of goals, and is vital to assisting the flow of information and delineating the responsibilities for the investigation, handling and follow-up of problems. (See Appendix 4-B for several examples.)

Policies and procedures. These are two different things, though often intertwined. Policies are general principles, or decisions to adhere to certain standards or strive for certain goals. Procedures are the specific means of carrying out the policies to eventually conform with the standards or achieve the goals.

Policies reflect the wishes of those in charge of an organization, program, department, or operation. Procedures are the guidelines for those hired to do the things that bring the policies to fruition (for example, the staff physicians).

For several reasons, every medical group should have an explicit set of policies and procedures. First, these clarify expectations. Second, there are then usable standards against which to measure performance. Third, when things are in writing, people are less able to evade responsibility by claiming, "I didn't know" or "I forgot." Fourth, it is far easier to train new personnel when the information is written down.

Job responsibilities. For the nondepartmental medical staff, there should at least be a statement of overall expectations and responsibilities (for example, timely visits, adequate documentation, and appropriate care).

For the departmental staff, there should be a fairly detailed job description for each role in the department (e.g., division head, education director, staff physician), that supplements the general departmental or medical staff requirements. This is especially useful at the time of annual personnel evaluations, as it provides some specific objective criteria against which to measure performance.

Other professionals or departments. For the nondepartmental staff, certain relationships with other LTC professionals (nursing, social services, dietary) should be clarified. For example, who notifies families in the event of changes in patient condition? Who makes arrangements for transfers to acute facilities? Who discusses with patients or families their wishes about care options or resuscitation efforts? Who documents what on the charts?

Relationships of departmental staff to other departments should be similarly clarified, but in more detail and in anticipation of more frequent interactions. For example, who is responsible for various aspects of monitoring infectious outbreaks, such as recording pertinent information, or reporting them to the health department?

Assignments. Each physician's assignments, including hours, units, and ancillary duties, should be specified in detail.

Expectations of employees–job descriptions and performance evaluations. For departmental staff, performance evaluations should be a time for the exchange of ideas and suggestions to help both the individual and the department or program. They should be based on as many specific criteria as possible.

General categories of such criteria might include:

- Medical knowledge and skill in geriatrics
- Compliance with institutional needs
- Cooperation and general reliability
- Documentation and recordkeeping
- Ancillary skills and achievements (publications, teaching abilities, research grants).

As always, the criteria for a competent performer depends on the standards and goals of a given program. Nevertheless, cooperation and reliability, including respect for the rights and feelings of others, are as important as clinical skills and academic accomplishments. Appropriate behavior and treatment of others are essential, and may be assessed under performance (see Appendix 4-C).

For nondepartmental staff or attending physicians, a list of general expectations such as those in Chapter 3 are very helpful in monitoring quality of care and in acting on privilege renewals.

Categories of Medical Policies

Policies pertinent to LTC medical staffing may be grouped as follows:

- General policies, department organization, and job descriptions;
- Admissions, discharges, and transfers
- Physician interactions with patients and families
- Physician interactions with other staff and departments
- Medical care issues
- Laboratory and other testing
- Documentation and medical records
- Infection control
- Consultant services
- Orders
- Provision of information
- Permissible privileges and practices.

These policies and procedures should cover basic organizational questions, such as those discussed in Chapter 3 and earlier in this chapter. How is the department or staff organized? What coverage is provided, how often, and to whom? Who has primary patient responsibility? During what hours are staff available? What is the coverage during off-hours? From where or whom are other consultative and support services obtained? How are emergencies handled? How often must physicians see patients, and what kinds of supporting documentation are required? What are policies on vacation and educational leave? How do physicians get reimbursed for expenditures? What are the prerogatives and restrictions for house officers, students, and other non-physicians in the department? What are special needs for specific or special units, like rehabilitation or psychiatric units? How should clinic or consultation requests be initiated and followed up? Appendix 4-D shows a categorical arrangement of long-term care policies as part of a manual.

Admissions, discharges and transfers. These include medical responsibilities on admission; patient transfer; discharge summaries; and patient leaves of absence.

Admission medical information should include at least certain basic items, discussed in more detail in Chapter 9, including:

- Primary admitting diagnosis

- Summary of current medical findings

- Current physical examination

- Diet, medication, activity, and treatment orders

- Functional status

- Pertinent past medical history

- Rehabilitation potential (good; fair; poor; none)

- Condition (good; fair; guarded; critical)

- Prognosis (good; fair; guarded; poor)

- Pertinent laboratory, X-ray and consultation reports.

Good care of the LTC patient also requires certain physician actions at the time of discharge and transfers, including:

- No patient should be discharged without a physician's order

- A discharge plan should be worked out collaboratively between medical, nursing, and social work professionals

- Necessary forms and prescriptions should be completed at the time of discharge

- Patients should not be transferred without the physician's first contacting the receiving facility
- Pertinent parts of the medical record should accompany the patient at the time of transfer.

Interactions with other staff or agencies. These should cover delineation of responsibilities, such as notification of information on patient status, interactions with acute hospitals, or requirements for reporting to regulatory agencies.

Patient and family interactions. As discussed in Chapter 5, these responsibilities include meeting with families, following up on questions, handling complaints, and completing forms (such as insurance or level of care justification forms).

Medical care. As discussed in Chapters 5 and 6, these include utilization and quality assurance issues, diagnostic or treatment protocols, and specialty-specific information.

Specific clinical protocols for the management of certain diseases, symptoms, or problems are helpful quality assurance tools, and also provide objective criteria for performance evaluation. These protocols should be particularly helpful in reducing the most frequent and widespread problems in LTC; for example, overprescribing of medications, too many drugs for the same condition, inadequate follow-up after treatment is instituted, poor response to notification of changes in condition, and failures to adequately evaluate potentially treatable conditions (such as acute changes in mental status). Relevant diagnostic and treatment protocols might cover management of: decubitus ulcers, incontinence, constipation, behavior changes, or the workup and management of anemias.

One problem in creating such protocols is the frequent lack of consensus about the treatment of conditions or problems, and the fact that there is often more than one way to achieve the same goals. Especially in the elderly population, adequate clinical data are often missing. Therefore, while any such protocols must be sufficiently broad to allow for individual physician decision making, they should at least promote some basic standards of good care.

Infection control. Policies should address medical ordering of antibiotics; monitoring of infections; vaccination; surveillance; prevention; and handling of communicable disease outbreaks (see Chapter 6).

Consultant services. Policies should cover the existence of various consultant services, and the procedures should detail how these are to be requested, how the forms should be filled out, how the consultant should be notified of the request, following up after the consultation, and authorization and transcription of a consultant's suggested orders or tests. As full a range as possible of medical and surgical consultations should be available to the attending medical staff of LTC facilities. Organized medical staffs should ask regularly called consultants to become members of the medical staff.

Another practical arrangement is to have a rotating schedule of outside consultants who cover for a period (such as a month or quarter) at a time. These consultants are available to assist attending physicians with patients who have problems relevant to their specialties. They can also be very helpful as a backup for the medical director in the event of inadequate response by an attending physician, or for a patient or family to choose from if they do not have a physician or specialist.

Handling phone information is a major concern in LTC. Though such calls are often for routine matters, they are often made to report changes in patient condition, concerns of patient or family, or problems or side effects with medications. Many such persons wind up being sent to emergency rooms, because the attending physician cannot ascertain the severity of the problem from the information provided by the caller. The purpose of such policies is not to make telephone diagnoses, but to improve the management and disposition of LTC patients with acute problems.

It is helpful to design protocols to assist nursing staff in evaluating, documenting, and reporting changes in patient condition. While they cannot be expected to make diagnoses, nurses should at least provide the most complete and accurate descriptions and information.

Whenever possible, the caller should have the chart available, as well as the following information: current vital signs, medication list, description of symptoms and observations, and current state of distress. The physician receiving the call should request any necessary information to help make a decision about proper disposition.

Verbal orders should always be read back to the authorizing physician to ensure accurate transcription. Such orders should be countersigned at the next visit.

Orders. Policies should include standards for correct and complete order writing; use of a formulary; drug utilization and review (see Chapter 6); signature requirements; verbal orders; abbreviations; p.r.n. orders; hold and stop orders; nasogastric and parenteral drug administration; emergency drug boxes; discharge medications; medications for leaves of absence; required admission and discharge order writing; and acceptable protocols for nondrug orders, such as diet, treatments, clinic visits, supplemental oxygen, activities, vital sign monitoring, consultation requests, and lab tests.

Restraints and protective devices are a special medical care issue. The use of restraints and protective devices in institutionalized individuals has always engendered considerable controversy. If judiciously used, they can help protect individuals from injury and lessen the requirement for psychotropic drugs, with their attendant side effects. When improperly or inappropriately used, they can cause injury and even death. Therefore, certain policies regarding their use are appropriate, including:

- A physician's order should be required for their use.

- The order must be rewritten daily for restraints, and monthly or bimonthly for protective devices, and should reflect the reasons for their use.

- The patient must be observed periodically for complications, and to ensure that other care needs are met.

- The patient should be turned and positioned periodically.

- Verbal orders for use of such devices should be cosigned promptly.

Laboratory and other testing, includes test ordering; diagnostic and monitoring equipment; and procedures regarding specific tests.

For example, policies on admission tests on LTC patients might require baseline CBC, chemistries, EKG, urinalysis, and chest X-ray. Copies of any of these studies done within the last six months may substitute for retesting, unless previous results were abnormal and should have been followed up. Some states also require screening for tuberculosis and enteric pathogens within a certain period before or after admission.

Most routine annual laboratory testing has not been shown to yield enough useful information, or significantly change patient treatment to justify the expense. Requirements for other "routine" periodic tests should be based on the situation; for example, diabetics should be followed with periodic blood sugars, anticoagulated patients with intermittent prothrombin times, and those on diuretics with periodic electrolytes. These should be written into the regular orders, and where possible placed under the problem for which they are being ordered. There are no absolute current recommendations as to how often any of these should be done. The medical director, in conjunction with staff, should decide on absolute minimums, or other appropriate standards.

Documentation and medical records. While most physicians abhor paperwork, documentation is critical to quality care, and essential for adequate facility reimbursement. Policies should cover release of information; chart use and organization; record completion requirements; provision of information on admission, discharge, and transfer; acceptable abbreviations; and instructions on the completion of specific forms (especially death certificates).

Permissible privileges and practices. A policy should cover those clinical privileges appropriate to a particular facility setting (See Chapter 3). Decisions on what to allow should be based not just on a physician's demonstrated skills and capabilities, but also on whether the facility has necessary supplies, equipment, and trained and available staff to assist and support those activities.

In most NHs, for instance, only minor surgery under local anesthesia, such as suturing of lacerations or debridement of wounds, is appropriate. Administration of general anesthesia, or performance of general surgery, is unsuitable.

Organized medical staffs should specifically delineate allowable clinical privileges for each physician. With informal medical staffs, a general policy should at least describe the boundaries of acceptable procedures and practices (for example, no insertions of arterial or central venous lines; no procedures under general anesthesia).

The Role and Organization of LTC Committees

In any organization, committees can help accomplish many things, but can also be just another source of confusion and disruption when improperly organized. Which committees are necessary, and their essential roles, depend on regulatory requirements as well as on our goals and objectives.

Important clinical responsibilities in LTC often handled by committees, for which medical input is helpful and important, include: quality assurance, infection control, documentation, drug prescribing and dispensing, diagnoses and treatment, proper utilization of beds and resources, environmental safety, emergencies, diagnostic services, and patient transfers and placement.

Committees for which medical staffs are often directly responsible generally include:

- Medical records
- Infection control
- Pharmacy and therapeutics
- Utilization review
- Patient care.

The teaching NH may also have education and research committees (see Chapter 13).

Medical Records Committee

This committee should be responsible for assuring patient medical records that are complete, timely, and clinically pertinent. The committee should selectively examine currently maintained medical records to assure that they describe the condition and progress of the patient properly, the therapy provided, the results thereof, and the identification of responsibility for all actions taken, and that they are sufficiently complete at all times to facilitate medical comprehension of the case in the event of transfer of physician responsibility for patient care. The committee should also review the records of discharged patients to determine the relevance, adequacy, and completeness thereof. It should also advise and recommend policies for the medical records department, and supervise the organization of the medical records to assure that sufficient details are recorded properly to permit evaluation of the care of the patients; oversee proper filing, indexing, storage, and availability of all patient records; and advise and develop policies to guide the medical record librarian, medical staff and administration regarding problems of privileged communication and release of patient information.

Infection Control Committee

This committee should oversee the surveillance for inadvertent infection potential, review and analyze actual infections, promote a preventive and corrective program designed to minimize infection hazards, and supervise infection control.

Pharmacy and Therapeutics Committee

This committee should develop and oversee all drug utilization policies and practices within the facility, to strive for optimum clinical results and a minimum potential for hazard. The committee should assist in the formation of broad professional policies regarding the evaluation, appraisal, selection, procurement, storage, distribution, use, safety, and all other matters relating to drugs. It should also advise the facility's medical staff and the pharmacist on the aforementioned matters.

Utilization Review Committee

This committee should evaluate the appropriateness of admissions and discharges, the lengths of patient stays, the use of medical services and all related factors which may contribute to the effective utilization of institutional and physician services. The committee should communicate the results of its studies and other pertinent data to the entire medical staff and should make recommendations for the optimum utilization of institutional resources. It should also formulate a written utilization review plan for the facility, which should be in effect at all times. Where appropriate, the committee should evaluate the medical necessity for continued services for particular patients, according to established criteria.

Patient Care Committee

This committee should adopt specific programs and procedures for reviewing, evaluating, and maintaining the quality and efficiency of a facility's patient care. It should also coordinate the findings and results of staff activities designed to monitor patient care practices.

Efficient Organization and Use of Meetings

How many committees there are is not as important as what they do. The medical director cannot allow his time to be used excessively on these committees, at the expense of his other responsibilities. Nursing and other staff, and attending physicians, who are represented on these committees obviously have limited time.

In addition, because of the difficulty of gathering and coordinating key personnel in LTC, the efficient scheduling of meeting time is essential. One solution is to combine quality assurance activities with other departmental and staff committee functions, to facilitate rapid transfer of information and assignment of investigative and problem-solving activities.

Physician and other staff time may be best utilized by organizing a single monthly quality assurance/staff committee meeting. Key personnel from the clinical services should be present. The work of various committees or departments should be presented consecutively. Quality of care reports and discussions should be worked in as well.

Figure 4-3 is an actual example of how a regular 1 to 2 hour monthly meeting can, on a rotating basis, accommodate the basic needs of both physicians and the institution.

The following are examples of the agenda items covered at these meetings, all of which can benefit from physician input:

- Summaries of the reviews of patients at Medicare skilled or chronic levels of care (UR)

- Prevention of employee injuries and reduction of sick time (risk management)

- Fire hazards in the institution (fire & safety)
- Incidents and accidents involving patients and employees (fire & safety)
- Actions necessary to reduce number of falls on a particular unit (patient care)
- Review of physician documentation deficiencies (medical records)
- More effective ways of treating decubitus ulcers (patient care)
- Review of quarterly drug and therapeutics evaluations (pharmacy & therapeutics)
- Preemployment TB testing among employees (infection control)
- Appropriate routine laboratory testing for patients (patient care)

Medical Committee/Quality Assurance Meeting Schedule

Month 1

1:00	QA Review/UR/Risk Management/Fire and Safety
1:30	Pharmacy and Therapeutics
2:00	Medical Records

Month 2

1:00	QA Review/UR/Risk Management/Fire and Safety
1:30	Patient Care
1:50	Infection Control

Month 3

1:00	QA Review/UR/Risk Management/Fire and Safety
1:30	Patient Care
1:50	Medical Records

Month 4

1:00	QA Review/UR/Risk Management/Fire and Safety
1:30	Patient Care
1:50	Infection Control
2:30	Pharmacy and Therapeutics

Month 5

1:00	QA Review/UR/Risk Management/Fire and Safety
1:30	Medical Records

Month 6

1:00	QA Review/UR/Risk Management/Fire and Safety
1:30	Patient Care
1:50	Infection Control

Figure 4-3 Example of a monthly meeting schedule.

In this way, in each 6-month span, essential committee functions are covered at appropriate or required times, with a minimum of staff disruption and travel time. The entire spectrum of problems and quality of care issues faced in LTC facilities may be addressed in a coordinated fashion. By insisting on objective investigation according to specific criteria and standards, behind-the-scenes data gathering and activities of all committees and departments gradually become more consistent.

Reports from these staff committee/quality assurance meetings are then channeled to the appropriate individual department heads or administrative persons for their input and action. Within the medical staff, they may go to the medical director and/or medical executive committee for their review or action, including recommendations requiring policy actions by the medical staff. That QA material pertinent to the physicians is evaluated and reviewed at staff meetings. Follow-up occurs at subsequent committee meetings.

The key to making this system work is the efficient organization of agendas and presentations, the adequate preliminary preparation of staff, and the use of subcommittees and individual departments to perform many investigations and data analyses before the scheduled meetings.

Summary: Establishing a Role as a Medical Director

In summary, each physician must consider a number of important questions in the process of establishing a role as a medical director. First and foremost is the question of, "What are my personal goals, including my commitment to long-term care?"

After deciding that long-term care is compatible with his or her objectives, and that he or she has enough of the training, knowledge, and skills for the position, the physician must evaluate the prospective situation. This requires asking questions about role, responsibilities, authority, staffing, support, expectations of others, job description, time commitment, compensation, and liabilities (see "Strategy Worksheets").

Having taken a position as medical director, a physician must then perform appropriate organizational and administrative functions. The first critical step is establishing a structure, represented by an organization chart. The organization chart, like the patient problem list, is an extremely effective and simple way of summarizing a complex situation.

The next step is to decide whether there will be any special programs, activities, or divisions that will require other medical administrative persons, such as an assistant medical director, or non-physician administrative coordinator. Such persons must be authorized, funded, hired, trained, and advised of their responsibilities and objectives.

At the same time, policies and procedures need to be established to cover areas of medical practice and interactions with others in a facility (see above). Lines of communication with other departments and programs need to be established, and areas of responsibility and cooperation delineated. Committees should be set up, and their membership determined.

Finally, the program, division, or department operates with the clear understanding that involvement with all the above steps will continue to be necessary as organizational structures change, new programs are instituted, and old policies must be modified.

Appendix 4-A Sample medical director's agreement

EMPLOYMENT AGREEMENT

THIS AGREEMENT is made as of the _____ day of _____, by and between _____ (hereinafter referred to as the "Home"), and _____ (hereinafter referred to as the "Physician").

In consideration of the mutual covenants herein contained, the parties agree as follows:

1. *Employment.* The Home hereby employs the Physician as the Medical Director on a full time basis and the Physician hereby accepts such employment upon the terms and conditions herein set forth.

2. *Term.* The term of this Agreement shall be for a period of one year and shall be renewed automatically each year thereafter, unless terminated as herein provided. The appointment is subject to the approval of the Board.

3. *Compensation.* For all services rendered by the Physician under this Agreement, the Physician shall receive the salary and benefits set forth on Schedule A attached hereto. Such salary and benefits shall be paid to the Physician in such installments as are determined by the Board of Directors of the Home.

4. *License and Duties.* The Physician at all times shall be qualified, professionally competent, duly licensed under the laws of _____, and have a current narcotics number. The Physician must apply for and receive a medical staff appointment and clinical privileges, and direct the regular medical staff activities and responsibilities including attendance at required meetings. The Physician agrees to make himself regularly available for such service at such times as shall be mutually agreed upon by the parties. The Physician further agrees to be physically present at the institution during those hours for which he is obligated or otherwise required for committee or staff attendance. The Physician agrees that, in performing the services, he will be governed by the standards and criteria prescribed by the Board of Directors of the Home and by the Medical Staff Bylaws.

5. *Medical Fees.* The Physician shall not bill or receive fees for medical services rendered to the Home's patients in the course of his employment hereunder. The Home shall determine whether a fee should be charged for a particular patient service and to prescribe the amount of any such fee. The Home shall have the exclusive right to bill and collect all fees and payments which may be generated by such services; in the event that payment for such services is available from the service patient's private insurer or from Medicare, Medicaid or a

similar government program, the Physician will sign such forms, certificates and/or documents as may be necessary to the Home's collection of such payment.

6. *Termination.* This Agreement may be terminated:

   a. By the Home immediately without notice in the event the Home, in good faith, determines that the Physician is not providing adequate patient care, or that the safety of patients is jeopardized by continuing the employment of the Physician;

   b. At the end of the initial or any renewal period by either party upon written notice delivered at least sixty (60) days prior thereto;

   c. By suspension, revocation or cancellation of the Physician's right to practice medicine in the State of _____;

   d. By a governmental authority having appropriate jurisdiction, placing or imposing of any restrictions or limitations upon the Physician so that he cannot engage in the practice of medicine;

   e. By the Home in the event the Physician shall fail or refuse to comply with the reasonable policies, standards and regulations of the Home.

7. The Physician agrees to comply and provide all necessary documentation or completion of the medical records within acceptable time limits.

8. The Home agrees to provide an adequate level of professional liability coverage on a claims made basis, and while performing administrative responsibilities for the medical staff or Home.

9. The Home agrees to provide an appropriate level of financial support for continuing education programs, and the Physician is responsible for maintaining currency in their specialty field to meet the normally acceptable standards as established by the State, or other licensing or certifying body.

10. The Physician is responsible for recommending or establishing additions or changes to the Medical Staff Bylaws to conform to the current acceptable practices of medicine, and to promulgate those practices as approved by the Board; and to represent the Medical Staff before the appropriate meetings and committees.

ATTEST:

_____   By: _____

WITNESS:

_____   _____(SEAL)

DATE: _____

Schedule A

To

Employment Agreement

1. Name: _____

2. Annual Salary: _____

    Beginning: _____

3. All personnel benefits currently received by other full time employees, such as vacation and sick time accrual, health and life insurance, and retirement plan coverage, etc., will be provided at no expense to the Physician.

Appendix 4-B Sample organizational charts for a long-term care medical staff

Medical Department Organization

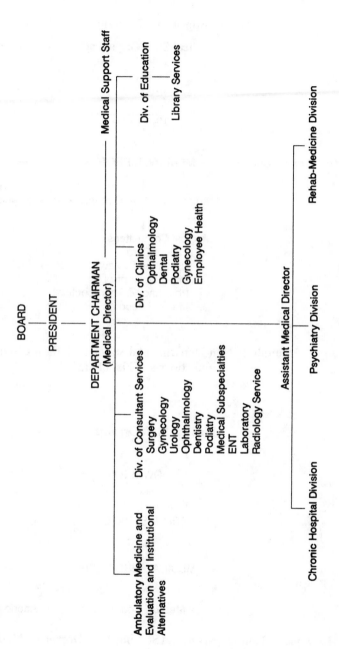

Example 1: Departmental Staffing

Appendix 4-B continued

Medical Staff Organization

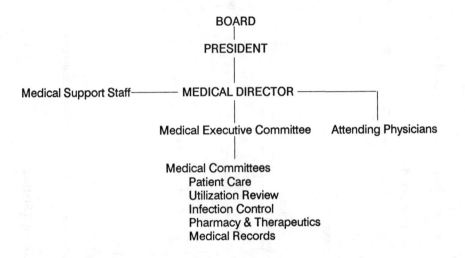

Example 2: Non-Departmental Staffing, Medical Director
Functions as Chief of Staff

Medical Staff Organization

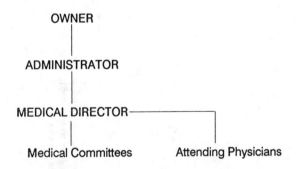

Example 3: Non-Departmental Staffing, Non-Organized Medical Staff,
Small Facility

Appendix 4-C Example of an evaluation tool for
salaried long-term care physicians

Employee's Name: _____

Job Title: _____

Date: _____

Type of Evaluation:

_____ probationary

_____ interim

_____ annual

_____ overall

CODE: 2 = more than satisfactory; 1 = satisfactory; 0 = not satisfactory

Responsibilities:

1. *Medical Care*

   a. provision of competent diagnosis and treatment of
      assigned patients   2   1   0
   b. handling of patient/family inquiries, problems   2   1   0
   c. sensitivity to needs/problems of assigned patients   2   1   0

2. *Knowledge*

   a. understanding of principles and facts which
      underlie geriatric medicine   2   1   0
   b. appropriate justification of medical decisions
      and actions   2   1   0

3. *Cooperation*

   a. cooperation with other department members   2   1   0
   b. willingness to accept assignments and assist
      where needed   2   1   0
   c. collaboration with other professionals   2   1   0

4. *Institutional Matters*

   a. attendance   2   1   0
   b. dress code   2   1   0
   c. compliance with policies and procedures   2   1   0

5. *Recordkeeping/Documentation*

   a. adequacy of written histories, physicals, and
      progress notes   2   1   0
   b. legibility of written documentation   2   1   0
   c. completeness and timeliness of documentation   2   1   0
   d. timeliness of discharge summaries and signatures   2   1   0

Comments:

_____

_____

_____

Overall Performance: 1 = Excellent; 2 = Very Good; 3 = Satisfactory;
4 = Marginal; 5 = Unacceptable (circle one)

_____   _____
Evaluator   Date

Appendix 4-D Example of a categorical arrangement of
long-term care medical policies

DEPARTMENT: MEDICAL

SUBJECT: CONTENTS - MEDICAL DEPARTMENT

POLICY MANUAL

SECTION NO.   500   General Services, including:
Organization/Job Description
General Personnel Policies Regarding Physicians
Medical Department Divisions – Long-Term Care
Medical Department Divisions – Psychiatry
Medical Department Divisions – Hospital
Medical Department Divisions – Rehabilitation
Medical Department Divisions – Clinics
Medical Department Divisions – Consultations
Medical Department Divisions – Continuing
    Education

510   Relations with Other Departments, Staff, Adminis-
    tration, Employees, Agencies, including:
Nursing
Other Departments
Administration
Other Hospitals
Regulatory Agencies/Health Departments

520   Admissions, Transfers, Discharges, including:
Attending Physicians and Others – Obligations and
    Privileges
Admissions – Physician's Role
Transferring Patients
Discharges
Discharge or Transfer to Hospital
MLOAs and LOAs (Special Problems)
Ambulance and Other Forms

530   General Interactions with Patients and Families,
    including:
Patient/Physician Interactions
Family/Physician Interactions
Incident Reports

540   Patient Treatment, Quality and Appropriateness
            of Care, including:
        Audits and Quality Assurance Reviews
        Utilization Review, Levels of Care

550   Specific Illnesses or Medical Needs – Their
            Treatment and Follow-up, including:
        Medicine (including internal medicine,
            dermatology, nuclear/radiotherapy)
        Surgical (including ophthalmology, ENT, urology,
            orthopedics, cardiovascular, neurology)
        Gynecologic
        Psychiatric
        Dental
        Specific Treatments – by objects, especially catheters
        Dietary

560   Laboratory and Diagnostic Testing and Monitoring
            of Illnesses
        Ordering Tests, including:
        Radiology
        Laboratory
        Diagnostic and Monitoring Equipment
        Procedures Regarding Specific Tests

570   Medical Records, including:
        Release of Medical Information
        Completion of Specific Forms
        Organization and Use of Floor Chart
        Completion of Records by Physicians
        Abbreviations

580   Infection Control, including:
         Prevention/Vaccination/Isolation/Precautions
        Employees
        Diagnosis and Follow-up
        Environment and Equipment
        Reporting Infectious Disease/Public Health Agencies

590   Medical Staff Matters, including:
        Appointments and Reappointments
        Clinical Privileges, Abridgement
        Suspension and Disciplinary Actions
        Hearings and Appeals

References

Bennett, A. C. 1978. *Improving Management Performance in Health Care Institutions.* Chicago: American Hospital Association.

For Further Reading

American Medical Association. 1977. *The Medical Director in the Long-Term Care Facility.* Chicago: AMA. A collection of articles on the role, responsibilities, and prerogatives of the LTC medical director.

National Foundation for Long Term Health Care. 1981. *Proceedings of a Conference Held May 23-24, 1981.* Washington, D.C.: National Foundation for Long Term Health Care.

Pattee, J. 1983. Update on the medical director concept. *American Family Physician* 28(6):129-133.

For additional information on medical administration and management, contact the following organizations:

American Medical Association, 535 N. Dearborn; Chicago, IL 60610.

American Medical Directors Association, 1200 15th St. N.W., Washington, D.C. 20005.

American Geriatrics Society, 770 Lexington Ave., NY, NY 10021.

National Foundation for Long-Term Health Care, 1200 15th St. N.W., Washington, D.C. 20005.

Chapter Five

General Medical Care Issues

Debra S. Wertheimer, M.D.

Chapter Objectives

This chapter will highlight important general care issues relevant to the practice of LTC medicine. These include:

- the importance of continuity and coordination of care
- the place of geriatric assessment services
- the physician role in care planning
- deciding on levels of care and service
- the involvement of family
- important principles of prescribing
- the value of preventive and screening measures
- important aspects of dealing with terminal illness.

Continuity and Coordination of Care

The elderly are major users of health care services (Cassel and Walsh 1984); almost everyone over 60 would benefit from a continuing relationship with a physician or other health care provider. Continuity of care is often difficult to achieve, as patients consult various specialists and use many levels of the health care system. As people age, they use all types of medical services (physicians, hospitals, chronic care facilities, nonphysician health providers, drugs, etc.), often resulting in fragmented care.

Those well elderly, who function independently in society, typically experience some symptoms related to aging which may require medical advice. But much of the time and attention of medical providers is focused on the frail elderly, who have numerous problems and who require multiple interventions. Their care must be coordinated and continuous. Patients, providers, and families must understand the health care system and know how to link services to improve coordination of care. Quality medical care requires that each professional in the system know relevant information about a given patient.

The primary care physician has an important role in ensuring that each patient's care is coordinated and continuous. Physicians are involved at many levels of care, as a primary outpatient provider, inpatient attending, or nursing home (NH) physician. The primary care physician also initiates involvement by specialists and services such as home care or day care. The physician can help improve continuity of care by the orderly and timely provision of information to other providers (see Chapter 9). Yet even when much of the patient's care is provided by a consultant, the primary physician should remain involved, since consultants frequently must depend on a primary physician's knowledge of the patient's condition, prognosis, desires, or quality of life.

Experience has shown that the use of case managers has improved patient and family satisfaction and allowed patients to remain in the community for a longer time. Because case managers are often not physicians, they need physician contact and input to adequately assess the individual's ever-changing condition. In most communities, physicians must fill the case manager role by informing patients and their families of the available services and alternative care sources.

In short, the LTC physician may increase coordination and continuity of care for the LTC patient by:

- becoming aware of the facilities, programs, and services available to the LTC patient for assistance with care, funding, and follow-up

- using the services of case managers as provided by government or private agencies

- referring the patient to appropriate places or persons to assist with the actual management and follow-up

- informing patients and families of necessary information about the LTC system

- completing appropriate forms and contacting appropriate agencies

- ensuring adequate communication and information exchange with other persons and programs in the LTC system.

Geriatric Assessments

Formal geriatric assessment programs (GAPs) are helpful in establishing proper diagnosis and appropriate therapy, placement, and referral of the elderly. Geriatric assessments can be performed in a variety of settings and with a variety of participants, depending on location of the programs, other secondary objectives (education or research), or the funding sources. GAP evaluations can be done on inpatient units, as consultation services in the acute hospital, as in-home evaluations, in LTC facilities, or as outpatient programs. Regardless of location and the differences inherent in the locations (e.g., home evaluations provide an insight into the social and community supports not obtained in other settings), all GAPs provide an in-depth evaluation of functional (mental, physical, and social) status. The goals of these geriatric assessment programs (GAPs) include:

- improving the functional status of the frail elderly
- improving the coordination of services and therapy
- improving the quality of life
- improving the functional, mental, and social diagnosis of impairments
- determining the most appropriate sources of care
- determining appropriate placement
- coordinating services and resources

Several studies suggest that GAPs do indeed help achieve these goals (Rubenstein 1987; Rubenstein et al. 1984; Williams 1987). As GAPs are a growing component of the American health care system, such programs are even more valuable because of the rapid growth of the "old-old" (over age 75), a segment of the population which has been shown to use a disproportionate amount of health care resources (Pawlson and Berenson 1986). As such, GAPs can help benefit both the individual and society as a whole.

Most GAPs restrict the participants to those over age 65, those functionally impaired individuals at risk for placement in NHs, those who make frequent emergency room visits or have repeated acute hospitalizations, those who have multiple medications and receive care from many different physicians, and those with possible rehabilitation potential. Clearly, the earlier someone is assessed and a care plan formulated, the more likely the intervention is to be successful. The timing of the assessment often depends on the ability of the referring physician, social agency, or family, to recognize the problems and know that such programs exist.

Regardless of the types or sites of assessments, the core assessment team usually consists of a physician, a social worker, and a physical or occupational therapist. Depending on available resources, other team members or consultants may include: nutritionists, pharmacists, psychiatrists, psychologists, lawyers, dentists, and nurses (see Chapter 7). After team members evaluate the patient, they discuss their assessment and propose a care plan or modifications to the current care plan, with the aforementioned goals in mind.

Such recommendations often include:

- further diagnostic studies to allow better definition of the medical condition

- changes to improve the medical regimen

- methods to improve the functional status

- suggestions for the use of community services not previously considered (such as day care, home health care, or companionship)

- consultations with a lawyer regarding guardianship or other protective services

- options regarding placement (such as LTC facilities or foster care).

Although GAPs are becoming more available, they are not widely accessible to most physicians who care for the frail elderly. In addition, they are time- and labor-intensive, and often cost more to perform than they generate in reimbursement. However, the elderly can be assessed even without an organized GAP. Individual physicians can obtain much of the relevant information, including:

- a mental status exam
- an assessment of the activities of daily living (ADLs)
- an assessment of the instrumental activities of daily living (IADLs)
- a critical review of all drugs (both prescription and OTC)
- dietary review
- financial review
- available family and community support systems.

With this information the physician can begin to offer a more comprehensive care plan oriented towards improved function.

Role of the Physician in Care Plans

"Care planning" is a term frequently used by nonphysician health professionals to indicate the goals and methods established by providers for all aspects of a person's medical care, including medications, nutritional needs, prevention of pressure sores, goals for ambulation, and discharge plans. While physicians ultimately establish many of these objectives, the medical orders and progress notes constitute a *medical* care plan rather than a *comprehensive* care plan.

Care plans allow all those involved with the care of the patient to have some input. Such plans should include:

- the medical goals

- the functional goals

- the short-term goals

- the long-term objectives

- when to transfer to a different level of care

- what to do in an emergency (e.g., intubation, antibiotics, use of emergency rooms)

- appropriate nutritional support

For his part, the physician must evaluate the patient's needs, medical condition, and ability to perform activities of daily living (ADLs) and instrumental activities of daily living (IADLs), and short- and long-term objectives. This evaluation should be shared with family and with the other health professionals caring for the patient, and realistic objectives developed, based on this additional input.

A formal method for establishing, reviewing, and changing care plans is essential. Regular review of care plans by all involved professionals allows for a more holistic approach to the patient and also provides a mechanism to change the plans as the patient's status changes. The physician should remain an active member of this interdisciplinary team.

The care plan must also consider the wishes of the patient and the family, both of whom often have strong opinions about quality and quantity of life. Physicians must ascertain these feelings, help advise as to a plan's risks and benefits, and help incorporate the desires of the patient and family into the final plan. After careful discussion and consideration, if the desires and goals of the patient or family cannot be reconciled with the physician's plan, the doctor ought to refer the care of this patient to another qualified physician.

Decisions on Levels of Care and Service

Transfers to or from a long-term-care site are very traumatic to both patients and their families. A previously well individual living at home who becomes acutely ill usually understands the reasons for, and adjusts better to, admission to an acute hospital than does a chronically ill patient at home or a NH resident. Perhaps most difficult of all is a transfer from home or the hospital to a NH for the first time.

Some of the disruptions of transfers can be reduced by establishing a care plan that addresses the possibility of a transfer, and by providing established care plans to the site of transfer. When an acute problem occurs, not all patients need to be subjected to the discomfort and expense of being transferred to an emergency room for evaluation, nor should they have to wait until the next appointment or routine physician visit to the NH.

In the outpatient setting, the primary care provider should ensure some form of coverage for emergencies, and the patient should know how to access the system. Many problems can be dealt with over the telephone.

Most NHs handle many medical problems by telephone. With a well-trained nursing staff, good knowledge of the patients, and a carefully worked out care plan, telephone communication is often sufficient (see Chapter 4). However, with the sicker populations now coming into many NHs, the number of acute problems is increasing.

Physician extenders, such as the nurse practitioner and physician assistant, can perform preliminary evaluations to ascertain the severity of acute changes. In response to this growing need for closer supervision of the residents of NHs, Medicare has recently authorized payment for the services of a physician assistant and nurse practitioner in LTC facilities. When such persons provide primary care, physician backup is also necessary.

When a transfer *is* necessary, the physician can help alleviate the anxiety of the patient and family by informing them of the move as soon as possible. The LTC physician should also transmit the patient's comprehensive care plan to the new facility, to prevent excessive or repetitive testing, provide information for decision making, and facilitate actions consistent with the existing comprehensive care plan.

The Costs of Care and Services

Chapter 8 reviews in detail the sources of payment for various LTC services. There is limited coverage for both ambulatory and in-home services. Few insurers, other than Medicaid, will cover a NH stay.

Furthermore, while many third-party payors reimburse for acute hospitalizations, they are trying ever harder to limit the reasons for, and lengths of, such hospitalizations for the elderly. Documentation of the reason for the hospitalization and the inappropriateness of providing services in another setting is critical to assuring third-party reimbursement.

Given these restrictions and the limited resources of many of the elderly, it is important to consider carefully our diagnostic and therapeutic approaches. Can a generic medication be substituted for a brand name product without a poor outcome? Are yearly Pap screens necessary for women over the age of 70 without risk factors and with multiple previously normal results? Are there indications for a hospitalized patient to have daily chest X-rays or blood work? Could a diagnosis be made with one rather than several diagnostic procedures? Could treatment be given on the basis of the physical examination and careful assessment of information by the provider, rather than by obtaining many diagnostic tests? Will the diagnostic and therapeutic maneuvers likely change the outcome? Are there alternatives to NH placement or acute hospitalization?

Family Involvement in LTC

Families play an important role in many aspects of the care of ambulatory, homebound, and institutionalized elderly. Regardless of the setting, it is important to understand the composition of the family and the relationships between family members, including the patient, and the roles they are likely to play under various circumstances.

If the patient is fully functional, then the only need is to have an emergency contact in the event of an acute problem or the patient's inability to make appropriate decisions during an illness. But if the patient is frail or impaired, it is important to identify a primary caregiver. Once that person is identified, regular communication with him should be established. If the patient is mentally intact but physically frail, then the caregiver's role may be limited to transportation and general support of ADLs and IADLs. If there is significant cognitive impairment, the family role is expanded to include involvement in some decision making (e.g., when to perform testing, who should participate in adult day care, when to transfer to another level of care) necessary in the care of the long-term patient in all settings. The family should feel they can reach the provider without undue difficulty when they have questions.

Communication among staff, providers, the patient, and the family is crucial. It is more difficult when a number of family members are involved, each of whom has different opinions about appropriate decisions in a given circumstance. When time is limited, staff must be able to deal with families expeditiously. Arranging family conferences or requesting the family to appoint a representative are two ways to limit the staff time commitment without conveying the impression of being uncaring or unavailable.

The family should be made aware of the staff's care plan. There should be general discussion of major decisions regarding transfer policies, therapeutic and diagnostic maneuvers, testing and limitations on treatment, and a broad agreement between the staff, patient, and family. Staff should be open to discuss and consider alternative care plans presented by the patient and the family. If agreement over the general issues cannot be reached, then other care options (e.g., another physician or NH) should be offered.

The family needs to be kept informed of the patient's problems, especially significant changes in condition or treatment. In the care of the frail elderly, unexpected problems often arise. Some of these problems are unavoidable and easily understood by families, while others—especially those which are treatment-related or iatrogenic—can cause families to become upset and frustrated. When such a problem occurs, it helps to inform the family as soon as possible about any complications, as well as the course of action to handle them, and any plans to prevent a recurrence. Likelihood of mistrust, or the threat of legal action, is probably greater when families find out about adverse events on their own or by accident, instead of from staff.

Making the Ultimate Decision

When a patient is cognitively impaired, questions arise as to who makes decisions regarding institutionalization, treatment, procedures, etc. An associated question is when to include both patient and family in these decisions, and when to exclude one or the other (see Chapter 12).

Families look to the physician to help them decide about many of these problems. Each question raises common sense, medical, ethical, and legal issues. If the patient is significantly impaired but not unaware of events, it may be necessary to involve both patient and family. If the patient is totally unable to respond to his environment (e.g., comatose), then the law provides for others to make treatment decisions. The question of nontreatment, or the withholding of treatment, has been adjudicated on many occasions but without uniform solutions. Nonjudicial resolution through consensus among physicians, patients, and families remains the preferred approach.

The physician may need to recommend that the family of a cognitively impaired individual seek legal advice on guardianship prior to a crisis. Sometimes, it also helps to hold conferences regarding impaired individuals without their presence, and then to have the recommendations explained to that individual by those family members in whom he has the most confidence.

Patients who are physically impaired, with or without mild cognitive impairment, ought to make decisions regarding all aspects of their care. In these cases, if there are significant conflicts between the wishes of the patient and the family, the physician should preferentially honor the patient's desires.

Principles of Prescribing

In prescribing for the elderly, physicians must consider those physiologic differences which result from normal aging and may cause significant problems even when using doses of medications considered normal for an adult (Cassel and Walsh 1984). In addition, between 12 and 17% of hospitalizations of the elderly are drug-related (Lamy 1986), and drugs have a role in the incidence of other complications, such as fractures (Ray et al. 1987). Medications should be considered in searching for the cause of any acute illness or change in mental or functional status.

Because several medical problems often coexist, the elderly often take several medications. Interactions between medications need to be considered. Though the elderly comprise only 11% of the American population at this time, they consume 25% of the medications sold (Lamy 1986). These include not only prescribed, but also over-the-counter (OTC) drugs. The physician must consider and ask about all medications being taken by the elderly to avoid adverse drug interactions.

The basic rule for the use of medications is *primum non nocere* (above all else, do no harm). Though true in treating anyone, it is particularly important in the elderly, because of the physiological changes of normal aging, numbers of medications, and the difficulties often encountered in administering drugs to the frail elderly. The LTC physician should therefore keep in mind the need to:

- maintain careful records and notations of all drugs (prescription and OTC)

- review constantly medications and schedules of drugs prescribed by all physicians

- limit the number of medications

- simplify the dosage schedule

- determine who will be administering the drugs and instruct them as to the schedule, side effects, and purpose of the medications

- consider the cost of the medication and whether there is an alternative

- ascertain whether a child-proof cap is a help or a deterrent to compliance.

Prevention and Screening

Some physiologic changes accompany normal aging. The primary care physician can prevent some problems resulting from these changes if he is aware of and monitors them. An example of these normal physiological changes is the decrease in the amount of light the retina receives with aging, resulting in poorer vision and an increase in the risk of falls (Ham 1983). By being aware of this problem, the physician can offer suggestions to improve lighting and minimize environmental hazards (e.g., loose rugs or electric cords).

While most elderly eventually develop irreversible health problems, good preventive care can probably "compress morbidity" into the shortest possible period at the end of life (Fries, 1980). However, no large-scale studies yet exist which clearly show that routine preventive care and large-scale screenings improve older persons' functional ability or decrease their mortality. It is therefore very important to consider the risks, benefits, and costs of each measure considered for a patient. As the goal of the LTC physician is to maximize individual function, it is important to use common sense to determine which preventive health practices and screenings are indicated.

Criteria for Preventive Health Care or Screening

While periodic routine examinations can reveal potentially treatable abnormalities, the appropriate use, frequency, and content of routine physical examinations, disease-specific screenings, and tests remains unclear (Kennie, 1986). In the elderly population, especially the "old-old" over age 85, cost, risk, and the likely benefit to the patient become important factors in the choice. Optimum frequency of such services to assure continuity of care is also an individual matter, depending on a person's physical and psychosocial needs. While some published guidelines suggest certain specific routine screenings in individuals of certain ages (e.g., colorectal examinations yearly over the age of 50) (Winawer et al. 1985), these guidelines have not been firmly established as valid in the geriatric population.

Frame and Carlson (1975) outlined the following six criteria to help the practitioner determine whether to perform routine preventive care:

- The disease must have a significant effect on the quality and quantity of life.

- Acceptable methods of treatment must be available.

- The disease must have an asymptomatic period during which intervention is effective.

- Intervention in the asymptomatic phase must yield outcomes superior to outcomes after the appearance of the symptoms.

- Detection procedures must be available at reasonable cost.

- The incidence or prevalence must be sufficient to justify the cost of detection.

These criteria are especially relevant to LTC, as they reemphasize the importance of such things as life expectancy, quality of life, cost, and discomfort in any clinical decisions for the elderly (Thomasma 1986). Until studies have proven the appropriateness of routine preventive care for the elderly, each practitioner needs to consider his patient in light of such criteria as the above.

It is also important to remember that age does not equal disease and disability. Therefore, regardless of age, our goal is to minimize each person's morbidity (Hazzard 1983), and to improve function at all times.

Terminal Care

It is important for the physician to inform a patient of a terminal illness, as people need time to settle affairs with their family. Most patients know there is a significant problem even before they are told, but even if the physician is simply confirming what has already been suspected, the patient still needs to hear that confirmation to facilitate moving on to the next step.

When patients deny so much that they neither hear nor comprehend the information they are given, the physician should not insist that they must accept such unsettling information. On the other hand, the physician should recognize the preeminent rights of the patient, and resist family requests to withhold the facts from their loved one, if the patient desires or needs such information in order to choose a course of action.

Families or caregivers also need to be informed of a terminal diagnosis (with the patient's permission, where indicated), so that support systems can be established to help with financial and other concerns.

Once the diagnosis of a terminal illness is made, the patient and family should feel that the physician is available to them to discuss problems, changes, and alternatives. The physician must also be able and willing to deal with the frustrations of not being able to cure the illness. The goal is to make the patient and the family as comfortable as possible. Close supervision of medications is important.

Since the goal is to relieve or prevent severe pain, one should not worry about possible addiction.

To handle the patient who chooses to remain an outpatient, the physician should be familiar with community-based systems to help the terminally ill patient and family, including:

- home care agencies

- durable medical equipment

- transportation services

- in-home pharmacy and nutritional services

- outpatient hospice services

- physician house calls.

In-home services can often be increased as the patient becomes more debilitated. However, all those involved must also be aware of alternatives so that they can make informed decisions about when and to what extent to use those services. If such a patient needs acute hospitalization, pertinent questions include: What are the circumstances for the hospitalization? Which diagnostic and therapeutic procedures should be performed, and how often? What should be done about resuscitation and life-support measures? The physician has a crucial role in ensuring that the acute hospital carries out the wishes of the patient and the family.

When community support systems cannot provide all the care a terminally ill person needs, inpatient hospice facilities for both short- and long-term stays are available, with staff specially trained to support a dying patient and his family. These are sometimes located in LTC facilities. Unlike ordinary care units, hospice units frequently offer greater accessibility to staff, fewer restrictions on visiting hours, an emphasis on increasing the time the patient and family spend together, and often even sleeping arrangements for family members. In these specialized units, as well as in regular LTC facilities where terminal care issues are so often relevant, routine meetings allow the physician and staff to support each other, to discuss problems, and to deal with both difficult patients or families, and with their own feelings about death.

Physicians are often asked about funeral arrangements, especially for a patient who dies at home. Families who do not ask these questions are often relieved when a physician raises these issues. It helps to suggest that family make arrangements prior to the death of their loved one; then a simple phone call after death is all that is necessary in this time of great stress. Physicians can help families understand by recommending to them such references as that by Nelson (1982).

Physicians should also advise about what to do in the event the patient dies at home. Discussion ahead of time can avoid the need for the police or fire department to arrive at the home at this difficult time. Depending on state law, death may be pronounced by a physician or nurse, or there need not be a pronouncement of death in the home; if the family is certain, they need only call a prearranged funeral home.

References

Cassel, C. K., and J. R. Walsh. 1984. *Geriatric medicine: fundamentals of geriatric care.* New York: Springer-Verlag.

Frame, P. S., and S. J. Carlson. 1975. A critical review of periodic health screening using specific criteria. *Journal of Family Practice* 2(29):123, 189, 283.

Fries, J. F. 1980. Aging, natural death, and the compression of morbidity. *New England Journal of Medicine* 303(3):130-135.

Ham, R. J. 1983. *Primary care geriatrics: A case-based learning program.* Boston: John Wright, PSG.

Hazzard, W. R. 1983. Preventive gerontology: strategies for healthy aging. *Postgraduate Medicine* 74(2):279-287.

Kennie, D. C. 1986. Health maintenance of the elderly. *Clinics in Geriatric Medicine* 2(1):53-83.

Lamy, P. P. 1986. Adverse drug reactions and the elderly: an update. *Geriatric Medicine Annual 1986.* Oradell, NJ: Medical Economics 128-154.

Nelson, T. C. 1982. *It's your choice.* Glenview, IL: Scott, Foresman & Co.

Pawlson, L. G., and R. A. Berenson. 1986. Financing and delivery of health care services: changes and more changes. *Geriatric Medicine Annual 1986.* Oradell, NJ: Medical Economics, 260-268.

Ray, W. A., et al. 1987. Psychotropic drug use and the risk of hip fracture. *New England Journal of Medicine* 316:363-368.

Rubenstein, L. Z., et al. 1984. Effectiveness of a geriatric evaluation unit: A randomized clinical trial. *New England Journal of Medicine* 311:1664-1670.

Rubenstein, L. Z. 1987. Geriatric assessment: An overview of its impact. *Clinics in Geriatric Medicine* 3(1):1-15.

Thomasma, D. C. 1986. Quality-of-life judgments, treatment decisions, and medical ethics. *Clinics in Geriatric Medicine* 2(1):17-27.

Williams, M. E. 1987. Outpatient geriatric evaluations. *Clinics in Geriatric Medicine* 3(1):175-183.

Winawer, S. J., et al. 1985. Surveillance and early diagnosis of colorectal cancer. *Cancer Detection Prevention* 8(3):373-392.

Chapter Six

Quality Assurance, Infection Control, and Utilization Review

Steven A. Levenson, M.D.

Chapter Objectives

This chapter will:

- Discuss the concept of quality care in LTC
- Discuss the general principles of quality assurance (QA) in health care, especially in LTC
- Review the components of QA: standards, criteria, and tools
- Consider quality assurance standards and criteria for different settings and situations in LTC
- Consider the medical role in setting quality standards in LTC, and in quality assurance
- Review aspects of medical quality assurance in LTC
- Suggest policies and procedures to support medical quality assurance
- Review infection control as a special facet of quality assurance
- Assess utilization management and review in LTC, and its relationships with QA
- Consider the medical role in utilization review in LTC
- Consider some specific medically-related utilization issues.

Quality Care and the LTC Setting

The difficulties in delivering quality services in LTC have been noted repeatedly. Various investigators have criticized many aspects of that care, from administrative to medical services, in many LTC facilities. For example:

Testimony at state and federal legislative hearings in the 1970s, while anecdotal, indicated that many residents of nursing homes infrequently saw physicians, although most of them were under active treatment for chronic disease. A relatively small fraction of physicians (14%), far fewer than the fraction of family practitioners or internists in the population (48%), make nursing home visits. Physicians, particularly in urban areas, apparently do not follow their patients into nursing homes, causing discontinuity in care at a critical time for the patient: a time when mortality and rehospitalization rates are high (Rabin 1981, 126).

One of the more recent of many such reports about inadequate NH care, issued in 1986 by the Senate Special Committee on Aging, reiterated many of the familiar medically-related problems, such as: insufficient physician visits; too many drugs (especially psychoactive medications) prescribed per patient; insufficiently documented indications for medications, and failure to watch patients for complications or side effects; and inadequate follow-up after a diagnosis is made or a treatment instituted (Senate Special Committee 1986).

Clearly, quality of care issues have become increasingly important and more widely discussed. It has, however, proven very difficult to establish criteria and standards for both professional and nonprofessional services, and for overall care. Problems have included definition, valid standards, and appropriate criteria for evaluations of care against those standards. In this chapter, we will explore some reasons for this situation, and propose some concepts and policies for QA in LTC.

Quality of Care: A Definition

Quality of care refers to the most appropriate care and decisions about care for an individual's needs, taking into account limits of time, cost, staffing, and patient goals and prognosis. Quality care is the primary goal of any health care service or facility.

Five major trends expected to influence future evaluations of the quality of medical care in long-term care have been identified (Pattee 1984, 46):

-the shift in responsibility and accountability for health from providers to consumers of health care;
-an emerging definition of health which is shared by both providers and consumers of long-term care and which identifies wellness concepts rather than illness concepts as its core;
-change in the focus of health care delivery from an emphasis on service sites to an emphasis on clusters of client needs;
-a broadening of long-term health care services to emphasis on quality of life rather than quality of medical care;
-reintroduction of cost/benefit models of health care evaluation. . . .

Unique Problems of LTC

Several unique features of LTC influence quality of care issues, especially in trying to translate the acute medical model:

- The residents are long-term, and their underlying conditions vary little over time.

- The care is usually low-technology, and even in LTC facilities equipped to do cardiac monitoring and resuscitation, there is little other high-technology equipment.

- Quality of life issues are an especially important part of quality of care.

- Relationships between process and structure (what we do and how we do it), and outcome (the ultimate results), are less clear.

- Patients generally have multiple chronic illnesses, rather than isolated acute illnesses.

- New onset of acute illness is often difficult to distinguish from exacerbations of chronic illness.

- Goals of care are generally not as clearcut.

- Unlike in the hospital, physicians are rarely present in the nursing home from day to day.

- Follow-up care is often minimal or absent.

- Patients tend to be on multiple medications, with great potential for iatrogenic illnesses.

- Patients often have extensive medical records, with care obtained from many different people and institutions.

- The appropriate degree of medical intervention is harder to determine.

- Patients are often incomplete historians, and information must frequently be obtained from families or staff.

In summary, appropriate long-term treatment must often be directed as much, if not more, towards maintaining current status, slowing deterioration, and preventing or treating acute exacerbations, than towards cure of isolated acute illness.

Some important differences specifically between NHs and hospitals include: NHs are smaller, have lower staff-patient ratios and higher personnel turnover, and often have less capacity to develop and implement care review programs. Quality of LTC recordkeeping systems varies, and such systems are often incomplete. Physician checks and balances are often not operational in NHs because of lack of medical organization or commitment. Diagnoses of LTC patients do not always predict their disability levels. On the positive side, the fact that LTC patients are longer-stay patients allows for direct observations and interviews with patients, rather than reliance on the record. Also, nonphysician personnel (e.g., aides, licensed practical nurses) can have major roles in improving care of LTC patients by greater attention to patient monitoring and quality of care, even though they can also contribute to negative or inadequate care if insufficiently motivated (Kane 1981).

Quality Assurance: A Definition

Quality Assurance (QA) refers to the defined and organized program by which health care professionals, administrators, and owners or boards strive to assure quality patient care. Increasing emphasis has been placed on an organized process, including establishing standards, objective assessment of various aspects of patient care, and the correction and follow-up of identified problems.

In short, then, QA in LTC requires *reasonable goals, review strategies, measurement methods,* and *corrective actions.*

In health care organizations, the quality assurance plan is an important starting point for this process because it defines the organization, function, and information sources used in any quality assurance program. It is through such definitions that the meaning of "quality care" emerges in a given LTC setting.

The QA process is summarized in Figure 6-1.

How Standards are Established

Quality assurance starts with *standards,* defined as broad statements describing expected degrees of performance or accomplishment. Standards establish acceptable norms, while, at the same time, specify acceptable deviations from those norms. They may be established either by authority (such as state or federal regulations), or by agreement (by the Joint Commission on the Accreditation of Hospitals or health professionals).

Quality assurance standards for LTC have been established at several levels:

- Voluntary professional (nurses, doctors, etc. agreeing through their professional organizations or institutional staffs to establish certain standards and to perform certain monitoring functions)

- Mandatory regulatory (standards are established by law or regulation, and are required for licensure or payment)

- Voluntary accrediting (standards are established by independent nonregulatory bodies to go beyond regulatory

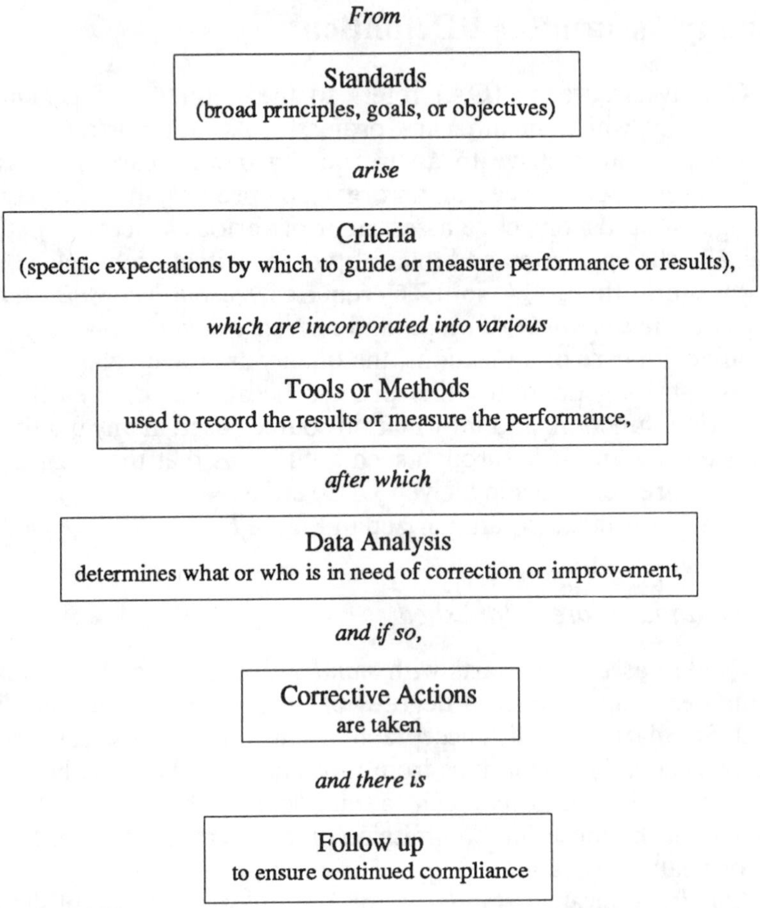

From

```
┌─────────────────────────────────────────────┐
│                 Standards                     │
│   (broad principles, goals, or objectives)    │
└─────────────────────────────────────────────┘
```

arise

```
┌───────────────────────────────────────────────────────────────┐
│                           Criteria                              │
│ (specific expectations by which to guide or measure performance or results), │
└───────────────────────────────────────────────────────────────┘
```

which are incorporated into various

```
┌───────────────────────────────────────────────────┐
│                  Tools or Methods                  │
│  used to record the results or measure the performance, │
└───────────────────────────────────────────────────┘
```

after which

```
┌─────────────────────────────────────────────────────────────┐
│                      Data Analysis                            │
│ determines what or who is in need of correction or improvement, │
└─────────────────────────────────────────────────────────────┘
```

and if so,

```
┌───────────────────────────────┐
│       Corrective Actions       │
│           are taken            │
└───────────────────────────────┘
```

and there is

```
┌─────────────────────────────────────┐
│              Follow up               │
│  to ensure continued compliance      │
└─────────────────────────────────────┘
```

Figure 6-1 Breakdown of the QA process in healthcare.

minimums, and are complied with voluntarily to demonstrate interest in higher levels of care).

The sources of these standards commonly include:

- State and federal laws and regulations
- Peer review and third-party payors
- Common practice

- State certification and licensure requirements

- Medical literature, reports of studies and collective experience.

For example, the LTC accreditation manual of the Joint Commission on Accreditation of Hospitals (JCAH, a voluntary accrediting agency) contains certain standards for medical staffs, focusing on staff structure and organizational processes, and quality monitoring activities. Many state health departments have certification and licensure requirements which concern the frequency of physician visits and the contents of progress notes and orders (process-oriented standards).

A changing emphasis. Most LTC standards have evolved from mandatory regulations. A growing body of opinion suggests that the standards and monitoring criteria of outside regulatory agencies may hamper efforts at quality of care, when they emphasize process at the expense of outcome. "In other words, the emphasis has been on compliance with carrying out the letter of the law rather than on implementing the law's intent, which is to insure that quality nursing care is delivered" (Gustafson, et al. 1980, 337).

Unfortunately, voluntary professional standards have faltered, in part because of lack of interest and time among the professions, including medicine. Voluntary accrediting standards, dependent on the willingness of institutions or professions to seek and comply with them, have similarly had limited success.

Recently, a number of attempts have been made to replace some required structure- and process-oriented standards, with more outcome-oriented surveys. The Department of Health and Human Services, for instance, authorized development of a Patient Care and Services (PaCS) appraisal system to examine an individual's medical, dental, psychosocial, and nutritional needs, and to periodically measure progress at achieving various goals relating to these needs. After each evaluation, time-limited goals are set for desired improvements. Unfortunately, the original instrument was long and fairly costly to use. Efforts are currently underway to simplify the process and reduce its cost.

Some states have begun to implement similar new survey formats, emphasizing observations of, and interviews with, patients and staff, as reflections of outcomes of care, with much less presence of a facility's administrative staff. Reviewers focus on paper compliance, structure, and process only if problems are found in the course of the review, or if the facility is a known prior offender.

A major remaining question is: which standards are valid and broadly applicable, and for which aspects of LTC? While previously derived mostly from common practice and regulations, it is hoped that these standards will in the future come more from professional consensus based on the systematic testing of ideas and theories. Such efforts will identify those standards which help accomplish the goals of quality care at reasonable cost, and those which are ineffective or too costly for the benefits provided.

Standards may be based on *structure* (how things are established and organized), *process* (activities and procedures), or *outcome* (observed results of activities upon patients), or some combination of these.

An example of a structural standard is one requiring an organized medical staff, or a specific set of procedures and bylaws. A process-oriented standard would be one which requires multidisciplinary QA plans with physician participation, including periodic committee meetings. Outcome-based standards would examine how physician actions affect a patient's physical, mental, or psychosocial status, according to certain desirable goals.

Structural measures of quality are the most objective, reliable, and easily measurable, but are not necessarily related to outcome of care (Vogel and Palmer 1982, 105-106).

While outcome-oriented standards may be the most desirable, such measurements are also the most difficult to establish reliably and consistently. This is especially true in LTC, because of the impact of the combinations of diseases and the consequences of normal aging.

What outcomes should we study for the LTC patient? Among the options are: physiologic measurements, levels of pain and discomfort, ADL performance, affect, cognition, social activities, social contact, and satisfaction with care and environment. In LTC, mortality rates are often not nearly as significant a measure as they are for younger adults.

In the outcome-oriented approach, sources of data are primarily either the chart or the patient. Types of data include value preferences, functional levels, incidents and accidents, incidence of new decubiti, vital signs, and lab test results. Outcomes may be categorized as expected versus observed.

In treating heart disease, for instance, desirable outcome may be fewer episodes of angina or pulmonary edema, improved endurance and sense of well-being, a better score on tests of cardiac output, an improved electrocardiogram, or greater ability to participate in social and personal care activities.

Because establishing outcome measures for LTC requires extensive data collection and analysis, and can be very costly, many have therefore advocated some mix between process and outcome as the most beneficial and cost-effective approach, at least until there is further validation.

Medical quality assurance in long-term care should thus be seen in the future as a tool for learning and planning changes to help accommodate new trends and expectations.

Examples of general standards. The following list provides some examples of general standards for LTC which could be used as the foundation for individual professional criteria for quality care:

- The greatest possible functional, mental, and social independence should be sought

- Various needs should be met by providing qualified professional staff

- These professionals should assess resident needs and document same.

- A care plan for each individual should be developed by interdisciplinary collaboration, including some input from resident or family

- These philosophies and standards should be made known to staff, residents, and interested outsiders.

- Discharge plans should educate where possible, or at least facilitate a smooth transfer to a new setting.

Another example of general standards for LTC quality assurance (QA) activities is provided by the JCAH LTC accreditation guidelines (Joint Commission 1986, 1-3), which require the following:

- An ongoing QA program designed to objectively and systematically monitor and evaluate the quality and appropriateness of resident care, to improve that care, and to resolve identified problems

- A broad multidisciplinary approach to QA monitoring, including medical staff participation

- Ongoing monitoring and evaluation activities using objective criteria reflecting current knowledge and clinical experience

- Identification of patient/resident problems and attempts at follow-up and resolution

- Coordination and periodic reevaluation of the facility's overall QA program.

Establishing Criteria

After we have standards, we next establish criteria to allow us to evaluate performance by matching it against those standards. Criteria should clarify the explicit behaviors expected, and of whom they are required. Truly valid QA criteria should take into account financial resources and time, and should be measurable, observable, and relevant. Criteria, like standards, may be structure-, process-, or outcome-oriented. Structural criteria, for example, would mandate that medical staff bylaws require certain numbers of meetings and the attendance of active staff, and cover specific QA topics. Process-oriented criteria would require guidelines for how often patients should be seen and progress notes written, and how drug utilization is to be monitored. Outcome criteria would propose guidelines for reducing mortality from hypertensive complications, or for helping people die comfortably.

Identifying the Tools

Having established standards, and the criteria for judging performance against those standards, we next need tools to help us with the actual measurements. Quality assurance tools should facilitate the most complete, accurate, and time-efficient collection of information as possible. Such tools may be:

- Patient-oriented (measurements or examinations of patient feelings, attitudes, responses, or characteristics)

- Facility-oriented (measurements or examinations of facility setup, organization, staffing, policies, procedures, etc.)

- Professional-oriented (measurements or examinations of the activities, decisions, prescriptions, conduct, or documentation of those caring for the patient or operating the facility).

Quality assurance tools may also be categorized as structure-, process-, or outcome-oriented.

Outcome-oriented tools are the most difficult to devise, but may be most likely to provide useful information. According to Dr. Robert Kane (Kane, R. L., R. Bell, S. Riegler, et al. 1983) it is possible to distinguish specific achievable outcomes for each individual, so that payment could be linked to how well the facility or program achieves these outcomes. The advantages of such a system are:

- Rewards and results are in the context of reasonable expectations.

- Innovation is encouraged.

- Many of the current costly regulations could be modified (e.g., staff/bed ratios).

- It encourages consideration of patient wishes and potential.

- It is more consistent with a rehabilitative outlook.

- It is compatible with incentive payments for heavy care admissions.

The Quality Assurance System

Participants

In every health care organization, the ownership or board of directors is ultimately responsible for ensuring that services provided are of high quality and reasonable cost. Because owners or boards usually consist primarily of lay people, and because their proper role involves more policy-making and oversight than day-to-day management, they generally delegate quality assurance responsibilities to the professionals in their institutions, and depend on the assurances and past performance of these professionals in reaching conclusions about proper quality of care.

Physicians are one of the main groups of participants in an overall LTC QA program, which includes:

- Ownership or board of directors

- Administration

- Departments of medicine, nursing, social services, dietary, rehabilitation, medical records

- Committees, including patient care, medical records, pharmacy & therapeutics, infection control, fire & safety, and utilization review.

In this system, each department is responsible for its own QA activities, *and* for the coordination of those activities with those of other departments.

General Concepts of Medical Quality Assurance in LTC

Today, LTC medical staffs should accept responsibility for developing and applying objective, performance-based programs for the ongoing monitoring of patient care and physician practices. There is a place for the participation of every physician caring for the elderly—even for community-based practitioners who do not participate actively in the data gathering or monitoring activities—in helping to discover, recommend and refine standards for care and practice. A knowledgeable and interested physician, preferably the medical director, should assume responsibility for medical participation in such a program.

Such medical participation should include:

Staff or Departmental

- Establishing standards, criteria, and measuring tools for practice in a given setting or institution
- Devising a program of monitoring, enforcement, and follow-up of compliance with those standards.

Institutional

- Advising and guiding other professionals regarding accepted standards and new knowledge of geriatric care and practice, which would contribute to their own standards and practices
- Participating in institutional QA programs and committees
- Advising and guiding administrations, owners, and boards regarding standards of quality care, and responding to questions or inquiries about such care or practice, which can help *their* policy-making.

In general, any medical quality assurance program, regardless of size, should contain:

- References to the standards on which the plan is based
- A set of explicit criteria for doing reviews
- Some evaluation of tools used in the review process
- The results of the actual case or chart reviews
- Summaries of trends, actions, follow-ups, and conclusions.

The 3 "S's" of Medical Quality Assurance

Medical QA in LTC may also be examined from the standpoint of *system*, *site*, or *subject*.

The *system* refers to the participants; the standards, criteria, and tools; and the plan for monitoring, enforcement, and follow-up. These standards, criteria, tools, and methods may be either *site-* or *subject-* specific.

In LTC the sites may be home, community, or institution. Subjects may be either *professional-* or *patient-*oriented. The former include such items as drug-prescribing practices and chart documentation; the latter, such things as falls or incontinence.

Medical Standards in Quality Assurance

Medical standards for LTC are both general (applicable regardless of site), and site-specific.

The following points are proposed as broad medical QA standards for LTC, from which we may in turn derive criteria for adequate physician performance (see Table 6-1):

- Each LTC patient or resident should have an adequate medical review of past history and current complaints, and an evaluation of physical and psychological condition and functional status. *Rationale*: Maximizing individual function and autonomy (a general quality of care standard) requires the greatest possible freedom from the debilitating effects of physical illness, and the greatest possible relief from pain and discomfort. The wider options for treatment, and our better understanding of the broader possibilities that many elderly have for improvement, make it important to separate treatable illnesses accompanying aging from irreversible chronic changes of aging. This approach has often been overlooked, to the detriment of the patients.

- The physician should take part in translating the patient assessments into a medical plan of care, and coordinate that plan with those of other professional disciplines. *Rationale*: Care of the long-term patient is a multidisciplinary effort, covering many services, sites, and professionals over a period of time. No one profession can act properly, independent of the others.

- The medical plan of care should be commensurate with an individual's physical and psychological needs, as well as represent, as much as possible, the wishes of the patient. *Rationale*: Medical therapies, including drugs, cannot be ordered in a vacuum, but rather in light of overall function and the prospects for improving that function. Newer concepts of health and quality of life take into account

Table 6-1 Proposed medical standards, criteria, and tools for LTC.

Standard	Criteria	Tools
There should be an adequate review of past and current medical history, physical and functional status	1. History and physical done within 2 days of admission, and on chart within 5 days of admission. 2. History and physical contain certain specific information (e.g., functional status, review of systems). 3. An effort is made to substantiate diagnoses.	Medical records and documentation reviews
There is physician participation in translating assessments into a medical care plan	1. There is documentation of physician involvement in the patient care plan. 2. Medical orders reflect the physician assessments, and are appropriate for medical diagnoses and functional status. 3. There is a physician problem list, coordinated with medical orders. 4. There is evidence of physician attention to staff mention of problems.	Medical records, documentation, pharmacy reviews
Medical plan of care should be commensurate with patient needs and reflect wishes	1. Physician medication orders should follow certain procedures. 2. Medication orders should avoid potentially hazardous drug interactions. 3. As few medications as possible should be prescribed.	Medical records, documentation reviews Pharmacy and therapeutics committee monitoring Health department visit reports

Table 6-1, continued.

Standard	Criteria	Tools
	4. Standing orders should be periodically reviewed, and unnecessary ones should be discontinued. 5. Documentation should reflect some involvement of patient and family in decision-making processes. 6. Frequency of patient visits should meet requirements, and be enough to handle patient problems. 7. Medical intervention is timely.	Utilization review records Occurrence screening of discharges, transfers, and readmissions
Documentation should reflect evaluations and plans	1. Documentation should reflect condition, prognosis, and rehab potential. 2. There should be some evidence that the physician is checking whether his orders and care plans are resulting in some improvements or maintenance of function; if not, that these plans are reconsidered. 3. Documentation should reflect goals and objectives, and changes in patient condition. 4. There is a deduction in disallowed stays, refusals of payment, health department citations, and UR challenges.	Medical records, documentation reviews Pharmacy and therapeutics committee monitoring Health department visit reports Utilization review records Occurrence screening of discharges, transfers, and readmissions

Table 6-1, continued.

Standard	Criteria	Tools
Plans for discharge, referral, and placement should consider current treatment, prognosis, and goals	1. There should be physician orders before patients are moved or discharged. 2. Levels of care should be adequate to meet patient needs. 3. Number of discharges home or into the community increases. 4. More patients can be treated less intensively or at lower care levels.	Medical records, documentation reviews Utilization review records Occurrence screening of discharges, transfers, and readmissions
Medical care and practice conforms to broadly accepted standards	1. Management of specific problems (such as incontinence or dementia) follows certain guidelines. 2. There is a reduction of such complications as falls or bedsores. 3. Unplanned discharges are reduced, as are transfers and retransfers to the hospital.	Audits Occurrence screening of those with specific diagnoses Utilization review records

patient desires as well as professional opinions about the "best" thing to do. The physician should, as always, retain the individual older patient's best interests at heart, but should not think of himself as the sole arbiter of what those interests are or should be.

• Documentation should adequately reflect these evaluations, deliberative processes, and communications. *Rationale*: Documentation is very important as evidence of adequate care, to reduce liability, as a communication tool with other professionals, and to comply with standards for licensure and reimbursement.

- Plans for discharge, referral, and placement should take into account current treatment, prognosis, and goals, as well as individual capabilities. *Rationale*: Functional independence is often best assisted by providing the right combination of services in an appropriate setting. Through his knowledge of an individual's prognosis and condition, the physician plays an important part in determining the best setting and the most appropriate services.

- Medical care and practice for the elderly should conform to the same broadly accepted standards applicable to all patients. *Rationale*: The elderly are entitled to the same quality of care as anyone else.

Medical Criteria for Quality Care

Compliance with these general standards requires criteria for their fulfillment. These criteria may be either structure, process, or outcome-oriented, and may also be either subject-specific or site-specific.

Subject-specific criteria. Among the subjects covered by general medical QA criteria are: medical orders (including treatments, lab tests, referrals, and manner of order writing); prescription of medications; patient visits; patient evaluation and assessment; documentation; and the medical management of specific problems.

Site-specific criteria. Certain LTC sites, such as the NH and the ambulatory care facility, and the situation of patients transferred between settings, present some special QA problems.

Let us examine some of these in more detail.

Subject-Specific Criteria

General Medical Orders

While medical orders represent the ultimate of physician involvement in any patient care, they are the source of many problems.

In LTC, typical problems have included orders that are: incomplete, not clearly related to patient problems, illegible, insufficiently reviewed, and inconsistent with the general care plan.

Structure- and process-related criteria. There should be some policies to govern the writing of orders in all settings of care for the elderly. These policies should cover all necessary standard pharmacy and therapeutics issues, such as the use of nonformulary medications, the giving and taking of verbal orders, and monitoring for possible drug interactions. A mechanism should exist for reducing medication errors and for preventing and monitoring for possible adverse and toxic drug reactions. Pharmacy and therapeutics review and policy recommendations should either be assumed by a separate committee, or within the functions of some other committee. The medical director or a medical staff representative should participate in drafting and enforcing these policies. Since iatrogenic illness, largely due to the effects and side effects of drugs, is a major problem in the elderly, there must be some systematic oversight of drug use in LTC if there is to be any reduction in the problems of prescribing for millions of elderly persons.

Orders should be legible and complete, and should somehow relate to the individual's conditions and problems. Standing orders should be reconsidered periodically. Wherever possible, the number of drugs per patient should be reduced. Patient and family preferences, available resources, patient prognosis, and likelihood of various risks and benefits, should at least be considered when deciding among options for palliation or cure. In all cases, at the least, measures should be prescribed for the patient's comfort, and the relief of pain. Where indicated, appropriate laboratory monitoring of drugs should be in evidence. Necessary diagnostic and therapeutic procedures should be undertaken, and unnecessary ones omitted. Documentation should reflect how such determinations about necessary and unnecessary procedures were made.

Outcome-related criteria. Desirable outcomes of medical order writing would improve patient management and reduce harmful errors and complications. The incidence of adverse drug reactions should decrease over time, as should the number of medication errors (wrong drug to a patient, right drug to wrong patient, errors in transcription, etc.) and undesirable side effects (cardiac arrhythmias, blood dyscrasias, gastrointestinal bleeding, etc.). In an institution, the number and frequency of drugs for each patient should be reduced where possible, to minimize cost and improve quality of life, without lessening appropriate medical management.

Patient Visits

The minimum frequency of patient visits is generally prescribed by law and regulation. There is no strong evidence to support an *optimal* number or frequency of patient encounters. What is important is that there be enough encounters to provide adequate assessment, treatment, and follow-up care. What is done during those visits (process and outcome) is probably more important than the visits themselves.

Structure- and process-related criteria. Physician visits must follow prescribed laws and regulations. Documentation should reflect the physician evaluation of condition, prognosis, rehabilitation potential, follow-up of acute problems, and ongoing management of chronic problems. In the NH, documentation should periodically indicate the continued need for the current level and intensity of care.

Outcome-related criteria. The outcome of a physician visit should be some enhancement or maintenance of patient well-being, comfort, dignity, or self-determination, according to realistic goals and objectives.

Patient Evaluation and Assessment

Physician evaluations should be sufficiently comprehensive and accurate to enable appropriate patient management.

Structure- and process-related criteria. Policies should cover the critical content of a LTC assessment in each setting (see Chapter 10). The assessments should be current and accurate. Information should be recorded and coded to facilitate retrieval and review.

There should be a mechanism for improving the accuracy and appropriateness of diagnostic labels. For example, the patient with a diagnosis of "dementia, Alzheimer's type" should not be so labeled until other reasonable measures have ruled out other causes of mental status alteration. Or, if we were reviewing proper diagnostic labeling of geriatric patients, one standard might be that "the diagnosis of diabetes should be appropriately made." But based on studies, relative glucose intolerance apparently occurs with advancing age. Therefore, the *criteria* for diabetes in the geriatric population necessarily differ from those of the younger adult population. Quality care would thus anticipate some evidence in the record that the diagnosis was established according to appropriate criteria. Absence of such evidence would represent a deviation from the standard. Assessment should focus on separating potentially treatable problems of the elderly from untreatable changes of aging, as well as on such relevant aspects as psychological and self-care function.

Outcome-related criteria. Desirable outcomes resulting from proper evaluation and assessment could include improvement of patient comfort and well-being, reduction of morbidity, and fewer acute hospital transfers or retransfers.

Documentation

Physician documentation in LTC should facilitate patient care, and justify utilization of services and payment for those services.

Structure- and process-related criteria. There should be policies regarding medical record documentation and the proper and timely completion of records. Chart documentation should be legible and complete, complying with both institutional policies and applicable regulations.

Some kind of problem list or problem-oriented documentation is almost essential for the LTC patient. Many things can happen over the years, and the older patient is often only a fair to poor historian. It is impractical to go through years of records to try to review or summarize problems. The problem list should at least include the date of onset and resolution and should be updated regularly. Proper terminology must be used, avoiding abbreviations (COPD, HCVD) that may not be understood by all (see Chapter 9).

Physician documentation should reflect goals and objectives, and the ongoing awareness of changes in patient condition. There should be evidence of the awareness and follow-up of ongoing problems.

Outcome-related criteria. It is difficult to relate documentation directly to patient outcome. Rather, patient care can indirectly improve because of the activities that the documentation *reflects*, such as more timely medical intervention, including follow-up of patients' complaints and problems, or more accurate diagnosis.

Medical Management of Specific Problems

Of all areas of medical QA, establishing QA principles for the management of specific illnesses or problems may be the most difficult. Especially in proprietary homes, where the attending staff may consist of many community-based physicians, there are many different individual ways of managing medical problems. Nevertheless, it is still appropriate to consider and enforce certain broad principles, applicable to all.

Structure- and process-related criteria. Some policies and protocols should cover medical management issues. These can be produced by the medical director, principal physician, or a committee representing the medical staff in conjunction with either of these two individuals. The sources of these standards and criteria should be sources of current medical knowledge of the illnesses and problems of the elderly.

Medical management should be consistent with generally accepted standards of geriatric medicine.

Outcome-related criteria. Desirable outcomes of appropriate medical management would include reduced flareups of, or complications from, specific chronic illnesses or problems, fewer medications and treatments, increased patient satisfaction, and fewer transfers or retransfers to the acute hospital (e.g., for uncontrolled diabetes or hypertensive emergencies).

Other Criteria

Some other examples of subject-specific criteria which might be applied include:

- Patient declassifications and changes of level of care

- Number of discharges home or into community

- Number of patients able to be treated less intensively or at a lower level of care because of medical intervention or support

- Number of patients successfully treated in the NH who would otherwise be discharged to acute hospitals

- Number and type of regulatory citations, such as for incomplete or unsigned orders, or for poor documentation.

Site-Specific Criteria

Several aspects of QA deserving specific mention by site include ambulatory care, and transfers between nursing home and hospital and between hospital and nursing home.

Ambulatory Care

Besides encouraging the generally accepted principles and standards of good medical practice, little has been done to provide standards for quality care in an ambulatory setting. Since much care of the elderly is provided in that setting (outpatient clinic, day care, day hospital, etc.), it is important to look at the quality of the medical contribution to that care.

One group of investigators (Heller et al. 1984) tried to establish quality of care guidelines for five different common conditions affecting the ambulatory elderly. Although the study's major objective was to identify deficiencies in the treatment of these problems, it was also useful in suggesting how conclusions can be reached about the quality of the care. Minimal standards of care can be established and applied for some common problems in the elderly.

Based on such assessments, the following are some potential standards for ambulatory LTC.

Patient assessment. A diagnosis (e.g., Alzheimer's disease, congestive heart failure, dementia, or depression) should be based on specific recorded clinical criteria.

Patient management. Minimal standards of care should be described, representing important diagnostic, preventive, treatment, or outcome measures. Compliance with these standards should be monitored.

Documentation. Documentation should explain apparent deviation from minimal standards. For instance, the record of a diagnosed elderly hypertensive whose diastolic blood pressure is >105 should have some documentation about attempted evaluation or treatment (e.g., refusal to take medications, or probable noncompliance) rather than no comment or no evidence that the problem was considered important.

Physician education efforts. Some attempt should be made to inform or educate the patient or family about the medical conditions and problems for which they are being treated, and about the prescribed medications.

Physician follow-up care. There should be some evidence of awareness and follow-up of lab tests – especially for abnormal values.

Transfers Between Nursing Homes and Hospitals

While NHs have often been faulted for the problems of transferred patients, acute hospitals are often guilty of similar infractions. Therefore, there must be some quality assurance standards at *both* ends.

Standards. The movement of patients between acute and LTC settings, which also involves the transfer of information, occurs quite regularly. The process itself is important to the care that an older person receives, and probably in the eventual outcome.

Acute to long-term care. Proposed standards for such transfers include:

- The patient's medical condition should not require more care than the NH can reasonably offer (*Rationale*: NHs are not staffed to deal with medically unstable patients, and often cannot get rapid physician evaluation. Therefore, acute hospitals should not transfer patients who are medically unstable unless specific arrangements have been made for their immediate and follow-up care and monitoring).

- The NH should receive accurate, complete and up-to-date information about the patient (*Rationale*: This is essential for adequate long-term patient management).

- Changes in patient condition should be evaluated and documented by the acute-care facility, and if not resolved before return to a LTC setting, adequate follow-up visits should be arranged (*Rationale*: Acute hospitals have an obligation to recognize the problems that hospitalization can cause in elderly patients, and to prevent or manage those problems).

Criteria. Based on these standards, the following are some proposed criteria for assessing the quality of care and services provided to LTC patients in the acute care setting:

- Patients transferred to a hospital without an indwelling urinary catheter should not be returned to the NH with an indwelling catheter unless there is a legitimate and clearly documented reason.

- Patients transferred to an acute hospital without decubitus ulcers, or with low-grade decubiti, should not be returned to the NH with such ulcers, or with the worsening of preexisting ones.

- Significantly medically unstable patients (febrile, septic, in active heart failure, etc.) should not be transferred to the NH until such problems are treated and stabilized.

- Transfers to the NH should be accompanied by medical and nursing discharge summaries, complete and current medication lists, copies of relevant documentation (lab test results, X-ray interpretations, consultant reports), and complete instructions regarding ongoing care and necessary follow-up care.

- Patients should not be transferred to the NH from the acute hospital with changes in mental status or functional status without some evidence of awareness and evaluation of such changes by those in the hospital.

Long-term to acute care. The NH also has certain responsibilities regarding patients sent to the acute hospital. Quality care requires that we find a new approach to helping those elderly persons whose condition deteriorates in the NH until they are finally transferred (often in the middle of the night) to a hospital emergency room, without background information and often beyond any real help. Therefore, the following standards are proposed:

- Adequate documentation and information should accompany the NH resident transferred to the acute hospital, including evaluations of patient decision-making capacity; previously expressed patient wishes; listings of pertinent family members; names and numbers of physicians; recent laboratory results; a description of the events surrounding the transfer; notes which reflect the extent to which the problem or illness has been evaluated or treated; a list of current medications; and recent functional status.

- There should be some communication between NH and hospital to prepare the hospital to receive the patient.

See Appendix 6-A for an example of a medical monitoring tool used by a NH to evaluate transfers from acute hospitals.

Medical Tools

The tools for medical QA are the instruments used by physicians to measure, record, analyze, and evaluate performance and care. These tools may be either profession-oriented, patient-oriented, or institution-oriented. In addition, they too may be structure-, process-, or outcome-oriented. The physician- and institution-oriented tools are much more related to structure and process, while the patient-oriented tools are more concerned with outcome.

Whenever any measurement tool is used by more than one person, the problems of interrater reliability arise, since the same test administered by different people can bring varying results. It therefore helps to standardize the tools, test them before use, and provide written instructions for all users.

Two major tools for medical QA have been the *audit* and *occurrence screening.*

Audits

These are formal, detailed studies of a specific subject (e.g., management of G.I. bleeders, or antibiotic selection in upper respiratory infection). A number of charts are selected and reviewed for the degree of compliance with specific standards (e.g., all G.I. bleeders must have a complete blood count).

These audits may be done *retrospectively* (e.g., on all discharged patients), *concurrently* (e.g., on selected patients still being treated), or *prospectively* (as future patients are admitted).

While audits do serve some useful functions, they have proven to be time-consuming, costly, and sometimes impractical. Therefore, current concepts of quality assurance have deemphasized the audit, in favor of occurrence screening, also called generic screening.

Occurrence Screening

This refers to a process by which information is selected and collected for analysis on the basis of certain occurrences or key indicators. Records are reviewed concurrently, based on specific objective criteria. For example, all patients who must be rehospitalized within 60 days of having been discharged from a hospital could be screened to see whether some of those rehospitalizations could have been prevented through changes in management, discharge planning, or postdischarge support services during the initial hospitalization period.

Quality assurance tools for LTC are most appropriately a mix of these different tactics: some concurrent, some retrospective; some review of all records meeting a specific criterion, and some review of selected records.

For example, if we want to monitor the transfer of patients between the NH and the acute hospital, we use as the key indicator the fact of admission to, or transfer from, an acute hospital. We would periodically (weekly, monthly, quarterly) want a list of all residents meeting this criterion. We then review the records according to established criteria (see discussion above).

As another example, antibiotic usage in long-term care patients is associated with certain risks and complications. By selecting from among all those patients on antibiotics, we can look at a specific issue (such as proper antibiotic prescribing and monitoring), according to specific criteria. A trained reviewer then applies these criteria to the charts of patients on antibiotics to check for compliance. Deviations from the standards are referred to the medical director, pharmacy committee, or medical executive committee (or equivalent) for discussion, review, and action, where indicated.

Putting the Pieces Together

In designing a QA program for a given long-term care setting, the ultimate goal is to assist in the provision of quality medical care for the elderly. Given the great diversity of the LTC settings around the country, and the substantial variability in medical participation, how realistic is it to establish and continue a QA program successfully in these settings?

The answer is—there is a place for a QA program in *every* LTC setting where physicians provide on-site care. Some programs will be small and simple, and others extensive and multifaceted. But it is neither possible nor desirable in the future to try to provide medical services in any setting without some means of monitoring them and trying to improve upon them. If physicians do not do so voluntarily, governments will force them to do so. The goal of the medical quality assurance program should be the best possible patient care, and physician education, not just paper compliance.

Every program has certain common elements, and could benefit from following these steps:

Approve and adopt standards. This may be done by the medical staff, the medical executive committee (where applicable), the medical director, a program director, a multidisciplinary committee (such as utilization review or patient care), or some combination thereof.

Select and approve criteria and measuring tools. Criteria must be established, and tools adapted. These, too, should be approved by physicians, and should reflect commonly accepted practice and understanding in geriatrics.

Collect the data. In most cases, data collection will be done not by physicians, but by a nonprofessional, or a QA coordinator, perhaps hired by the institution to assist all departments in their QA activities. Nevertheless, physicians should design and approve the data collection tools.

Important sources of information for QA reviews include:

- care plans
- medical records
- patient care policies and procedures
- reports from such outside agencies as PROs, JCAH, or health departments.

Data may also include reports of outside review agencies and third-party payors, who themselves look at such things as documentation and follow-up care.

Analyze and summarize the data. The information is of little value until it is evaluated and matched against accepted criteria. Today, computers can save much hard work by performing data analysis and generating reports (see Chapter 9), even for small staffs in small facilities.

Identify problems and trends, and determine causes. Isolated incidents should be distinguished from trends, and justifiable deviations from the standards should also be distinguished from deficiencies or violations. Trends may concern individuals or many or all physicians. The former may require individual counseling; the latter, changes in department or staff policies or procedures.

Assess the causes and scope of these problems and concerns.

Report the conclusions to the physicians. Hours of data collection and analysis serve no purpose unless the information is reported to professionals. This may be done through memos or letters from the chief of staff or medical director, reports to medical staff meetings from the medical executive committee or medical director, and direct communication with individual physicians.

Implement mechanisms and policies to deal with the problems and trends. These, too, may be done by medical directors, medical staffs, or committees, or a combination thereof. Follow-up discussion is as critical as the initial monitoring if practices are to be modified. The challenge is to devise tactics that have the desired impact on medical practice, and some handling of those who may not conform to broad guidelines of accepted practice. The medical director often has a critical role in QA analysis, performance measurement, and corrective action, but must have adequate authority as well as responsibility.

Though the successful quality assurance activity is truly institution-wide, much of the responsibility for developing and implementing patient-care-related policy changes involving quality assurance rests with the medical staff. Patient care-related policy recommendations derived from quality assurance reviews must generally be acted upon through such channels before they are adopted. Other recommendations for policy changes are channeled through the appropriate department heads and the administration.

Pursue individual accountability. Individual accountability is an increasingly important issue. More and more health care facilities are making compliance with QA principles a prerequisite for maintaining privileges, and failure to comply grounds for revocation or denial of privileges. In the small LTC facility with community-based physician staffing, this is notoriously difficult to achieve. Unlike acute hospitals, NHs and other LTC facilities often do not have formal privilege requirements.

In the past, LTC administrators feared alienating physicians by placing too many demands on them. This is beginning to change, however, as general public expectations about the quality of NH care are rising. In addition, since NH residents are usually referred by families or social agencies, not by physicians, some leverage in dealing with attending physicians via those patients and relatives is possible. For example, some facilities insist that families of patients whose physicians repeatedly fail to comply with standards find another doctor.

Examples of Medical Standards and Their Quality Assurance Implementation

Since physician drug prescribing and monitoring is considered a major source of concern in LTC, and deficiencies in monitoring have been repeatedly criticized, the examples presented here are of an actual medical pharmacy and therapeutics QA monitoring program, and of a plan for monitoring one particular kind of drug therapy: antibiotics.

General Pharmacy and Therapeutics Review

Much of the medical therapeutics QA review in LTC can be accomplished with the assistance of a pharmacist consultant. Drug review in a long-term care facility by a pharmacist was first mandated by the federal government in 1974, as part of the conditions for homes participating in Medicare programs. This has subsequently been broadened to also include all homes participating in the Medicaid program, and currently covers virtually any nursing facility with Medicare or Medicaid patients. Such reviews have been hampered by the virtual absence of helpful guidelines for a drug regimen review.

A typical drug regimen review is performed monthly on all patients in the facility. Both technical and therapeutics reviews are relevant to medical practice.

The *technical review* looks at whether the right patient receives the right drug at the right time in the right dose. This may be assessed by comparing all current physician orders with the medication kardexes and looking at such things as the drug, the dose, the directions, the dosage form, the times of administration, and the documentation to see that physician orders agree with the kardexes. Standards and criteria for this come from institutional policies and procedures, and state and federal regulations.

The monthly inspection report notes such technical problems as discrepancies between the physician orders (indicating how the drug was ordered) and the nurses' medication kardex (indicating how the drug was actually being given). The monthly report is generated for each nursing unit, and contains all the information found during the inspection on that nursing unit that month. Copies of these detailed reports are distributed throughout the facility to administration, medicine, nursing, and pharmacy. When problems are identified, they are also communicated verbally to the unit nurse coordinator or to others, as indicated. For example, errors in nursing transcription might be due to illegible or improperly written physician orders. A policy insisting that orders cannot be filled unless they are written clearly could therefore help reduce such errors.

Other aspects covered by the technical drug regimen review include: Are practices in compliance with policies; for example, are the orders being reviewed frequently enough? Are all state and federal regulations being met? Are the proper personnel accepting orders from physicians?

The *therapeutic review* examines whether drug therapy is optimal in the facility. This includes such things as indications (is this the best drug for this patient and for this condition, considering the cost of the medication, as well as its efficacy and its side effects?); whether drug therapy is necessary; and whether the drug ordered is consistent with documented diagnoses and goals for the patient. Medication dosage is reviewed, taking into account such things as the patient's body weight, sex, age, and renal and liver functions.

Patient allergies are also checked against medication lists for conflicts or incompatibilities. The pharmacy's use of detailed computerized records of patients' drug allergies permits identification at the time the drug is ordered. Also evaluated are possible interactions between drugs; between drugs and various lab tests ordered for the patient; and where possible, between drugs and diet. Monitoring for drug toxicity involves checking for documentation of the various indicators of toxicity for a given drug, such as vomiting, hallucinations, or dizziness.

As a result of these reviews and trend assessments, the medical staff has adopted several tactics to improve and monitor physician performance, which have helped keep major drug-related problems to an absolute minimum, including:

Problem-oriented ordering. Every order should be preceded by a word or phrase offering a problem or reason for its prescription

(See Appendix 6-C). For instance, a bedtime order for Halcion must read something like: "*Sleep*: Halcion 0.125 mg. p.o. q.h.s. p.r.n.," rather than just naming the drug and dosage. This has proven extremely valuable, for several reasons:

1. The prescribing physician is forced to clarify in his own mind reasons for ordering medications.

2. Staff are instructed in all cases as to why patients are receiving various medications.

3. More than one medication being given for the same reason becomes much more readily apparent, especially when medication lists are arranged by problems.

4. Correlation between medication lists and problem lists becomes much easier.

5. Quality assurance reviewers can much more readily determine that medications are being prescribed for their proper indications.

Illegible orders. Illegible orders should be clarified with the prescribing physician before they are transcribed, filled, or dispensed. This is preferable to the potential iatrogenic problems, or liability risks, of misinterpreted orders that result in adverse consequences.

Use of a formulary. Formularies are commonly used in hospitals, but not so often in long-term care facilities. They are, however, valuable quality assurance tools, by facilitating better control over the sum total of drugs used in the facility; some consideration of cost factors in drug selection; and some control over drug selection with an eye towards safety and efficacy, specifically in the elderly.

Compliance with policies. The medical director should work to ensure compliance with the established policies and procedures related to drug prescribing and administration. Adequate compliance with these should be one of the conditions upon which renewal of physician privileges is based.

Monitoring of Antibiotic Usage

Antibiotics are one specific category of drugs used in LTC which present special problems. Infections have been shown to be a major cause of morbidity and mortality in LTC patients, and the prompt treatment of febrile infections a significant factor in reducing morbidity and mortality. In addition, antibiotics are among the most commonly prescribed drugs in NHs. Much criticism has been leveled at what some consider their injudicious use and inadequate monitoring. Therefore, a protocol covering the use of antibiotics in LTC can be a valuable educational and QA tool.

- There should be some reasonable clinical indications for beginning antibiotic therapy, which should be documented somewhere in the record.

- A clearly indicated reason or problem (e.g., "urinary tract infection" or "possible pneumonia") for starting the antibiotics should be documented.

- Response to the treatment should be documented, and failures to respond should be followed up.

- Antibiotics should be ordered according to commonly accepted standards concerning dosage, duration, and route of administration.

- Appropriate laboratory monitoring for complications or side effects of certain antibiotic treatments should be ordered.

Appendix 6-B is an example of an actual monitoring tool based on similar criteria.

In the institution using the aforementioned criteria, an average of two charts a week of patients on antibiotics are reviewed by a pharmacy consultant, providing an adequate sample over a year's time. Reviews are both concurrent and retrospective to permit examination of follow-up care (e.g., cultures). Deviations are coded by both type of violation and physician involved. Results are reported to the medical director. Problems of individual practice are discussed with individual physicians. Trends or problems involving more than one physician are reviewed with the entire staff at medical staff meetings. At the same time, articles from the literature are presented periodically at staff meetings, or distributed, to attempt to educate staff and alleviate future problems. Quality assurance thus becomes an educational as well as a monitoring tool.

Infection Control In LTC

Antibiotic usage monitoring is one part of a LTC infection control program. The purpose of any such program is to protect the health of both the patients and the employees. The medical staff and medical director should play a key role in adopting the standards and criteria and in approving the tools used for such a program.

Infection control programs in NHs are required by the JCAH as well as in the Medicare and Medicaid standards for participation (Smith 1984, 224-228). In addition, state and local health departments invariably have rules and regulations or policies pertinent to LTC programs and facilities. Among other things, such standards cover infection control committee requirements, surveillance, reporting, aseptic techniques, and environment and sanitary conditions.

Participants in Infection Control

A LTC infection control program has three critical components: an infection control coordinator; an infection control committee; and infection control advisors.

Infection control coordinator. Someone with interest, experience, and understanding of the facility needs to coordinate the infection control program in the NH. While many facilities can manage with a part-time person in this capacity, "It has been suggested that nursing homes with greater than 150 beds warrant a full-time infection control practitioner" (Smith 1984, 145).

The infection control committee. Representation should include administration, nursing, medicine, dietary, housekeeping, maintenance, laundry services, pharmacy, and the infection control coordinator. These meetings, like those of other committees, can be held as part of a joint meeting session (see Chapter 4). The chairman should be either the medical director, or someone with special interest or training in the subject.

The committee *responsibilities* include review of policies and procedures for isolation, prevention, environmental control, and employee health, in addition to the detection, control, and reporting of infections and outbreaks. Among other topics for review are: food handling, safety, waste disposal, laundry, and pest control.

Physician Participation in Infection Control

Physicians do not have to do the surveillance and data collection, but their input is critical in specific areas, including:

- Infection surveillance and data analysis

- Analysis of antibiotic prescribing, culture results, and lab sensitivity studies (see discussion above)

- Developing tools for data collection and review

- Advising the infection control coordinator on proper policies and procedures

- Assisting in the investigation, management, and reporting of epidemics

- Education

Surveillance. A key question in any infection surveillance is, "What constitutes an infection?" This is often very difficult to ascertain in a NH patient. Therefore, some medical criteria are needed, such as: fever, indwelling catheters, antibiotic use, temperature records, X-ray reports, and antibiotic culture results (Smith 1984, 147). In addition, definitions of various infections are important, but often hard to come by. (For example, when is bacteriuria a urinary tract infection? When does a cough and fever become pneumonia, rather than just an upper respiratory infection?) It is also important to define "nosocomial infection;" that is, when do we consider an infection to have arisen during or because of a person's stay or residency on a particular unit or in a given institution?

Data analysis. The culture reports, sensitivity data, and antibiotic usage reviews must be considered carefully in infection control studies. Among the questions requiring medical opinion are whether physician management of infections is optimal; whether antibiotic usage needs to be changed because of development of resistant strains; whether information about culture results or antibiotic resistance is transmitted accurately and in a timely fashion; and whether there is appropriate follow-up of treatments. If necessary, recommendations for new or revised policies and procedures should be made by or to the infection control committee, and from there to the MEC or medical director for their approval and implementation.

Tools. While an infection control coordinator can use tools to perform data collection, the actual tools should be designed by physicians. Two examples are the infection report form, and the antibiotic usage surveillance tool (see Appendices 6-D and 6-E). These tools should be reviewed periodically, and modified according to changes in accepted standards or practice in geriatric medicine and infection control.

Epidemics. Specific criteria exist to help differentiate sporadic cases from true epidemics. Medical input is essential to determine the presence of an epidemic, manage the affected patients, prevent the spread to other patients or units, record information about the outbreak, report the outbreak to appropriate public health authorities, educate staff and public, guide administration, follow up for recurrences, review the management after the outbreak has subsided, and recommend new or revised policies to handle similar events in the future.

Education. Medical input in this area includes education of the infection control coordinator, the medical staff, nursing personnel caring for patients, patients and families, employees, administration, and the general public.

Policies and procedures. Policies and procedures for infection control in the following areas should be designed by, or with the assistance of, physicians:

- Surveillance

- Reporting to public health agencies

- Environment control

- Identification, confinement, and management of outbreaks

- Prevention (such as catheter care, handwashing techniques, and work restrictions on employees with infections)

- Isolation

- Screening (such as for TB or intestinal pathogens, like salmonella)

- Vaccination

- Antibiotic monitoring.

A comprehensive view of this subject, including discussions of many infectious disease issues, and detailed suggestions about standards, protocols, policies, forms and evaluation tools, and personnel, is available in *Infection Control in Long-Term Care Facilities* (P. W. Smith 1984), listed in the references.

Utilization Management and Utilization Review

Utilization management (UM) is defined as "the planning, organizing, directing, and controlling of the health care product in a cost-effective manner while maintaining high quality care and contributing to the overall goals of the institution. This is accomplished through the judicious use of resources to control inappropriate inpatient admissions, lengths of stay, and use of ancillary services" (Connor, et al. 1983, 7).

Utilization review (UR) is the monitoring arm of utilization management, and refers to the process of evaluating the use of medical care, services, and resources according to certain criteria.

"The AHA [American Hospital Association] policy on 'Utilization Review in Health Care Institutions,' adopted in 1975, states: 'Health care institutions should evaluate the medical necessity, appropriateness, and efficient use of health care services and facilities for all patients as a valuable mechanism for improving the cost effectiveness of the health care delivery system'" (Connor, M. D., Mack, B. A., and E. V. Handelman 1983, 5).

In the past, UR has been emphasized in the acute hospital setting, but little UR has been implemented in the LTC setting. The only real mandate for UR has arisen from the federal Medicare and Medicaid regulations. LTC, especially the geriatric specialty hospital and the NH, today faces many of the same issues that hospitals have long faced, including: questionable or inappropriate admissions or placement, continued stays, or transfers and discharges to or from hospitals; patients transferred between NHs and other settings without adequate evaluation or information about their conditions; and the need to provide services to adequately care for an ever-growing group of sick and functionally impaired individuals.

Given the rapidly increasing costs of long-term institutionalization, and the fact that third parties will pay an increasing portion of LTC costs, it is only a matter of time before more of the same criteria and standards for acute care are applied to LTC.

Quality care in the future will demand cost-effective utilization of those resources. LTC utilization will necessarily encompass more than just institutional care, extending also to the whole spectrum of community-based and home-based services rendered to the elderly. The issue of bed utilization is not as important in the NH as in the hospital, because the bed is part of the NH resident's home. More important are the services provided to that individual in that bed, and the results of such services.

Nevertheless, many of the same kinds of data collection and analyses are as helpful in LTC as in the acute setting. In addition, the same multidisciplinary approach for the effective treatment of geriatric patients is necessary for effective UR and QA programs in LTC.

The problems of *overutilization* and *underutilization* are present in LTC as well as in the acute setting, even though the specific criteria for appropriate utilization certainly differ.

Overutilization in the acute hospital setting focuses on such medically related issues as length of stay, timeliness of test results, and excessive ordering of ancillary services. In LTC, overutilization refers to placement of patients in beds for which they are receiving more nursing and ancillary services than they need for their given functional levels, prognosis, and psychosocial problems.

In contrast, *underutilization* in the acute setting refers to situations in which the patient receives less medical care than needed for the proper diagnosis or treatment of an illness or injury. Underutilization in LTC refers to placement of patients at a level of care less than optimal for their functional impairments, or their needs for proper diagnosis, assessment, treatment and follow-up care.

Assessments of over- and underutilization in the LTC setting must be highly goal-oriented, consistent with the broader range of possible goals for individual patients: for example, cure of acute illness, palliation of chronic pain, or a comfortable and dignified death.

Clearly, quality assurance and utilization review go hand-in-hand, since the expectations for the care affect the selection of services and resources, and the services and resources provided affect the quality of care rendered. Studies (such as O'Brien, et al. 1983; Fottler, et al. 1981) have suggested that quality care and cost-effective care are compatible. The more efficient approach to diagnostic assessment and testing focuses on using fewer and more specific tests, and ordering treatments which offer the best resolution of a problem at the lowest possible cost.

Therefore, although UR may be used because it is mandated, it should nonetheless be seen as one component of an overall medical QA program, part of the effort to improve patient care, reduce liability risk factors, and help ease the burden of compliance with external regulation.

Pertinent UR Standards

Standards and criteria for UR come from third-party payors, especially the federal government, and from independent agencies or organizations, such as the JCAH and American Hospital Association (see Chapter 11 for additional information).

Medicare. Every hospital (including the geriatric specialty hospital) and SNF are required under Title XVIII to have an effective utilization review plan. This must provide for at least the timely review of the medical necessity of admissions, extended durations of stay, and professional services rendered. The objectives are high quality patient care and effective and efficient utilization of health facilities and services.

The SNF must have a written UR plan, which must include a description of: frequency of meetings; type of records to be kept; methods and criteria used to define periods of continuous extended duration and to assign dates for continued stay review; relationship of the plan to filing claims; arrangements for committee reports and their dissemination; and responsibilities of the SNF's administrative staff.

Written records of the meetings must be kept, including attendance, date and duration of the meeting, ongoing review and quality-of-care studies and evaluations, and a summary of cases reviewed.

The SNF must also maintain a centralized, coordinated discharge program, and written discharge planning procedures.

Medicaid. Medicaid UR regulations are found in the Code of Federal Regulations, Title 42, part 456.

Each state must have a continuous program requiring review or screening of each admission in accordance with criteria established by medical and other professional personnel. The federal government can reduce Medicaid fund payments to any state without an effective UR program.

A physician must certify at admission, and must recertify periodically, an individual's need for inpatient care. Services must be furnished under a plan established and periodically evaluated by a physician. Prior to admission, there must be a written care plan and plan of service, which must provide for periodic inspections and reports by professionals of the care provided each recipient.

Elements of Utilization Review Programs in LTC

The UR process, like QA, requires attention to structure, process, and outcome.

Structure refers to the utilization management plan, written policies and procedures, and utilization management personnel.

Process includes procedures used for concurrent review; time periods for review; screening criteria to be used, and the methods for selecting those criteria; mechanisms for discharge planning or transfer; methods for identifying cases to be reviewed; data analyses to be performed; and the reports to be generated.

Outcome is determined both on an individual, case-by-case basis, and on a more general, policy-oriented basis. The former is established by the professional staff; the latter by the professionals in conjunction with administration, board, and community.

Key Participants in the UR Process

As with QA, key participants include: administration, medical staff, a coordinating (utilization management) committee, and the management staff of ancillary departments. In addition, outside agencies or individuals might be involved as reviewers.

Outside reviewers. UR is often turned over to outsiders, under contract. *Delegated review status* means that the institution conducts its own UR activities. *Nondelegated status* means that the institution has review conducted by an outside review organization or third-party payor.

PROs. The *Peer Review Improvement Act*, included in the Tax Equity and Fiscal Responsibility Act (TEFRA) of 1982, substituted Peer Review Organizations (PROs) for the existing PSRO programs. These PROs were authorized to participate in additional areas of quality assurance and utilization review, including appropriateness of admissions and discharges; validity of diagnostic information; and completeness, accuracy, and quality of care.

The federal Health Care Financing Administration (HCFA) awards Peer Review Organization (PRO) contracts to designated agencies for each state, to review the care given those individuals covered by Medicare in acute and specialty hospitals. State Medicaid programs were also authorized to enter into contracts with PROs.

The PRO reviews a representative sample of admissions, for necessity of length of stay and compliance with certain generic quality screens. The retrospective review looks at whether length of stay and specialized services rendered were necessary and appropriate. Generic quality screens may include adequacy of discharge planning; patient's medical condition at discharge; unexpected deaths; nosocomial infections; trauma suffered in the hospital; and major adverse drug reactions or medication errors. If the PRO reviewer decides that services were unnecessary or were not those covered under Medicare, a denial letter is sent by the PRO to the patient and the facility.

Thus, even when UR is done by others, the facility and its staff must be responsible for the accuracy, completeness, and validation of its information and documentation.

The Medical Role in UR

General JCAH standards for medical staff participation in acute care UR include expectations for periodic review of bed utilization, and use of diagnostic, nursing and therapeutic resources, considering both the availability of these resources to patients needing them, and physician responsibility for health care costs. This review should include admissions, lengths of stay, professional services furnished, and the availability and alternate use of out-of-hospital facilities and services. These general standards are applicable, with modifications, to the LTC setting, as well.

The utilization management (UM) plan. The medical director or medical staff should assist in drawing up or refining the UR plan, including: defining lines of authority, the organization of the UR committee, physician responsibilities, the review process to be used, reporting mechanisms, coordination of resources, protection of confidentiality, and responsibility for periodic review of the UR plan.

In the hospital, physicians, through their orders, are the primary purchasers of services. In the NH, residents and families are the primary purchasers of ongoing services, but physicians order tests and treatments which affect placement and overall cost. Physicians must therefore be prepared to review, justify, and perhaps modify their practices and care plans, based on changes in individual situations, and the requirements of outside agencies and third parties.

Documentation is a key medical function in UR in LTC. It should clarify the reasons why someone is admitted to, or should continue at, a particular level of care, reflect some thought to the possibilities of providing equivalent care at a less costly level, explain the medical reasons for changes in the plan of care, and give evidence that the physician is aware of the goals and objectives for the individual.

The medical director and medical staff must furthermore devise and review the criteria for such utilization decisions, whether of their own design, or that of outsiders.

A physician representative should work closely with outside review agencies under contract with the institution to conduct utilization studies and reviews, to follow up on their decisions, correct misunderstandings, assure adequate and appropriate documentation, keep abreast of new requirements and modifications of old ones, and analyze the rate of and reasons for denials of continued stay.

The medical role on the UR committee. At the least, the medical director or a medical staff representative should sit on the UR committee.

A *physician advisor*, who may be the medical director, another medical staff member, or an outside physician, acts as consultant to the UR committee, to advise and recommend on how well individual cases conform to established criteria, as well as to support and review the deliberations of the committee. This person cannot have any financial or professional involvement in the individual cases under review.

Based on its data collection and analysis, the medical staff should reach conclusions about the appropriateness, timeliness, and cost-effectiveness of medical care, according to criteria such as those below.

The medical staff should review care practices, to assure that these are appropriate, timely, cost-effective, and reflect new understandings in geriatric medicine. Medical policies should reflect the results of these care reviews.

The medical director or medical staff should also be prepared to address questions of the administration, owners, or board concerning utilization issues, including those uncovered or investigated by the UM committee or outside payors or review agencies. In this context, the medical director or medical staff can offer invaluable advice concerning appropriate personnel, programs, equipment, or services needed to provide adequate patient care at various levels. This can assist in planning for bed expansion or closure, additional community services, and improved occupancy.

Medical Utilization Criteria

Criteria for various levels of care, including skilled and geriatric specialty hospital (chronic), have been established by HCFA (see Appendix 6-F). In addition, however, there are other criteria by which the medical staff can review its performance and practices, including review of whether:

- A resident's documented condition is consistent with the criteria for a given level of care

- Placement takes into account an individual's personal wishes and needs, and involves family in the process

- Adequate and appropriate preadmission assessments allow for correct placement decisions, and are consistent with early postadmission findings

- Patient stays were retroactively or prospectively denied, and why

- Appropriate justification is documented for ordering expensive care items such as Clinitron beds

- Appropriate transfers of critically and terminally ill persons are arranged, and appropriate provisions for care within the NH are made before transfer to an acute hospital

- Attending physicians make timely assessments, and document adequate evaluation and follow-up of changes in patient condition.

Other medical UR criteria include:

- How many patients were transferred to the acute hospital in a given time period, for what reasons, and with what eventual outcome? What happened to their beds while they were gone, where were they placed after hospitalization, and how many of these transfers might have been prevented by earlier physician intervention or better staff observation?

- How quickly and appropriately were discharge or transfer plans made and implemented for persons found to no longer need their current levels of care?

- How many individuals were discharged appropriately into the community, or moved to a lower level of care? Was money actually saved in the long run, and what was the outcome?

Summary

In this chapter we have examined the medical role in LTC quality assurance, infection control, and utilization management. While physicians have been involved in these activities in acute hospitals, their participation in the NH and other LTC programs has been minimal. Many of the acute hospital-oriented standards, criteria, and methods are at least partially applicable to LTC, but invariably must be modified to accommodate the special characteristics of the LTC system and patients.

Physicians not only have an important role to play in monitoring the quality of *medical* care, but also in advocating and supporting rational standards for the entire LTC system, and in providing the facts that will justify and clarify such standards. Hopefully, quality assurance, currently enforced by mandatory regulations and viewed as an obligation, will become a major, vital educational tool for the LTC professional.

Appendix 6-A Example of a NH monitoring tool for hospital to NH transfers

Quality Assurance Review of Problems with Admissions

Patient name _____   Admission Date _____

Discharging
Hospital _____   Is this re-admission?   Yes   No

Person reporting _____   Unit _____

Patient admitted:

                                          No   *Yes* (if yes, please describe)

1. With urinary catheter without
   apparent justification
_____

2. With decubitus ulcer (if readmission
   change in stage)
_____

3. Significantly medically unstable
_____

4. Fever (undocumented/untreated
   while in acute hospital)
_____

5. Symptomatic for infection without
   appropriate treatment
_____

6. Without adequate information
   A. With incomplete d/c summary
   B. Incomplete medication lists
_____

7. Mental status change (undocu-
   mented/unevaluated)
_____

Please return this form to the quality assurance coordinator

Appendix 6-B Example of quality assurance criteria for antibiotic usage
in a geriatric hospital and nursing home

Antibiotic Usage Screening

Appropriateness of Empiric or Therapeutic Antibiotics

A. *Empiric* — initial therapy for suspected infection prior to final culture
results applies, in general, for the first 1, 2, or 3 days of antibiotic therapy.
Thereupon, if the results of initial cultures and the clinical course are supportive of a diagnosis of infection, *therapeutic* antibiotics (definitive) are continued for prescribed doses and duration.

B. *Appropriateness of Antibiotics for Specific Infectious Syndromes*

1. UTI (for patients with 2 of the following signs/symptoms with Foley):
   a. fever or flank pain
   b. > 10 WBCs in urine
   c. > 10,000 WBCs in blood with shift to the left (increased bands
      and polys)
   d. > 100,000 bacteria/ml. urine culture

2. UTI (for patients with 2 of the following signs/symptoms without
   Foley):
   a. dysuria
   b. fever
   c. > 10 WBCs in urine
   d. > 10,000 WBCs in blood with shift to the left
   e. > 100,000 bacterial/ml. urine culture

3. Pneumonia with 3 of the following:
   a. fever
   b. polys in sputum (micro)/purulent sputum (gross)
   c. predominant sputum Gram stain bug
   d. decreased ABGs
   e. infiltrate on chest X-ray
   f. sputum culture (+) for predominant bug
   g. leucocytosis
   h. positive physical findings

4. Wound infection or phlebitis with 2 of the following:
   a. redness or warmth
   b. swelling or pain
   c. purulent drainage (gross) or polys on smear (micro)
   d. positive culture or predominant bug by Gram stain

5. Meningitis with *all* of the following:
   a. CSF culture
   b. CSF Gram stain
   c. CSF glucose, protein, WBC
   d. blood culture

6. Endocarditis or sepsis *with* blood culture

7. Septic arthritis with *both*:
   a. blood culture
   b. Gram stain and culture of joint fluid

8. Osteomyelitis with Gram stain and culture of needle aspiration or biopsy specimen within first 3 days of therapy

Appropriateness of Nonformulary (N.F.) Antibiotics Administered for More Than 48 Hours

Was a N.F. antibiotic given for more than 48 hours without a legitimate reason, such as:

A. neutropenic cancer patient
B. multiply resistant bacteria
C. infectious disease recommendation

Effectiveness of Empiric or Therapeutic Antibiotics

A. Was reason for starting antibiotics documented in chart, i.e., suspected or proven infection?

B. Was the patient's response to antibiotics evaluated and documented?
   1. fever pattern
   2. repeat culture
   3. repeat WBC count
   4. reevaluation of other signs, symptoms or tests

C. When the results of cultures and sensitivities became available, was the antibiotic(s) in use effective against the bacteria? (not applicable if more than 2 bacterial species from urine or sputum culture).

D. If patient failed to respond to therapy or had a recurrence of infection, was a change in therapy documented?

Safety of Empiric or Therapeutic Antibiotics

A. General Considerations

1. Was drug given to patient with known allergy or known adverse reaction to that drug class, e.g., penicillins, cephalosporins, aminoglycosides, or other individual agents?

2. Was drug given for more than 14 days (except in such cases as endocarditis, osteomyelitis, lung abscess or serious staph infections)?

3. Were more than 2 parenteral drugs being given at the same time?

B. Specific Safety Issues (Selected)

1. *Aminoglycosides IV, IM* (Gentamicin, Tobramycin, Streptomycin, Amikacin, Netilmicin)

   a. Was creatinine checked before beginning of therapy?
   b. If creatinine rose during therapy (by at least 50%), was the dose modified?
   c. Was creatinine checked at least weekly?

2. *Chloramphenicol* – CBC weekly?

3. *Penicillins, IV, IM* (Ampicillin, Penicillin G, Naficillin, Methicillin, Ticarcillin, Carbenicillin, etc.) – Were 2 penicillins given simultaneously?

4. *Trimethoprim - Sulfamethoxazole (Bactrim)* – being given simultaneously with another antibiotic?

Appendix 6-C Example of the "problem-oriented" arrangement of medical orders for nursing home patients

NAME:		BIRTH DATE:	03/07/08
CHART NO:	19-34-96	DATE ADM:	10/23/57
LOCATION:	B-2	LATEST READM:	02/02/84
ROOM:	B292		

PHYSICIAN'S ORDERS FOR ONE MONTH BEGINNING
03/31/87

Discontinue All Previous Orders

This Patient is Certified as Needing ICF/SNF Services

Level of Care: Intermediate   Condition: Fair
Rehab Potential: Poor   Prognosis: Fair

Diet: Soft NAS
Activ: OOB in chair ad lib - ambulate c walker
Lab:

	Due Date
HB (P8) Every 3 months	04/12/87
HCT (P8) Every 3 months	04/12/87
FBS (P7) Every 3 months	04/12/87

Allergies: No known allergy

Medication and Treatments

1. ASCVD (429.2)
   Furosemide (Lasix) 40mg: 1 Tab p.o. each morning

7. Diabetes Mellitus (250.0)
   FBS: Every 3 months
   Chlorpropamide (Diabinese) 250 mg: 1 Tab p.o. each morning

8. Anemia (285.9)
   Trinsicon - M : 1 cap p.o. 2 x daily
   Ascorbic acid - vit c 250 mg: 1 tab p.o. 3 x daily
   HB: every 3 months
   HCT: every 3 months

21. HX Constipation (564.0)
    Phosphate Enema (Fleet's Enema) : As needed
    MOM/Cascara Conc 15cc (= 30/5) : 15 cc p.o. at bedtime as needed

27. Degenerative Joint Disease - Knee (715.9)
    Darvocet-N (Propoxyphene NAPS/APAP) 100mg: 1 tab. p.o. at 6
    AM 12 PM 6 PM & 12 AM as needed

Other Drugs
    Maalox (mag/alum hydroxide) 30cc: 30 cc p.o. every 4 hrs as
        needed for abdominal discomfort
    Cocoa butter lotion: apply to skin 2x daily as needed for dryness
        (may keep at bedside)

Other Orders
    In-house routine eye clinic prn
    In-house routine dental clinic prn
    In-house routine podiatry clinic prn

            Signed:
            Date:

Appendix 6-D Example of a long-term care infection report summary form

Report to the Committee on Infections for the Month of: _____

CENTER STATISTICS

	PATIENT CARE DAYS	NUMBER OF DISCHARGES	MEAN STAY (DAYS)
Hospital	_____	_____	_____
Long Term Care	_____	_____	_____

SURVEILLANCE STATISTICS

DISTRIBUTION BY PATIENT CARE UNITS

UNIT	Nosocomial Infections	Pathogens	Pathogens	Pathogens
Stein	____	____	____	____
H I	____	____	____	____
H 2	____	____	____	____
B 2	____	____	____	____
B I	____	____	____	____
BG	____	____	____	____

DISTRIBUTION BY INFECTION SITES

UNIT	RESP.	URINARY	EYE	WOUND	ENTERIC	OTHER	TOTAL
Stein	____	____	____	____	____	____	____
H I	____	____	____	____	____	____	____
H 2	____	____	____	____	____	____	____
B 2	____	____	____	____	____	____	____
B I	____	____	____	____	____	____	____
BG	____	____	____	____	____	____	____
TOTAL							

(Reprinted by courtesy of Levindale Hebrew Geriatric Center and Hospital, Baltimore, Md.)

Appendix 6-E A long-term care infection surveillance tool

INFECTIOUS DISEASE SURVEILLANCE LOG

MONTH: _____

YEAR: _____

PATIENT NUMBER	DATE OF REVIEW	RM#	AGE	SEX	DATE OF ADM.	STATED DIAGNOSIS	SITE INFECTED	SIGNS AND SYMPTOMS	DATE OF ONSET	DATE OF CULTURE	RESULT OF CULTURE	PHYSICIAN'S ORDERS	ACTIONS/RESOLUTION	M.D. CODE

Reprinted courtesy of Levindale Hebrew Geriatric Center and Hospital; Baltimore, Maryland.

Appendix 6-F Typical utilization criteria for various levels of long-term care

TYPE OF FACILITY

1. Home Health

   The home setting is both practical and effective in improving and/or maintaining the patient's health status. Visiting home care services must be physician prescribed.

   Patient Needs

   - Skilled nursing care, skilled supervision of Physical Therapy needed on an Intermittent basis.
   - Physical Therapy and Speech Therapy needed a minimum of one time per week.
   - Skilled services needed two to three times per week for treatment and instruction. Examples of such services would have to meet Medicare's definition: dressing changes, catheter changes, medication monitoring, blood pressure monitoring, injections, inhalation therapy.

2. Foster Care

   A non-licensed, non-medical facility that provides room and board.

   Patient Needs

   - Patients do not need an attendant at all times.
   - Only need room and board
   - Capable of independent ambulation (either self or with assistive device).
   - Should not be confused.

3. Domiciliary

   A non-medical facility for personal care and general supervision of the elderly who are physically or mentally disabled. A licensed protective environment with care provided by non-licensed personnel.

   Patient Needs

   - Essentially independent with ambulation (either self or with assistive device).
   - Social needs with very minimal medical needs (could take some long standing oral medication)
   - Mild confusion
   - Minimal assistance with Activities of Daily Living (A.D.L.)
   - Needs more protection than a foster home can provide.

4. Intermediate

A medical facility for the treatment of patients having convalescent or irreversible medical or surgical problems who require direct care by licensed nurses 24 hours/day, rendered under the supervision of a registered nurse. Specialized rehabilitative services for the restoration of normal form and function needed on a less than five-day-a-week basis, by or under the supervision of a licensed therapist.

Patient Needs

- Needs institutional level of protection that can't be provided in a foster home or domiciliary home.
- Rehabilitation (physical or speech).
- Has medical needs greater than what a domiciliary facility can provide.
- Needs are greater than for ADL:

Administration of complex oral medication or combination thereof; subcutaneous medication when patient is too senile or too physically incapacitated to perform the act himself. Intramuscular injection; irrigation, indwelling catheter; prescribed medication for intermittent bladder irrigation, routine catheterization for incontinence; skin lesions requiring sterile dressings; administration of O_2 or compressed air on a continuous or as-needed basis; care of patients with braces, casts, or splints without complications; aspiration of tracheotomy tubes on an as-needed basis; routine gastrostomy feedings.

5. Skilled

A medical facility for post-hospital care of patients with medical, surgical and multiple nursing problems which can, for practical purposes, only be provided on an inpatient basis. Care needs to be provided by RN's on all shifts seven days a week. Specialized rehabilitative services under supervision of a licensed therapist are needed on a minimum of five days a week. If rehabilitation needs are the only qualifier for this level, the patient must require treatment a minimum of five days a week to maximum potential.

Patient Needs

- Each service must be provided at least five days a week or combination of several skilled services provided on a total of five days a week.
- Needs observation for modification and initiation of medical procedures.
- Condition is unstable.

- Needs are usually short term at this level.
- Examples of skilled services. Administration of medications for observation when response is unpredictable, administration of IV fluids or IV meds, insertion of catheter every four-six hours for bladder training, needs a catheter for resolving problem with urinary tract post surgical, decubiti extending into subcutaneous tissue or other wide-spread skin disorder. These require applications of medication, irrigation and/or sterile dressing, administration of O_2 on a regular and continuing basis in the presence of pathology, post-acute care of patients with Bucks traction or pelvic traction, post-acute recurrent aspiration of nasopharynx and tracheotomy tubes, initial phase of levine or gastrostomy feedings when high probability of complication and/or deterioration exists.
- Needs are subject to contract exclusions by various Federal programs.

6. Chronic

A specialty hospital for the diagnosis and treatment of chronic disease and medical and physical rehabilitation on a daily basis (min. five times a week) including OT, PT, speech and/or hearing therapy.

Patient Needs

- Needs are multiple medical problems
- Care of complex terminal stage of illness
- Needs require daily physician observation and management
- Needs intensive nursing services on a continuous basis
- Combination of several skilled services (each daily) where management is too complex for a nursing home environment
- Severe incapacitating problems.
- Recurrent bouts of severe respiratory or cardiac failure.
- Frequent acute exacerbations of chronic condition with intractible pain, difficulty breathing or continuous ascites.

References

Connor, M. D., G. A. Mack, and E. V. Handelman. 1983. *Dynamics of utilization management.* Chicago: American Hospital Association.

Fottler, M. D., H. L. Smith, and W. L. James. 1981. Profits and patient care quality in nursing homes: Are they compatible. *The Gerontologist* 21:532.

Gustafson, D. H., C. J. Fiss, J. C. Fryback, et al. 1980. Measuring the quality of care in nursing homes: a pilot study in Wisconsin. *Public Health Reports* 95:336.

Heller, T. A., F. B. Larson, and J. P. LoGerfo. 1984. Quality of ambulatory care of the elderly: an analysis of five conditions. *Journal of the American Geriatrics Society* 32:782.

Joint Commission on Accreditation of Hospitals. 1986. *Long-Term Care Standards Manual.* Chicago: JCAH.

Kane, R. 1981. Assuring quality of care and quality of life in long term care. *Quality Review Bulletin* (Oct.) 7(10):3-10.

Kane, R. L., R. Bell, S. Riegler, et al. 1983. Predicting the outcomes of nursing home patients. *The Gerontologist* 23(2):200-206.

O'Brien, J., B. O. Saxberg, and H. L. Smith. 1983. For-profit or not-for-profit nursing homes: Does it matter? *The Gerontologist* 23(4):341-348.

Pattee, J. J., and J. M. Gustafson. 1984. Quality in long-term care: Challenge of self-evaluation. *Minnesota Medicine,* 67(1):45-50.

Rabin, D. L. 1981. Physician care in nursing homes. *Annals of Internal Medicine,* 94:126-128.

Senate Special Committee on Aging Staff Report. 1986. *Nursing Home Care: The Unfinished Agenda,* May 21, 1986.

Smith, P. W. 1984. *Infection control in long-term care facilities.* New York: John Wiley & Sons.

Vogel, R. J. and H. C. Palmer. 1982. *Long-term care: Perspectives from research and demonstrations.* Washington, DC: HCFA.

For Further Reading

Gottlieb, T. W. Quality assurance in a long-term care facility. 1984. *Quality Review Bulletin,* 10(2):51-54.

Joint Commission on Accreditation of Hospitals. *Long-Term Care Standards Manual.* Chicago: JCAH. Published annually, this accreditation manual includes information on utilization review and quality assurance expectations and standards.

Joint Commission on Accreditation of Hospitals. *Quality Review Bulletin.* Published 12 times a year, offers practical assistance on QA activities and patient care evaluation techniques.

Joint Commission on Accreditation of Hospitals. *Infection Control and Drug and Antibiotic Review.* Chicago: JCAH. Presents methods of infection and antibiotic surveillance.

Meisenheimer, C. G. 1985. *Quality Assurance: A Complete Guide to Effective Programs.* Rockville, MD: Aspen. A comprehensive review of the components, design, implementation, and management of effective QA programs.

Pattee, J. J., and J. M. Gustafson. 1984. Quality in long-term care: Challenge of self-evaluation. *Minnesota Medicine* 1:45-50.

Schwartz, T. 1982. How to install a first-rate doctor in a third-rate nursing home. *New England Journal of Medicine* 306:743-44.

Shaughnessy, P., et al. 1983. Case mix and surrogate indicators of quality of care over time in freestanding and hospital-based nursing homes in Colorado. *Public Health Reports* 98, 5 (Sept-Oct):486-492.

Stevens, J. E. 1983. Quality assurance in long-term care. *Quality Review Bulletin* 9(8):229-230.

Williamson, J. W. 1978. *Assessing and improving health care outcomes.* Cambridge, Mass: Ballinger.

Educational material on QA, risk management, medical staff issues, accreditation, and standards for care are available from the JCAH, 875 N. Michigan Avenue, Chicago, IL 60611.

Chapter Seven

Physicians and the Long-Term Care Team

Elizabeth L. Rogers, M.D.

Chapter Objectives

This chapter will:

- Review the importance of the team approach in LTC
- Explain the roles and expertise of the members of the LTC team
- Discuss the physician's role and responsibilities as a member of this team

Introduction

When physicians become involved in long-term care, especially in long-term care of the elderly, preexisting expectations often shade their responses to the stresses of caring for the patients, as well as to other professionals, paraprofessionals, and lay people involved in such care. Medical school and postgraduate medical training frequently occur in acute medical centers, where the house staff is protected from activities which would "distract" them from efficiently diagnosing and treating acutely ill patients in expensive inpatient facilities. Even when properly supervised, with access to capable subspecialty consultants, the physician-in-training frequently feels alone, and often solely responsible for the patient's outcome. Other professionals are judged as helpful or difficult based on their ability to expedite orders and patient discharge.

Involvement in geriatrics and long-term care involves different perspectives about what constitutes good patient care (see also Chapters 2 and 13). Goals shift toward rapidly treating those processes which may lead to deterioration of the patient, to attempted prevention of the development of disabling processes, and to maximizing function, comfort, and independence.

Robert Kane (1982, 72) has described the major problems of the frail elderly as "incontinence, incoherence, instability, immobility, infection, inanition, isolation, impecunity, and iatrogenesis." As the frail geriatric patient, with his numerous problems and disabilities, moves more slowly, the time and expertise necessary to adequately care for such an individual increases.

With these chronic medical problems, LTC patients are often at high risk of developing complications both from the diseases themselves and from various prescribed and nonprescribed medications. Poor eyesight and balance, and lack of safety awareness leave them vulnerable to falls. Altered urinary and respiratory function, combined with decreased immunocompetence, leave them vulnerable to infection. They therefore require more frequent medical supervision and intervention than does a healthy population.

Good long-term care is manpower intensive. In addition, compassionate, quality long-term care requires us to maximize a patient's socioeconomic support systems as well as the functional and emotional abilities. As pointed out earlier (see Chapter 2), physicians alone cannot deliver all the necessary care. With close communication and the identification of goals and approaches to therapy, many other people can work with the physician toward this end.

In short, optimal quality of care demands development of a team approach.

The Team Approach in LTC

Much of the development in the specialty of geriatrics has benefited from the development of the specialty of pediatrics several decades earlier. From these roots come the concepts of comprehensive, compassionate care of the patient as an individual, attention not only to treatment but also to primary and secondary prevention, reinforcement of the social support systems, minimization of isolation or dependence, and attention to rehabilitation. Achieving these goals requires the involvement of a multidisciplinary team. Table 7-1 lists alphabetically the minimum areas of expertise required of a multidisciplinary geriatric team.

Effectiveness in each one of these areas can best be achieved by people with extensive knowledge and skills. Specialized training in such areas as gerontologic nursing and social work, physical and occupational therapy, clinical pharmacology, dentistry and oral hygiene, psychology and psychiatry, neurology,and geriatric medicine is fundamental because the information base and necessary skills in each area are so vast. Although one well motivated person may develop expertise in some of these areas, few can fully master all of them. Truly, to formulate an adequate treatment plan, more than one person's involvement is needed. This concept – that of the treatment team – has become one of the hallmarks of geriatric medicine.

The size of a treatment team can vary with the patient's needs and the financial resources of the patient and of the treating unit. The levels of skill and time commitments of the individuals involved will also affect the size of the team.

All the team members must act as patient advocates. This demands repeated empathetic communication with patient and family to ensure that goals of treatment are appropriate. Each team member needs to analyze critically and repeatedly whether the team is functioning to achieve these goals and is succeeding in making the LTC patient physically and socially comfortable and maximally functional.

Table 7-1 The geriatric multidisciplinary team expertise required.

Expertise Required
Clergy/Ethical
Clinical Pharmacology
Dental/Oral Hygiene
Medical
Nursing
Nutrition Support
Ophthalmic/Podiatric/Surgical
Psychiatry/Psychology
Rehabilitation Therapy
Social Work

Role of the Team Members

While the number of LTC team members will vary, there are certain essential functions and roles to be filled. Whether these roles are carried out by a physician or by others, as described below, depends on individual circumstances. The list is alphabetical, rather than in any order of importance, because each of these roles may be vital in the care of any one patient, yet not always necessary for all patients in all settings.

Clergy and Ethicists

Care of the elderly involves many stresses, each requiring careful handling. The wishes and expectations of the patient, the family, and the members of the treatment team may vary. The resources of the patient or the community may not support unlimited options. In addition, the benefit of some treatments may or may not outweigh physical discomfort and social alienation. Issues of restraints for safety, involuntary feeding, and cardiopulmonary resuscitation, are among the recurring ethical crises which must be addressed differently for each patient (see also Chapter 12). Likewise, the elderly, their families, and the treatment team must cope with disabilities, losses, institutionalization, and death. There is a great need for one or more people to be the "conscience" and the emotional stabilizer of the team.

Clinical Pharmacists

Major pharmacologic issues inherent in the care of the elderly, especially the frail elderly, include:

- Polypharmacy
- Efficacy
- Side effects
- Drug-nutrient interactions
- Compliance.

With multisystem illnesses, the elderly often require several medicines. Since the average number of appropriately written prescriptions per geriatric patient may range from five to fifteen, special problems can arise for both the physician and the patient. One problem is to differentiate desired effects from cross-reactions and unwanted side effects. Another is to recognize that a new or recurrent symptom may be related to a drug reaction instead of to additional disease processes. Such understanding can help reduce complications, limit unnecessary diagnostic interventions, and improve therapy. The clinical pharmacist can help with these as well as in the recognition of drug-nutrient interactions and nutritional deficiencies. Other contributions of the pharmacist include assessment of the efficacy of a given medication at a certain dose and recognition that one medication would reduce the need for two or more others.

Medication compliance is often poor in the elderly because of the number of bottles, the differing dosage regimens, the unwanted side effects, and the cost. Compliance can be worsened further by confusion, limited mobility, or visual or manual dexterity impairments. The clinical pharmacist can both determine the degree of compliance and work with the patient and support system to suggest innovative and alternative methods to improve compliance.

Dentist or Oral Hygienist

The elderly, like much of society, frequently wish to avoid dentists. Preservation of dentition, maintenance of adequate oral hygiene, development of bridgework, and proper fit of dentures are necessary, however, to help the elderly continue to eat solid food and maintain adequate nutrition. The lack of dentures, because of high cost or the often painful alteration of fit with change of weight or illness, may contribute to social isolation and to eventual malnutrition.

Nurse

Much of the day-to-day care of LTC patients is vested with the nursing staff because of their training in patient assessment and compassionate clinical care. Issues facing the nursing staff daily include:

- Medication supervision
- Mobility maintenance
- Activities of Daily Living (ADL) support
- Skin Care
- Nutritional support
- Communication and orientation
- Coordination of activities
- Identification of new problems
- Adequate supervision and control of dysfunctional behavior.

Additionally, the role of the registered nurse, nurse practitioner, or physician assistant as the primary practitioner of health care has been explored in various settings. Ebersole (1985) points out a major difference between the roles of institutional and community-based nurses. While institutional nurses are part of a well-developed system of regulations and support services, community nurses have more flexibility in defining their roles and limitations, and usually work where support services must be actively sought.

In home health care, the nurse's role involves:

1. Direct nursing care
2. Evaluation of the patient and the caregiver's abilities and limitations
3. Monitoring of the patient's progress, regression, or complications
4. Instruction and supervision of patient and family
5. Communication with other disciplines and agencies.
6. Initial evaluation of the patient in his home. Usually performed by a nurse, with or without other members of the healthcare team. The home care nurse must often act as a physical therapist, aide, dietician, social worker, and laboratory technician, as well as a nurse (Birenbaum and Figlioli 1983).

Community geropsychiatric nurses need to perform mental as well as physical assessment and must be able to offer therapy, crisis intervention, and case management skills as needed within the multidisciplinary team (Ebersole and Hess 1985).

Supervision of medication dose and timing is frequently necessary for homebound patients, and may include removal of the individual's hoarded supplies of outdated or unnecessary medications.

Other common nursing activities include assistance in feeding the patient who is unwilling or unable to feed himself; assessment of adequacy of intake, and the usefulness of supplements; and administration of tube feedings.

Without frequent and constant stimulation and prompting, patients in LTC facilities may lose interest in exercise, resulting in reduced muscle tone and slow deterioration of function.Therefore, day-to-day maintenance of mobility—whether ambulation, wheelchair mobility, or bed movements—becomes the responsibility of the nursing staff.

Similarly, the nursing staff assess, encourage, and assist the patient's participation in the activities of daily living (ADL). Maintenance of, or improvement in, ADL allows the patient more independence and control over his/her environment.

Avoidance of decubitus ulcers in malnourished, bedbound patients is difficult and time consuming. Patients must be turned frequently, and their extremities positioned on pillows, wedges, or protective blankets to reduce pressure on bony prominences. Careful attention to skin color, application of local salves, and early application of wet-to-dry dressings may prevent or delay the development of decubitus ulcers.

Disorientation, confusion, and isolation are also common in nursing home residents. Frequent encouragement, conversation, and the establishment of schedules by the nursing staff may help reduce such isolation and disorientation.

Nutrition Support

Malnutrition is common in the elderly living at home, because of financial, social, and mobility constraints, as well as prescribed dietary alterations and personal idiosyncracies. In addition, approximately 80% of institutionalized elderly have some evidence of malnutrition. The vital role of the nutritionist or clinical dietician is therefore to both recognize and respond to mild dietary irregularities, as well as to recommend appropriate changes. The dietitian can work with the patient to translate diet terminology into a tolerable and palatable diet (Levenson 1985).

Intellectually intact ambulatory homebased elderly are frequently preoccupied with nutrition, and respond positively to well-informed advice. The nutritionist can also work with patients to discuss how food preferences and eating habits affect their health.

When oral intake is inadequate, dietary supplements, tube feedings, or parenteral nutritional support may be necessary. Skilled professionals can guide the process by accurate review of caloric and nutrient intake, and optimal use of supplements.

The role of the dietician or nutritionist in home care includes both direct nutritional and dietary counseling of the patient as well as assistance to the family and treatment team (Birenbaum and Figlioli 1983).

Optometrists and Ophthalmologists

Loss of visual acuity in the elderly contributes to further isolation, as well as decreases in mobility, contact with friends and family, and stimulation. While many of the visual problems of the elderly are not reversible, many others are subject to improvement. The development of intraocular lenses, for example, has greatly enhanced the lives of many LTC patients. Simple reading glasses and lenses to correct astigmatism can increase patients' interactions and safe maneuvering. Although ophthalmologists may be needed only periodically, their presence as part of the evaluation and treatment team will increase the function of the LTC patient.

Surgical/Podiatric Specialists

Many home care and nursing home programs have incorporated the skills of the podiatrist into the treatment team. Whether evaluating for supportive shoes or braces, correcting painful lesions, or simply maintaining nail hygiene in the diabetic, the podiatrist has become an important resource for the LTC team. Other surgical specialists frequently consulted by the multidisciplinary team include the urologist and the orthopedic surgeon.

Psychologists and Psychiatrists

Depression, dementia, and disorientation are common occurrences in the LTC setting. Neuropsychological evaluation, depression assessment, establishing treatable causes of depression, separating the depressive symptoms from those caused by dementia, and helping the patient, family, and support staff to deal with the stresses of chronic disease and death are all part of the psychologist's and psychiatrist's role.

Rehabilitation Therapists

Rehabilitation therapy is central to geriatric and long-term care. Maintenance or improvement of function are necessary to prevent further deterioration of the patient. Depending on the facility, rehabilitation therapy may be provided by some or all of these staff:

- Audiology
- Occupational therapy
- Physiatry
- Physical therapy
- Recreational therapy
- Speech pathology.

Central to any rehabilitative program is periodic evaluation of the patient's progress, including the degree of joint range of motion, muscle strength, gait, ability of the patient to perform the activities of daily living, sensory and perceptual assessment, and cognitive functional assessment.

Physical therapy of disabled patients in LTC involves therapeutic exercises to strengthen weakened muscles, improve endurance, maintain or increase joint range of motion, improve coordination of skilled motor function, and restore functional gait (Steinberg, 1983).

Progressive rehabilitation after stroke, for example, entails the greatest possible restoration of function, adaptation to the residual disability, and prevention of secondary disabilities (Steinberg 1983).

Activities will include active exercises and control of muscle tone, passive range of motion and positioning to prevent contractures; reeducation of speech processes and alternative methods of communication; progressive gain in mobility and function, including the activities of daily living; development of fine muscle coordination; assessment of the usefulness of assistive devices; and more positive use of free time.

Physical therapy also assists in the management of prosthetic and orthotic devices, and in patients requiring cardiac and pulmonary rehabilitation.

While the role of the occupational therapist in LTC varies across regions of the country, some general goals apply in all situations. These include: 1) the provision of rehabilitative treatment when functional limitations prevent the individual from performing activities requiring upper extremity or fine motor function, and 2) early intervention to minimize dysfunction in the areas of self-care, work, and leisure time activities (Mann 1983). In some centers, the development of assistive devices and concentration on ADLs are the domain of the occupational therapist, while the physical therapist deals mainly with antigravity and major motor problems.

The speech pathologist's role is to evaluate and develop a comprehensive rehabilitation program to improve a patient's communication, including verbal speech, telephone communication, money handling, and the ability to associate date and time.

Rehabilitation therapy plays a role not only in the institutionalized patient but also in evaluation of the patient in his home environment. Safety features of the house, availability of assistive devices, and ability of the family to help the patient function on stairs, in the kitchen, or in the lavatory can also be assessed by the therapist.

Social Workers

Clearly, social casework expertise is needed in many areas of the LTC patient's environment. Help is frequently needed to straighten finances, use available social services, define resources necessary for long-term care, improve housing, and establish social support systems in the community.

The personal, emotional, social, financial, and environmental difficulties related to or resulting from the patient's illness are the particular concern of the social worker to the extent that such problems may further complicate the illness or hinder the maximum response to medical care and therapeutic treatment (Birenbaum and Figlioli 1983, 597).

Social workers frequently help expedite communication with community nursing homes and home health care programs for the elderly. Supportive interaction with family members can assist both family members and other health team members to understand the patient's emotional and psychologic response to illness or disability, and can help the team members understand their own emotional responses to the patient (Birenbaum and Figlioli 1983). Perhaps as much as half of the social worker's time can be spent usefully in dealing with the emotional problems of support staff (Kane 1983).

The social worker is also the major coordinator of discharge planning for the older patient, explaining the goals and alternatives of returning home or going to other institutions. In addition, the social worker must often help arrange payment of the bills and alternative methods of health care reimbursement (see Chapter 8).

Role of Assistants and Volunteers

Many LTC patients need total care, 24 hours a day. Much of this care is common sense, and much of the remaining routine care can be learned easily. With proper emotional and educational support, family members, neighbors, religious groups, and other volunteers can care for many long-term care patients in their homes. Indeed, the bulk of care given to long-term care patients is provided by family, friends, and neighbors. Because this caring is offered with love and compassion, it is frequently superior to that which can be bought in an institutional setting.

In many LTC institutions, the majority of direct service is provided by the nursing aides, a group which is the least trained and the least rewarded. Nursing aides also form the backbone of many home care programs. As personal home care assistants, they help relieve the burden of the primary caregiver, especially when that caregiver is too weak, sick, or otherwise unable to cope. Under the direction of a qualified professional, the home health aide can assist the patient with personal hygiene, dressing, meal preparation, light housekeeping, grocery shopping, and similar tasks (Birenbaum and Figlioli 1983).

Nonphysician Primary Providers

Relatively few physicians are trained to deal with the multi-dimensional problems of the elderly. Adequate compassionate skilled care will require recruitment of more physicians and other primary care providers into the discipline. Shared responsibility between physicians, nurse practitioners, nurse clinicians, social workers, and physician assistants has been suggested as a practical proposal for care of the aged (Kane 1982), which could help decrease the need for trained LTC physicians over the next 15 years from the astonishingly large number of 54,000 to a still substantial 34,000.

The registered nurse (RN) has served the homebound patient as patient advocate, clinical assessor, and therapeutic administrator, when physicians were preoccupied with delivering care in acute care facilities and busy ambulatory care clinics.

Gerontologic nurses, especially in community programs, are involved in direct patient care activities, teaching patients and family members, medical and psychosocial assessment, and arranging for paraprofessional and other support services (Ebersole and Hess 1985). With appropriate telephone and physical support from the physician, this process can work very well. Unfortunately, however, the nurse is often left with the uncomfortable situation of either having no physician accepting responsibility for the patient or inadequate medical decision-making support.

Because many nursing homes have long had trouble attracting capable medical support for its frail residents, care models using RNs, nurse practitioners, and physician assistants have been developed. Adequate physician backup is essential for their success. Without such support, other professionals have found it harder to assert power and mobilize resources. With it, however, nonphysician primary care providers can render care with minimal on-site supervision, follow protocols for care, or even prescribe medications supported by appropriate consultations.

Some have suggested that care of the elderly be directed by socially oriented professionals, with physicians and nurses acting as technical advisers. Although this approach may work with the problems of the well elderly, its success in LTC has yet to be shown.

More likely, maximal care is offered when the nurse, social worker, and physician work together as part of a team, sharing both authority and responsibility. Because LTC has so many facets and information needs, it demands these multiple skills.

The Physician's Role on the Team

Eidus (1981) has said that the physician on a long-term care team must assume four relations: to the patient, to the family, to the institution, and to himself. The physician must know the patient, his ethnic and personal background, his desires, concerns, expectations, and intimacy with family and friends. He should be able to define the patient's level of functioning and current mental status. Diagnoses should be critically reviewed and verified, prescriptions reviewed and simplified, and symptoms or findings that might represent side effects of the medications investigated. The use and side effects of nonprescription medications must also be assessed. At this point, evaluation by the appropriate members of the multidisciplinary treatment team should be sought and preliminary orders developed.

Levenson (1985, 101) has noted that, "As part of any person's struggle for self-determination, reliable information is needed to help in making health care decisions." Thus, one physician role is to present such information so that the patient and other team members can understand it.

The physician should assist the team in dealing with family members, and help assure the family role in decision making.

The physician's role with the family may be complicated by the family's guilt, anger, or hostility. Explaining to them the realistic limitations of their resources and capabilities for handling the disabled person may help ease the guilt and frustration. Also important is clarifying what the family desires and establishing reasonable expectations. Future placement, intensity of treatment, desire for transfer for acute illnesses, and the desirability of cardiopulmonary resuscitation all need to be discussed before the crises occur.

The physician's role within the institution includes support and education of the multidisciplinary health team members and administrative staff, and participation in problem solving and strategic planning to improve the quality of long-term patient care (see chapters 4, 6, and 10). This support includes active participation on utilization review, quality assurance, and strategic planning committees (see Chapters 3 and 4).

The physician should also support agencies and health care workers by certifying the need for therapies; certifying and recertifying the need for home, institutional, or other care; reviewing medical records; providing necessary and appropriate medical information; and providing interim reports on the patient.

Ideally, the LTC physician should serve as the coordinator, arbitrator, and adviser of the patient's health care, and should seek to resolve medical, ethical, financial, or personal issues. As part of the team, the physician needs to attend or otherwise have input into team conferences (see Chapter 5).

Distant supervision of nurses and physician extenders can be successful if it is ongoing and supportive, rather than simply neglected responsibility.

In summary, important physician roles include:

- coordination of the multidisciplinary team

- supervision of development of a treatment plan

- coordination of communication with the patient and family for decision-making purposes

- acceptance of ultimate responsibility for the health care of the patient.

Physician as Gatekeeper

The physician is responsible for certifying and recertifying the need for direct medical service; appropriate admission to an acute, chronic, or rehabilitative hospital; appropriate admission to a state psychiatric institution; appropriate placement in a skilled nursing facility; and home health care. The LTC physician's role is to minimize unnecessary services while still assisting patients in receiving the most appropriate level of care. In the conflicts between prescribing necessary services versus the constraints of third party payors, physicians should always try to do what is best for the patient.

Consistent with the principle of maximizing independence and avoiding institutionalization wherever possible, the physician should evaluate the need for institutionalization carefully, counsel family and patient, and propose alternative methods to deliver care and support the patient and family, especially in trying to postpone or prevent institutionalization.

Those frail elderly who want to stay home will benefit by the physician prescribing and certifying necessary home care services or special equipment. Other patients will have no desire to stay in their homes, while still others will be unable to stay in their homes because the intensity of needed care cannot be given at home. These latter two categories of patients may be appropriate for day care centers, day treatment programs, conjugal living programs, or admission to nursing homes.

Availability of community resources is often a more important factor in disposition decisions than the patient's functional status. Unavailability because of geographic or financial reasons may preclude the use of existing community and home care programs, while distance and resources may preclude institutional services.

Studies have shown that about 70% of decisions about use of health care resources are dictated by the physician (Vogel and Palmer 1982). While this percentage is somewhat less in the elderly, both individuals and their families still often surrender their control because of the physician's superior medical knowledge or control of access to such key elements of the LTC system as physical therapy or third party reimbursement. Acting as agent for patient, family, and society, "gatekeeping" is thus a substantial LTC physician responsibility.

Multidisciplinary Care Plans — The Physician's Role

Table 7-2 illustrates that a number of actions must precede development of an effective multidisciplinary care plan. The physician, in conjunction with rehabilitation therapists and psychologists, should ascertain the patient's current physical and mental functional status. This should include at least the equivalent

Table 7-2 Steps prior to formulation of care plans.

1. Ascertain Patient Function
2. Assure Accurate Diagnoses
3. Minimize Medications
4. Determine the Patient's Goals
5. Determine the Family's Expectations
6. Ascertain Available Resources and Options
7. Develop Multidisciplinary Care Plan Based on Steps 1-6

of the "mini-mental" examination (Folstein et al.1975), assessment of possible depression, and evaluations of motor function, mobility, and ability to perform ADLs and instrumental activities of daily living (IADLs).

Diagnoses should be verified, as discussed earlier, to make sure that treatable processes are being treated, and that side effects of medicine have not been misdiagnosed as new diseases. Because the elderly suffer more side effects from medications than do younger adults, and because these side effects are less tolerated, the fewest possible medications with the best tolerated side effects should be selected.

After discussion with the patient and family, and after the team members have each had a chance to evaluate the patient, the physician should coordinate a multidisciplinary conference including representatives from the various members of the health care team caring for the patient.

After review of the information obtained from each team member, goals should be established to define expected medical and rehabilitative, as well as nursing, nutrition, psychological, and social work issues. Goals should be realistic, and should take into account the expectations and resources of the patient and family (see also Chapter 5).

Timely review of the multidisciplinary treatment plan allows for renewed input from various observers, reappraisal of goal accomplishment, definition of new issues, and establishment of new goals.

Enhancing Teamwork

Clearly, physician participation is essential to the success of any multidisciplinary LTC team. When the physician is too busy or too insecure to participate, or when the views of each team member are not open to critical scrutiny, the team ceases to function effectively. As Blues and Zerwekh (1984) have noted, the members of effective teams invariably believe in shared responsibilities and prerogatives.

For a team to function well, members must understand the group purpose, the importance and definition of the roles played by the individuals, how and why leadership is developed, how to develop effective vertical and horizontal communication, and how to define the patient goals and convert them into actions.

In the establishment of roles there should be both flexibility and overlapping of responsibilities. All team members must participate in a multidimensional functional assessment of the LTC patient which considers the physical, cognitive, emotional, social, economic, and environmental aspects of the patient and how these affect maximum function.

Physician recognition of the skills and contributions of the multidisciplinary professionals, the resource limitations of the patient and the community, and the complex needs for coordination will further the delivery of health care to the long-term patient.

References

Birenbaum, A., and M. Figlioli. 1983. Coordinated home care, in *Care of the geriatric patient in the tradition of E. V. Cowdry*, edited by F. U. Steinberg, pp. 592-604. St. Louis: C. V. Mosby Company.

Blues, A. G., and J. V. Zerwekh. 1984. *Hospice and palliative nursing care*. New York: Grune and Stratton.

Ebersole, P., and P. Hess. 1985. *Toward health aging: human needs and nursing response*. St. Louis: C. V. Mosby.

Eidus, R. 1981. The physician and the nursing home patient. In *The geriatric imperative: an introduction to gerontology and clinical geriatrics*, edited by A. R. Somers and D. R. Fabian, pp. 269-280. New York: Appleton-Century-Crofts.

Folstein, M. R., S. E. Folstein, and P. R. McHugh. 1975. "Mini-mental state." A practical method for grading the cognitive state of patients for the clinician. *Journal of Psychiatric Research* 12(3): 189-198.

Kane, R. L. 1982. Manpower requirements in providing services for the elderly. In *The hospital's role in caring for the elderly—a series on aging from the office on aging and long term care*, pp. 64-78. Chicago: The Hospital Research and Educational Trust.

Levenson, S. A. 1985. The physician. In *Care of the elderly: a health team approach*, edited by G. Maguire, pp. 95-112. Boston: Little Brown.

Mann, W. C. 1983. Occupational therapy. In *Care of the geriatric patient in the tradition of E. V. Cowdry*, edited by F. U. Steinberg, pp. 562-568. St. Louis: C. V. Mosby.

Steinberg, F. U. 1983. Rehabilitation medicine. In *Care of the geriatric patient in the tradition of E. V. Cowdry*, edited by F. U. Steinberg, pp. 530-550. St. Louis: C. V. Mosby.

Vogel, R., and H. Palmer. 1982. *Long term care: perspectives from research and demonstrations*. Washington, D.C.: Health Care Financing Administration.

Chapter Eight

Economic and Financial Issues in Long-Term Care

A. J. Lucco, M.D.

Chapter Objectives

This chapter will:

- Outline federal spending on the elderly, particularly as it relates to health care expenditures

- Discuss current financing mechanisms for informal care, nursing home care, home health care, and adult day care

- Review Medicare and Medicaid, particularly as they relate to reimbursement for long-term care services

- Outline alternative proposals for financing long-term care services

- Discuss LTC physician responsibilities in assuring adequate reimbursement for care and services

- Consider physician role in judicious cost-effective utilization of health services for the elderly.

The Physician Role

Direct physician service is not the cornerstone of long-term care for the elderly. The great majority of this care is provided informally and without charge by families, friends, and neighbors. Formal services (e.g., those provided by nursing homes, adult day care centers, home health care programs, and congregate living facilities) operate primarily under the supervision of licensed nurses, with the majority of hands-on care being provided by skilled therapists and unskilled and semi-skilled aides and homemakers.

The single largest source of funds for LTC services is the government, with Medicaid and Medicare covering most expenditures involving nursing homes. More than half of expenditures for home health care services are also paid by these two programs. Besides paying much more for institutional care than home care, Medicaid and Medicare favor noninstitutional care with health-related services provided by licensed nurses under physician supervision. Both Medicare and Medicaid require that a physician authorize services and monitor patient progress and results of services, either in person, as with visits to nursing homes, or by reviewing progress notes and care plans of those who receive services in their homes, while continuing to provide primary care.

Thus, the physician has been made the gatekeeper and supervisor for the system. Even though physician involvement in long-term care, particularly in the institutional setting, has not been viewed favorably (Kane, Hammer, and Byrnes 1977; Solon and Greenawalt 1974; Willemain and Mark 1980) and some reports have raised questions concerning the quality of care rendered in nursing homes (Garibaldi, Brodine, and Matsumiya 1981; Ray, Federspiel, and Schaffner 1980), the physician nonetheless determines the need for LTC services, provides information from which levels of care are determined, prescribes which services will be provided and to what extent they will be provided, and decides when services are no longer needed.

The need for LTC services, both institutional and noninstitutional, is frequently the result of a person's sociodemographic characteristics rather than medical condition (Brody, Poulshock, and Masciocchi 1978; McCoy and Edwards 1981; National Center for Health Statistics 1977, 5-6; National Center for Health Statistics 1986a, 2; Palmore 1976; Vicente, Wiley, and Carrington 1979; Wachtel, Derby, and Fulton 1984). As a result, many physicians may not be qualified or feel comfortable justifying in physical terms the need for care prompted by socioeconomic problems (Kane 1984, 387). It has been proposed that physicians should make such judgments in collaboration with others (Ruchlin, Morris, and Eggert 1982, 105).

Since the nature of the current financing system determines which services are paid for and who is eligible to receive them, physicians who care for the elderly should be familiar with the basic financing mechanisms involved in long-term care. More importantly, an understanding of the current system, as well as its problems, is essential to the development of proposals designed to improve that system, either by modifying current programs or by determining the need for additional programs and services. Long-term care physicians should be at the forefront of these efforts.

The need for long-term care, the escalating cost of that care, and the demographic changes in the population combine to create major, long-range issues. This chapter will attempt to provide the most current information, although what is current at the time of this writing can change rapidly with time.

The discussion will focus on the financial aspects of long-term care within nursing homes, adult day care centers, and home health care programs. For a review of special housing for impaired older persons other than nursing homes, see Lawton (1980, 75-103).

Current Status of LTC Financing

Between 1960, when 9% of the population was 65 and over, and 1984, when 12% of the population was elderly, the share of the federal budget spent on programs serving the elderly nearly doubled from less than 15% to nearly 30%. This increase resulted primarily from the enactment of Medicare and Medicaid. In 1960, 90% of all federal spending on the elderly was for retirement income, while only 6% was for health and health-related services. In 1984, two-thirds of federal spending for the elderly was for income, and nearly 30% was for health. This health expenditure for the elderly represents a third of the country's total health care expenditures for all sources, excluding research (Senate Special Committee 1986, 103, 122).

Forecasts for the next 50 years indicate that the share of the federal budget spent on pension-related programs for the elderly will decline somewhat and remain below current levels in the future. Meanwhile, without some changes in the methods of financing health, the share of that budget devoted to health care spending will continue to rise and may eventually surpass the cost of pensions.

These dramatic increases in the proportion of all federal spending on the elderly occur despite a declining elderly support ratio (number of persons 65 and over to number of persons of working age, 18 to 64). This ratio is important because, in economic terms, the working population can be thought of as supporting the nonworking age group. It is, however, a crude measure, since many younger and older people are in the labor force and not dependent, while persons of labor force age may not be working. There were only 7 elderly persons for every 100 persons of working age in 1900, while in 1984 there were 19 elderly per 100. Estimates for 2020 are 29 elderly per 100 persons of working age and for 2050, 38 elderly per 100 (Senate Special Committee 1986, 20).

While the total support ratio (number of persons under age 18 plus number of persons 65 and over to the number of persons of working age) is declining, the effect of the increasing number of elderly has been masked by the declining number of children. This is important because the elderly are served primarily by publicly funded programs, while mostly private (i.e., family) funds (except for education) support the young. Using a broad measure of public spending, it has been estimated that government expenditures are at least twice as great for older dependents than for children (Clark and Spengler 1978, 71-73).

Spending for personal health care for the elderly was projected to reach $120 billion in 1984. Figure 8-1 details the sources of payment involved. Two-thirds of the expenditures came from public programs. The hospital insurance and supplementary medical insurance programs of Medicare combined to account for nearly half of the elderly health bill. Federal and state Medicaid payments absorbed another 13%, and other government programs, mainly the Veteran's Administration, paid 6%. The remaining third of expenditures were paid by elderly consumers. About one-quarter—consisting of deductibles, coinsurance, and noncovered services and goods—was paid with out-of-pocket funds. Private health insurance covered 7% of total spending.

Figure 8-2 illustrates how the money was spent. Two-thirds went for institutional care (45% for hospital care and 21% for nursing home care). Physician services accounted for 21%, and the remaining 13% went almost evenly for services of dentists and other health professionals and for consumer goods (Waldo and Lazenby 1984, 8).

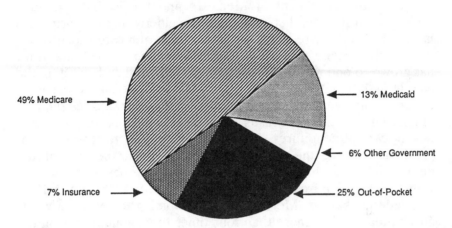

Data from Waldo and Lazenby 1984, table 13.

Figure 8-1 Distribution of personal healthcare expenditures for the elderly by source of funds: United States, 1984.

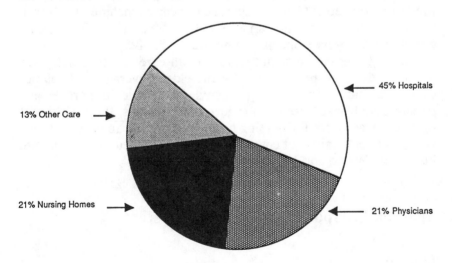

Data from Waldo and Lazenby 1984, table 14.

Figure 8-2 Distribution of personal health care expenditures for the elderly by type of service: United States, 1984.

While the enactment of Medicare and Medicaid triggered a rapid growth in federal spending for the elderly, the two programs have not effectively reduced the burden of health care expenses for the elderly. From a program spending $7 billion in 1970, Medicare has grown to one with $58.5 billion in federal outlays benefiting the elderly in 1984. Over the past 12 years, Medicare outlays have increased at an average annual rate of 18%, more than twice the rate of inflation and one-third faster than the growth in national personal health care expenditures. These are projected to grow at approximately twice the rate of inflation through the end of the decade. Medicaid has also grown rapidly in the past two decades, with outlays rising from $4.9 billion in 1970 to $35.5 billion in 1983. The federal share of Medicaid payments going to the elderly was $6.4 billion in 1983, more than four times the amount spent on the elderly only a decade earlier. The portion of total Medicaid spending attributed to the elderly has increased from 31% in 1972 to 36% in 1982, largely because of the rapid growth in the cost of nursing home care. Despite spending more than $73 billion dollars on the elderly in 1984, these programs have not kept pace with rising health costs, and health care expenditures not paid by Medicare or Medicaid equaled 15% of the average per capita income of a person 65 and over in 1984—the same as before Medicare and Medicaid were enacted (Senate Special Committee 1986, 125).

In 1984, per capita spending for health care for the elderly was $4,202, with out-of-pocket costs for the elderly averaging $1,059 per capita (excluding premium payments for Medicare part B and private health insurance). As Figure 8-3 indicates, the majority of these expenses were for nursing home care, physician visits and services, and health aids not covered by Medicare, Medicaid, or private insurance (Waldo and Lazenby 1984, 25).

Selected Components of the LTC System

Informal Care

The majority of services offered to the elderly in the community are provided by informal networks. This subject has been reviewed in detail by Horowitz (1985).

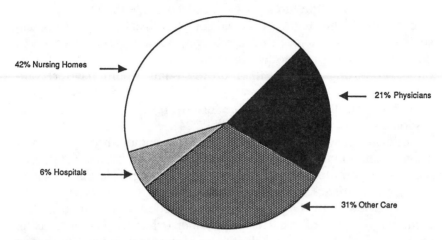

42% Nursing Homes

21% Physicians

6% Hospitals

31% Other Care

Data from Waldo and Lazenby 1984, table 14.

Figure 8-3 Distribution of out-of-pocket expenditures by the elderly by type of service: United States, 1984.

Families provide 80% of all home health care for older people, with one family member usually occupying the role of primary caregiver. That primary caregiver will be a spouse, if available, or a child, with female caregivers predominating. As a result, and because of the difference in longevity between men and women, the usual caregivers for elderly men are their elderly wives, while the usual caregivers for elderly women are their daughters.

Both the elderly and their caregivers believe the responsibility for financing services should rest with government agencies, and while some financial contributions are made to the elderly by their families, the greater costs are in time and the loss of other wage-earning opportunities. Exhaustion of family revenues, excess burden on family members, and changes in family circumstances are more often the primary precipitants of nursing home placement than a change in the older person's health status.

While informal and formal services frequently coexist, the latter do not supplant the former. The concern that increasing formal non-institutional services will lead to a decrease in informal caregiving is not supported by research. Having family available not only reduces the probability of institutionalization, but also reduces the probability of utilizing formal services in the community. When formal services are used, the family continues to provide the major portion of care, and higher levels of formal service utilization tend to be associated with higher levels of family care. Family caregivers tend to be very selective and modest in their requests for formal services, often requesting far less than professionals would have recommended. The types of services families report as most needed and desirable typically represent some form of respite from the ongoing responsibility of care (Horowitz 1985, 224).

Informal services are not limited to the community setting, and a significant amount of informal participation continues after people have been admitted to institutional care settings (National Center for Health Statistics 1977, 9-14; Smith and Bengtson 1979).

As reviewed by Day (1985), this situation will change as the demographics of informal care providers change. The increasing number of elderly—especially those 85 and over, who have the highest incidence of chronic illness and disabilities—and the decreasing fertility rates have contributed to a decrease in the ratios of offspring to elderly and offspring to dependent elderly. The higher percentage of older women working and the trend toward having children later in life will place more competing demands on the female caregiver—demands of a frail parent, a dependent child, and a job. The age of caregivers in increasing. The average age of spouses providing care is 65, with over 30% being 74 and over; most adult children providing care are over age 50.

The subject of funding for informally provided home care has not been studied systematically. Currently, no official public or private funding mechanisms exist to support informal caregiving, unless the elderly person in question qualifies as a dependent. Demonstration projects have been limited primarily to those offering financial incentives in the form of cash grants for providing care for the elderly and service support programs providing direct housekeeping services, institutional respite, and counseling and support groups. Since these programs have not been subject to controlled evaluation, their cost-effectiveness is unknown.

Meanwhile, it is generally felt that Medicaid gives strong disincentives to continued informal home care: Entitled benefits under the Supplemental Security Income program are decreased if an elderly person lives as a dependent in someone else's home. The determination of eligibility to receive home care services is based on the income and assets of both the impaired elderly and spouse, while eligibility for institutional care is based only on the independent assets and income of the applicant.

Alternative programs, which will be discussed later, include filial financial responsibility laws, tax credits, LTC individual retirement accounts, and home equity conversion.

Formal Care

Nursing Homes. According to the 1982 National Master Facility Inventory of nursing and related homes, there are 17,819 nursing homes in the United States, excluding residential facilities, hospital-based facilities, and 238 nonresponding facilities. These homes account for 1,508,732 beds. Homes that are certified as skilled nursing facilities (SNFs), including those certified as both skilled and intermediate by Medicare or Medicaid, represent nearly 40% of the total number of facilities. Homes certified as intermediate care facilities (ICFs) account for 31% of facilities, while the remaining 29% are not certified or their certification status is not known. Of the total number of beds, 45% are certified as skilled, 28% as intermediate, and 27% are not certified or unknown (National Center for Health Statistics 1986b, tables 1-2, 14, 16).

Total nursing home expenditures have risen from $4.7 billion in 1970 to $35.2 billion in 1985, a growth attributable to price inflation, increased numbers of elderly, and changes in the number and types of days of care per capita for the elderly. Over this period, there has been little change in the sources of funding for nursing home care. In 1985, 51.4% of costs were paid directly by patients, 1.7% by private health insurance and other private funds, 1.7% by Medicare, and 41.8% by Medicaid (Waldo, Levit, and Lazenby 1986, table 7).

Medicare will reimburse for one physician visit to the same patient in a nursing home per calendar month, on the presumption that such a visit is medically necessary for a person whose condition requires residence in such a home. More frequent visits are reimburseable only in situations where the physician has adequately substantiated the need.

If a physician visits a single patient in a nursing facility, reimbursement will not exceed the normally applicable, customary, and prevailing charge for a routine house call. If a physician sees more than one patient during a single visit to a nursing facility, the reimbursement is based on an amount not to exceed the normally applicable, customary, and prevailing charge for follow-up office visits. The physician must submit a claim that indicates a single patient visit, or the carrier will assume that the claim involves a multiple visit situation.

Prompted by the belief that a significant proportion of people in nursing homes are inappropriately placed, states have tried to decrease nursing home expenditures by establishing certificate-of-need laws to restrain the growth in the number of nursing home beds. While the decrease in the rate of growth in the number of nursing home beds between 1979 and 1983 may in part be attributable to these laws, it is not known whether that has had the desired effect on inappropriate bed use (Lave 1985, 12-13; Rango 1982).

Many states mandate preadmission screening of Medicaid-eligible patients prior to nursing home admission, in an attempt to decrease inappropriate utilization and thereby reduce cost. It is unclear whether either of these objectives have been met by the programs, and it is possible that it has caused an increase in the use of community services (Lave 1985, 11-12; Preadmission screening survey 1986). To the same end, geriatric evaluation units and assessment clinics have been established. In one randomized study, the experimental group of frail elderly assigned to an inpatient geriatric evaluation unit was less likely to be discharged to a nursing home than a matched control group who received standard acute hospital care. During one year of follow-up, the study group, which received continued care at a geriatric outpatient medical clinic, used fewer acute-care hospital and nursing home days, resulting in lower total cost for institutional care, than did the control group receiving continued care at general outpatient medical clinics. In addition, the study group had a lower mortality rate (Rubenstein et al. 1984). The financial feasibility of such units outside of Veteran's Administration facilities or other academic settings is untested.

Alternatives to the current system of financing nursing home care include LTC insurance and continuing care retirement communities, changing the reimbursement method for nursing homes, and social health maintenance organizations.

Home Health Care. In 1981, there were 3,014 Medicare/Medicaid-certified home health agencies (HHAs), with only 6% being operated by proprietary agencies (Lloyd and Greenspan 1985, 152).

By 1985, the number of HHAs had increased to approximately 6,100 and, with the elimination of the federal statute prohibiting Medicare/Medicaid certification for proprietary HHAs without prior state licensure, the percentage of proprietary HHAs grew to 32% (Waldo, Levit, and Lazenby 1986, 11).

Using a sample of the Department of Health and Human Services' Long-Term Care Survey of 1982, Liu, Manton, and Liu (1985) identified 5,582 persons of approximately 36,000 screened as being dependent in one or more activities of daily living (ADLs) or instrumental activities of daily living (IADLs). This represented a population of 4.6 million disabled elderly, 18% of the total elderly population in 1982. Of that group of disabled elderly, 74% were receiving help from nonpaid persons (informal care), 6% were receiving help from paid helpers only, and the remaining 21% were receiving assistance from both paid and nonpaid helpers. The percent paying for help varied from 19% of those with limitations of only IADLs, to 35% of those with five or six ADL limitations.

The source of payment for formal care varied, depending on the type of services required. Table 8-1 indicates the sources of payment for all purchased services, as well as for purchased nursing services (visiting nurses, nurse aides, home health aides). These data are only an approximation, since the data were adjusted for that 26% of the respondents claiming they received some paid care, but who did not have complete payment source information. Only 25% of persons who received paid services were receiving nursing services. This, together with the differences in sources of payment by type of service, suggests that many persons are paying out of pocket for services not covered by third-party payors. As may be expected, the percentage of persons receiving services paid for by Medicare, Medicaid, and private insurance increased with level of disability from 15% of those with limitations of only IADLs, to 48% of those with five or six ADL limitations.

Total expenses for home-based services in 1982 were approximately $4.2 billion, with the majority from public sources: $1.3 billion from Medicare, $495 million from Medicaid, and $950 million from other public programs (e.g., Title XX of the Social Security Act, Title III of the Older Americans Act). Of those surveyed who paid for at least some part of their care, out-of-pocket spending averaged $164 per month. Projecting this monthly amount

Table 8-1 Percent of disabled persons with all paid helpers and nursing helpers, adjusted, by payment source: United States, 1982.

Payment source	All paid helpers (N = 1,151,762)	Nursing helpers (N = 290,181)
Sample person only	55.0	16.1
Medicare only	11.4	38.5
Medicaid only	8.1	14.8
Other organization only	6.5	7.3
Sample person and Medicare	3.6	3.9[a]
Other private persons	2.8	<1.0
Medicare and private insurance	2.7	7.1
Sample person and other private persons	2.6	<1.0
Sample person and other organization	1.6	<1.0
Medicare and Medicaid	1.4[a]	2.3[a]
Insurance only	<1.0	3.0
Other patterns	4.3	6.8

Source: Adapted from K. Liu, K. G. Manton, and B. M. Liu. 1985. Home care expenses for the disabled elderly. *Health Care Financing Review* 7(2):51-58.

[a]Relative standard error greater than 30%.

annually implies that the disabled elderly spent approximately $1 billion out of pocket.

The cost of home-based services and products was approximately $5 billion in 1982. This increased to $9 billion by 1985 and is expected to grow to $16 billion by 1990 (Waldo, Levit, and Lazenby 1986, 11).

There are no requirements or restrictions on physician services to persons receiving home-based services. Both Medicare and Medicaid require that a person receiving services reimbursed by these programs be under the care of a physician, and that initially, the physician certify the need for home care and formulate a written plan of care. Continued need must be recertified by the physician and the care plan reviewed every 60 days. The physician cannot bill just for establishing or reviewing a plan of care or for a certification, as time for these activities is calculated into the charge for home or office visits related to such patient's care.

While much of the research in home health care has been motivated by the desire to demonstrate that it is more cost-effective than institutional care, verifying studies have been difficult to undertake for a number of reasons. Different home health care programs have different objectives: intensive home health care is utilized to shorten acute hospital stays; intermediate home health care is intended to prevent acute hospitalization or to postpone institutionalization; and maintenance home health care's purpose is to keep frail elderly in their own homes, instead of nursing homes. Matching comparable patient populations is difficult. Data on costs for home health care (reported per visit or service unit) are not provided in the same way as those for nursing home care (reported in per diem rates), and frequently do not include costs of food, housing, transportation, program administration, and the contribution of informal care providers.

Research comparing home health care with nursing home care tends to assume an inverse relationship between the two; that is, the cost of expanded home health care services will be offset by reductions in institutional costs. However, if beds emptied as a result of available home health care services are filled quickly by other patients, it is not clear whether home health care has saved money or has simply added to the total of LTC costs and services. Intensive home health care to shorten the duration of acute hospital stays is probably cost-effective, as is home health care for those with low levels of dependency needs (Palmer 1985a).

Adult Day Care (ADC). ADC centers offer varying degrees of health and social services, assistance with activities of daily living, opportunity for social interaction, at least one congregate meal daily, and transportation to and from the center. As of 1980, there were 617 ADC centers in 46 states, an increase from 200 in 1977. Funding for ADC centers is fragmented, and not often directly reimbursed by a single public financial support program. Instead, many different programs provide for various services. Funding from Medicaid, Title XX of the Social Security Act, and Title III of the Older Americans Act combine to support 467 ADC centers. The remaining 150 are funded either privately or through other sources, including voluntary agencies, mental health departments, and philanthropic organizations.

Utilization figures for ADC centers are reported based on the average daily census. In 1980, this was 13,426, or an average of 22 persons per program per day. This number does not accurately reflect the total number enrolled in ADC centers, because many attend less than five days per week.

Since the funding sources do not sort this information by use of specific services, no national expenditure data are available. Ten states cover ADC as a Medicaid service under "adult day health care service." ADC provided under Medicaid requires authorization by the enrollee's physician. Title XX programs finance ADC in 38 states, classifying it as a social service providing a protective setting to promote self-sufficiency and to decrease institutionalization. Nineteen states include ADC under Title III plans, which provide for medically- and socially-oriented ADC (Lloyd and Greenspan 1985, 162-65).

Studies of ADC seek to discover if it can reduce inappropriate institutionalization significantly and serve as an alternative to nursing homes. One controlled experiment, performed under Medicare waivers, randomly assigned elderly persons who were assessed as likely to benefit from ADC to two groups. Members of the study group were enrolled in ADC centers in addition to receiving their existing Medicare and Medicaid services. The control group continued to use solely Medicare and Medicaid services. After one year of follow-up, ADC had not affected nursing home admission or length of stay significantly, nor had it provided any substantial health care benefits. Medicare-reimbursed costs, including the cost of ADC, were 71% higher for the study group. Moreover, even if ADC had been effective, the use of nursing homes was so low in the control group that it could not have prevented much use. It was concluded that most persons used ADC as an additional service rather than as a substitute for nursing homes, resulting in increased costs overall (Weissert et al. 1980). Criticisms of this study are reviewed by Palmer (1985b).

Major Federal Programs Supporting Services to the Elderly

Medicare

Medicare, a program for financing health care for the aged, was enacted in 1965 as Title XVIII of the Social Security Act. All persons 65 and over who are entitled to Social Security or railroad retirement benefits are eligible to participate, as well as Medicare-qualified federal employees (since 1983, federal employment is treated as private employment for the purposes of entitlement to Medicare benefits). Also covered are disabled beneficiaries of the Social Security and railroad retirement programs, and persons requiring dialysis or a kidney transplant for end-stage renal disease.

Medicare is a federal program administered by the Health Care Financing Administration (HCFA) within the Department of Health and Human Services. It consists of two insurance programs: hospital insurance (part A) which helps pay for inpatient hospital care, inpatient care in a SNF, home health care, and hospice care; and supplementary medical insurance (part B) which helps pay for doctors' services, outpatient hospital services, outpatient physical and speech therapy, home health care, and other health services and supplies not covered by part A.

Funding for part A for those entitled to participate is through enrollee cost sharing (in the form of deductibles and coinsurance), a compulsory payroll tax, and interest from past program revenues. Part B is paid through enrollee cost sharing (in the form of premiums, deductibles, and coinsurance), matching contributions by the federal government out of general revenues, and interest from past programs.

Part A eligibility automatically accompanies a person's receipt of Social Security or railroad retirement benefits. Part B is also automatic, but since it requires payment of a $15.50 per month premium (all dollar values are as of January 1, 1986), the individual has the option of not participating.

Most persons 65 and over ineligible for Medicare hospital insurance coverage may enroll voluntarily by paying a monthly premium ($214). Premiums paid by those not eligible for part A who choose to enroll meet the entire cost of their protection. Such enrollees are required to also enroll for part B. Elderly persons not eligible for Medicare part A may choose to enroll only in part B. All but four states pay the Medicare premiums for their Medicaid-eligible elderly and disabled who are also eligible for Medicare.

About 95% of the elderly are enrolled in part A, and, of these, nearly all choose to enroll in part B. Medicare serves predominantly the aged, who comprise 90% of all enrollees and receive 87% of all reimbursements (HCFA 1983, 1, 5).

As noted previously, Medicare was the source of 49% ($58.5 billion) of the health care expenditures for the elderly in 1984 (Waldo and Lazenby 1984, 15). Figure 8-4 shows where the Medicare dollar goes.

Medicare payments are handled by private insurance organizations under contract with the government. Organizations handling claims for part A are called intermediaries; for part B, carriers.

Hospital Insurance. Coverage for inpatient hospital care and medically necessary inpatient care in a SNF is based on benefit periods. Each benefit period begins with the first day of hospitalization and ends when the beneficiary has not been an inpatient in a hospital or

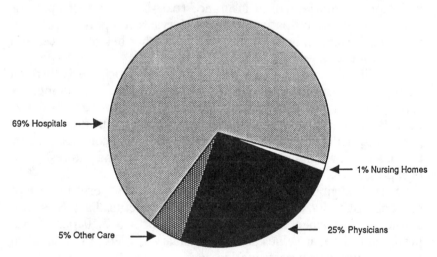

Data from Waldo and Lazenby 1984, table 14.

Figure 8-4 Distribution of Medicare expenditures for the elderly by type of service: United States, 1984.

SNF for 60 consecutive days. There is no limit to the number of benefit periods a beneficiary may use.

Inpatient hospital care is covered for 90 days per benefit period. After paying an initial deductible of $492 at the start of the benefit period (the deductible is based on the average per diem rate for inpatient services during the preceding year), hospital insurance pays for all covered services from days 1 through 60. Hospital insurance pays for all covered services for days 60 through 90, except for a daily copayment equal to one-fourth the deductible ($123). Hospital days need not be consecutive within a single benefit period. In addition to 90 days of covered inpatient hospital care per benefit period, each beneficiary has 60 nonrenewable, lifetime reserve days that may be used as needed (i.e., if the hospital stay in a benefit period is longer than 90 days). For reserve days, hospital insurance pays for all covered services except for a daily copayment equal to one-half the deductible ($246).

Hospital insurance can help pay for no more than 190 days of care in a participating psychiatric hospital during a beneficiary's lifetime. These days are not renewable, and reserve days cannot be used in psychiatric hospitals.

In 1983, Medicare instituted a prospective payment system (PPS) based on diagnostic related groupings (DRGs) to reimburse acute hospital services for Medicare patients. The new system did not change Medicare's hospital insurance coverage. The PPS does not determine length of stay in the hospital or the extent of care received. Hospitals are required to accept Medicare prospective payments as payment in full, and hospitals may not bill Medicare patients for anything other than the applicable deductible and copayment amounts, plus any amounts due for noncovered services. The background, development, and mechanisms of the PPS are reviewed in Vladeck (1984). It is too soon to predict the full impact of the PPS for Medicare-reimbursed acute care on the LTC system. Early indications are that the downward trend in hospital length of stay has been accelerated (Pawlson and Berenson 1986, 262), and preliminary data indicate that there has been a slight increase in Medicare SNF utilization (Schieber et al. 1986, 80). It can be expected that demand for most LTC services will increase.

Inpatient SNF care is covered for 100 days per benefit period. Medicare pays for all covered services from days 1 through 20.

Hospital insurance pays for all covered services for days 21 through 100, except for $61.50 per day (one-eighth the deductible).

Medically necessary inpatient care in a SNF can be covered if the following five criteria are met:

1. The beneficiary has been an inpatient in a hospital for at least three consecutive days (not counting the day of discharge) within 30 days of admission to a SNF (if patient then leaves the SNF and is readmitted within 30 days of discharge, there is no need for a new three-day hospital stay).

2. Admission to a SNF is for continued care of a condition which was treated during that preceding hospital or SNF stay.

3. A physician certifies the need for skilled nursing or skilled rehabilitative services on a daily basis.

4. The SNF participates in Medicare.

5. The SNF stay is not disapproved by the Utilization Review (UR) Committee or the Peer Review Organization (PRO) (see Chapter 6).

Major services covered during an inpatient SNF stay are a semi-private room; all meals, including special diets; regular nursing services; drugs furnished by the SNF during the stay; blood transfusions after the first three pints (the beneficiary is liable for cost or replacement of the first three pints of blood per benefit period); medical supplies, such as casts and splints; the use of appliances, such as wheelchairs; and rehabilitation services.

Services not covered during an inpatient SNF stay are requested personal convenience items, such as television, radio, or telephone; private-duty nurses; and extra charges for a private room, unless it is medically necessary.

A patient needing skilled nursing or rehabilitative care can be admitted to a SNF only upon the recommendation of, and while under the care of, a physician. If the patient is receiving skilled nursing services, the attending physician must visit at least every 30 days for the first 90 days; thereafter, the physician may adopt an alternate schedule of visits, but must visit at least every 60 days. If the patient is receiving skilled rehabilitative services, the attending physician must visit at least every 30 days throughout the entire course of treatment.

State-contracted PROs must conduct a review of extended duration cases with regard to the efficiency, appropriateness, and cost-effectiveness of care (this function may not be delegated to a SNF, unless that facility is attached to a hospital).

On admission, each patient's need for admission is evaluated, and a length of stay is determined, which is either the same number of days (but not more than 30) for all cases or a different number of days for different diagnostic classes (the period may exceed 30 days if the average length of stay for a specific diagnostic class or category based on functional capability exceeds 30 days).

At each periodic review, if the PRO finds that the individual continues to need inpatient skilled nursing care, an additional stay is approved for an appropriate number of days, with review at least every 30 days for the first 90 days and at least every 90 days thereafter.

If the PRO determines at any time that continued skilled nursing care is not necessary or appropriate, they must inform the attending physician, who is permitted to present his/her view and any additional information relating to the patient's need for extended stay.

If, after reviewing the physician's appeal, the determination is reversed, the attending physician is notified and the date for subsequent review is set. If the initial determination is not reversed, written notice of final determination must be sent to the attending physician, the patient (or next of kin, if the patient is not able to comprehend), and the facility administrator, no later than either two days after determination is reached or three working days after the end of the assigned extended stay period. Payment to the SNF may be made for up to two days after the SNF receives notice of the PRO finding, if the PRO has determined that additional time is required to arrange for post-discharge care. If the review is conducted by a hospital-based SNF's UR committee, payment may be made for care furnished before the fourth day following the day the SNF receives notice of the finding. If HCFA determines that a hospital-based SNF has failed to make timely UR of extended stay cases, payment may not be made for care furnished after the twentieth consecutive day after the effective date of HCFA's determination.

Physician visits to a patient are reimbursable if such services are reasonable and necessary to the treatment of the patient's illness, even if a finding has been made that SNF services are not justified.

Special benefit periods apply to hospice care. Hospital insurance can pay for two 90-day periods and one 30-day period. During a hospice benefit period, hospital insurance pays for all covered services for the terminal illness except for the cost of outpatient drugs (the beneficiary is responsible for 5% of the cost of outpatient drugs or $5 toward each prescription, whichever is less) and inpatient respite care (the beneficiary is responsible for 5% of the cost or $492 [amount equal to inpatient deductible], whichever is less, during a period that begins when the hospice plan is first chosen and ends 14 days after such care is cancelled). Inpatient respite care is limited each time to stays of no more than five consecutive days. If, while receiving hospice care, the beneficiary requires treatment for a condition not related to the terminal illness, Medicare still pays for all necessary covered services under the standard benefit program.

Hospice care can be covered if the following criteria are met:

1. A physician certifies that a patient is terminally ill (life expectancy less than six months).

2. The beneficiary chooses to receive care from a hospice program instead of standard Medicare benefits.

3. The hospice program participates in Medicare.

Covered hospice services include: nursing services; physician services, if the attending physician works for the hospice program; drugs; rehabilitation services; home health aide and homemaker services; medical social services; medical supplies and appliances; inpatient respite care; and counseling.

The first 90-day period must be certified by a hospice physician (either the hospice medical director or a physician member of the hospice interdisciplinary group) and the patient's attending physician. The second 90-day period and the 30-day period must be certified by the hospice physician.

Medicare pays the full approved cost of all covered home health care services.

Home health care will be covered if all of the following criteria are met:

1. The necessary care includes part-time skilled nursing care, physical therapy, or speech therapy.
2. The patient is confined to home.
3. A physician determines the need for home health care and sets up the home health plan.
4. The home health agency participates in Medicare.

Covered home health care services include part-time skilled nursing care, physical therapy, and speech therapy. If any of these three services are needed, Medicare can also pay for occupational therapy, part-time home health aides, medical social services, medical supplies, and 80% of the approved cost of durable medical equipment.

Uncovered home health care services include full-time nursing care, drugs and biologicals, home-delivered meals, homemaker services, and blood transfusions.

Physician responsibilities have been described previously in the home health care section.

Supplementary Medical Insurance. Part B coverage is based on the fiscal year. After the beneficiary has paid an initial $75 deductible for covered charges per year, supplementary medical insurance will pay 80% of all covered charges during the rest of the year. The beneficiary is responsible for the remaining 20%.

Medicare supplementary insurance payments for physician services are based on reasonable charges. For each service provided, Medicare considers three amounts: the customary charge (generally the charge most frequently made in an area for that service in the previous calendar year), the prevailing charge (the amount high enough to cover the actual charge in three out of four bills submitted in an area for that service in the previous calendar year), and the actual charge (the charge submitted by the physician for that service). The Medicare carrier then approves the lowest of these three charges.

A physician may choose to either accept or not accept assignment. By accepting assignment, the physician agrees that the total charge for the service will be that approved by the Medicare carrier. Medicare then directly pays the physician 80% of that approved charge (assuming the yearly deductible has been met by the beneficiary), and the physician can bill the beneficiary for the remaining 20%. Physicians bill beneficiaries directly for the actual charge of services not covered by part B. If assignment is not accepted, Medicare pays the beneficiary 80% of the approved charge (assuming the yearly deductible has been met). The physician bills the beneficiary for the full actual charge. Seven out of ten physicians accepted assignment in 1966, compared with less than one out of three in 1986 (Pepper 1986, 144).

Major services excluded from coverage include routine physical examinations for a purpose other than the treatment or diagnosis of a specific illness, symptom, complaint, or injury; diagnostic tests and procedures related to routine examinations; eye examinations, eyeglasses, or contact lenses, except for postsurgical lenses customarily used during convalescence from eye surgery in which the lens of the eye was removed, or prosthetic lenses for patients who lack the lens of the eye because of congenital absence or surgical removal; hearing examinations and aids; immunizations, except for vaccinations or inoculations directly related to the treatment of an injury or direct exposure (e.g., antirabies treatment, tetanus antitoxin, immune globulin) and pneumococcal vaccinations; orthopedic shoes or other supportive devices for the feet, except when shoes are an integral part of a leg brace; cosmetic surgery and related services, except as required for the prompt repair of accidental injury or to improve functioning of a malformed body member; foot care other than the treatment of warts, the treatment of mycotic nails (limited to one treatment per 60 days, unless medical necessity for more treatment is documented by the physician), or routine care, if the patient has a medical condition of the lower extremities requiring such care to be performed by a podiatrist; chiropractic services, except for manual manipulation of the spine to correct a subluxation that can be demonstrated by X-ray; and dental care, except that involving surgery of the jaw or related structures, reduction of fractures of the jaw or facial bones, services that would be covered if provided by a doctor of medicine (e.g., treatment of an oral infection), and inpatient hospital services when required because of the patient's underlying medical condition and clinical status or the severity of the dental procedure.

Supplementary medical insurance coverage for the outpatient treatment of mental illness is limited to $250 per year, assuming the deductible has been met.

Supplemental Medicare (Medigap) Insurance. According to the 1980 National Medical Care Utilization and Expenditure Study of the civilian, noninstitutionalized population 64 and over who are enrolled in Medicare, 21% are covered by Medicare only. Ten percent are covered by Medicare and Medicaid. The remaining 69% have some form of private health insurance (excluding dread disease policies) in addition to Medicare (or Medicare and Medicaid). The likelihood of having additional private coverage is greater for those with more years of education, better perceived health status, or a higher income, or who are white or younger (HCFA 1983, 3-5). Thus, almost four out of five elderly Medicare enrollees have some form of additional insurance coverage.

In 1986, approximately 21 million elderly owned supplemental Medicare policies at an estimated annual cost of $13 billion, or an average of more than $600 per person. In return, private insurance pays about 7% of the elderly's health care bill, in contrast to Americans under the age of 65 who pay about $112.4 billion per year for private health insurance coverage, which pays approximately 86% of their health care bills. According to the House Select Aging Subcommittee on Health and Long-Term Care, at least $3 billion spent on Medigap insurance will be wasted because of widespread abuses in the sale of individual policies (Pepper 1986, 143).

Since 1980, state-enforced regulations have required that Medigap policies meet certain minimal standards. Such policies must cover the part A deductible, part A coinsurance for Medicare-eligible expenses for hospitalization from days 60 through 90, part A coinsurance for Medicare-eligible expenses for hospitalization for lifetime reserve days, coverage of 90% of all Medicare-eligible expenses for hospitalization for up to an additional 365 days, and part B coverage of 20% of approved costs, subject to a maximum calendar year out-of-pocket deductible of $200 and a maximum benefit of $5,000 per calendar year. The sale of multiple Medigap policies is outlawed, and there is a minimum loss ratio (the percentage of each premium dollar that goes to pay claims) of 60%.

In addition, many Medigap policies include coverage of the part B deductible for an extra premium charge, outpatient prescription medications, and medical appliances and equipment not covered by Medicare. The premiums increase with age. Most do not cover the difference between the actual charge and the approved charge of physicians who do not accept assignment. Policies may exclude coverage for preexisting conditions during the first six months of the policy. Also, "coordination of benefit" clauses may invalidate duplicate policies.

Although they are not strictly Medigap policies (since they do not purport to fill the Medicare gaps), there are several other types of insurance, including:

1. *Group insurance* – Some insurance available to the elderly before retirement continues to be available after retirement, but the retired beneficiary may have to pay all of the premium. Medicare law requires that employers offer working persons over 64 and under 70 the opportunity to join the health insurance plan offered to employees under 65.

2. *Hospital income policies* – These are limited policies which provide cash payments directly to a beneficiary while hospitalized or during a period of sickness or accident. Payments may fail to keep pace with inflation and the rising costs of Medicare deductibles and copayments (which have climbed steadily since 1966).

3. *Specific disease policies* – These policies provide insurance against medical costs resulting from specific diseases, such as cancer.

As their name implies, Medicare supplementary policies attempt to fill the gaps resulting in out-of-pocket expenditures for the acute care services towards which Medicare is primarily oriented. Like Medicare, Medigap policies do not pay a significant portion of LTC costs.

Health Maintenance Organization (HMOs). Health maintenance organizations are community health organizations which provide facilities and professional services and supplies for a prepaid annual fee. In a controlled study in which 1,580 nonelderly persons previously receiving fee-for-service care were randomly assigned to receive free care either from their fee-for-service physicians or an HMO, the rate of hospital admissions and number of hospital days were about 40% lower for the HMO group, while ambulatory-visit rates were similar. The calculated expenditure rate for all services was about 25% less in the HMO group (Manning et al. 1984).

Since 1972, HMOs have been able to contract with Medicare, either on a cost basis or a risk-contract basis. To qualify, an HMO had to be certified by the federal government, have enrollments of at least 5,000 prepaid members, and (to enter into a risk-contracting agreement) make available to enrollees all of the Medicare services normally available to fee-for-service Medicare beneficiaries in its service area.

A post-audit adjustment determined the savings or losses of each HMO enrolled under risk-contract, by comparing its actual costs per Medicare member with a retrospectively determined adjusted average per capita cost (AAPCC), representing the hypothetical cost for enrollees if they had been in the fee-for-service system. If HMO costs were more than the AAPCC, it was required to absorb the loss. If HMO costs were less than the AAPCC, it shared in the savings with the Medicare program, with the HMO permitted to reserve savings of up to 10% of the AAPCC.

By 1979, 31 HMOs with 23,498 beneficiaries had cost contracts with Medicare, but only one HMO with 19,268 beneficiaries had a risk contract. Attributing this failure to attract HMOs to insufficient financial incentives, other methods of contracting that might increase HMO participation were tested. Among the findings of these demonstration projects was that HMOs were most likely to enter the Medicare market if they were located in an area where the AAPCC level was high. Beneficiaries who enrolled were more likely to not have supplemental Medicare policies, to be less satisfied with their usual source of fee-for-service care, and to describe themselves as healthier than nonenrollees.

Many of the concepts tested in the demonstration projects were implemented programmatically in 1985 under the Tax Equity and Fiscal Responsibility Act (TEFRA) of 1982.

Under the TEFRA regulations, payment to HMOs for each Medicare enrollee is based on two methodologies—the AAPCC and the adjusted community rate (ACR).

The AAPCC, calculated annually by HCFA, is based on national data on expenditures under the Medicare program, and is adjusted to the area. This rate takes into account the characteristics of HMO membership, including age and sex, and disability, institutional, and welfare status. The ceiling for payment is 95% of the AAPCC per beneficiary. The ACR, calculated annually by each participating HMO, reflects the HMO's expected cost of providing Medicare-covered benefits to Medicare enrollees. The ACR is compared with the AAPCC. If the ACR is lower, the HMO must convert the difference into additional benefits or reduced cost-sharing for Medicare enrollees, or the HMO may choose to receive less than 95% of the AAPCC.

As a result of the new risk-contracting program instituted in 1985, the number of participating HMOs has increased dramatically. As of March 31, 1986, 119 plans with 556,191 beneficiaries had signed TEFRA risk contracts.

Considerable controversy remains regarding further refinements of the HMO risk-contracting system. One major question is the appropriateness of current rate-setting policies. Levels of reimbursement must be high enough to attract HMOs into the Medicare market, but reimbursement must reflect differences among beneficiaries' expected expenditures. If Medicare beneficiaries who enroll in HMOs use fewer services than those who remain in the fee-for-service sector, then Medicare will pay greater costs under capitation. The current methods of reimbursement do not completely control for this possible selection bias. For example, Medicare HMO enrollees tend to be younger than nonenrollees, and age is related to health status and the use of services; but this potential selection bias is controlled by the adjustment in AAPCC for age. At present, there is no adjustment with regard to the beneficiaries' previous history of service use—a factor which may forecast future use patterns. Continued demonstration and research projects are currently being conducted by HCFA (Langwell and Hadley 1986).

Medicaid

Medicaid, Title XIX of the Social Security Act, was enacted in 1965 as a program of medical assistance for the impoverished aged, blind, or disabled, or members of families with dependent children. The aged and disabled make up less than 29% of all recipients, but are responsible for over 67% of all payments (HCFA 1983, 5). Medicaid was the source of 13% ($15.3 billion) of health care expenditures for the elderly in 1984 (Waldo and Lazenby 1984, 23-24). As Figure 8-5 indicates, 68% of Medicaid expenditures is assigned to nursing home care, covering the cost of the 5% of the elderly population in nursing homes at any one time. Medicaid plays a larger role than any other public program in covering nursing home costs.

Medicaid is administered on the federal level by HCFA. The states administer Medicaid within broad federal guidelines, which allows them considerable discretion in determining income and other resource criteria for eligibility, covered benefits, and provider payment mechanisms. As a result, the characteristics of the program vary greatly from state to state.

The Medicaid law requires federal payments to states, on the basis of a medical assistance percentage, for part of their expenditures for medical services provided under their approved Medicaid plans. The federal percentage is based on a state's per capita income and can range from 50% to 83%. In addition to federal payments made for medical services, payments are also made for state expenditures for administration of their plans.

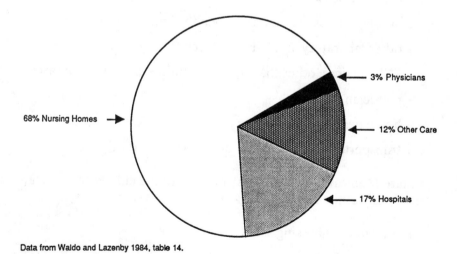

Data from Waldo and Lazenby 1984, table 14.

Figure 8-5 Distribution of Medicaid expenditures for the elderly by type of service: United States, 1984.

Medicaid must cover "categorically needy" individuals who are given public assistance under the Social Security Act because they are poor and either aged, or blind, or disabled, or specified members of families with dependent children. The states may also optionally cover other categorically needy persons who would qualify for such public assistance if they applied and "medically needy" persons who do not qualify for public assistance because of their income or resource levels, but who have medical bills that are large enough to reduce their income below a medically needy maximum. The states may also cover other individuals not associated with public assistance, but federal financial participation is not available.

State Medicaid programs must provide a basic set of services to all categorically needy persons. States receive federal financial reimbursement for these basic services, as well as certain optional services they may elect to cover. States may limit the scope of coverage for both required and optional services, as long as service coverage is uniform throughout the state.

States must cover the following basic services for all elderly categorically needy recipients:

- inpatient hospital services, other than in an institution for mental diseases
- outpatient hospital and rural health clinic services
- other laboratory and X-ray services
- SNF services, other than in an institution for mental diseases
- physician services
- home health services
- transportation to and from providers of medical care.

State Medicaid programs may provide to the elderly categorically needy any of the following services:

- private-duty nursing services
- clinic services
- dental services
- physical, occupational, and speech therapy

- prescribed drugs, dentures, prosthetic devices, and eyeglasses
- other diagnostic, screening, preventive, and rehabilitative services
- inpatient, SNF, and ICF services in an institution for mental diseases
- ICF services
- any other medical care and any other type of remedial care recognized under state law, including emergency hospital services and personal care services in the individual's home.

If a state's Medicaid program covers the medically needy, it must provide at least ambulatory services for individuals entitled to institutional services, and home health services for any individual who is entitled to SNF services.

Cost-sharing (e.g., deductibles, coinsurance) may be imposed on elderly categorically and medically needy recipients, excluding the following services:

- services furnished to an individual who is an inpatient of a hospital, SNF, ICF, or other medical institution, if the individual has been required to spend all his/her income for medical expenses, except for his/her personal needs allowance
- emergency inpatient or outpatient services necessary to prevent the death or serious impairment of the health of the recipient
- HMO services furnished to categorically needy individuals enrolled in an HMO.

Participation in the Medicaid program is limited to providers who accept, as payment in full, the amounts paid by Medicaid, plus any deductibles and copayments required by the state plan to be paid by the individual. Payments are made directly to the provider.

Physician responsibilities for Medicaid-reimbursed SNF services are the same as for Medicare. If the physician determines that a patient receiving skilled nursing services does not need to be seen every 30 days (after the first 90 days), the interval between visits may be increased up to 60 days; however, any interval greater than

30 days automatically leads to a review of the patient's need for monthly visits and the continued need for SNF services.

Regarding ICF responsibilities, a patient may be admitted only upon the recommendation of a physician and must remain under the care of a physician, who must visit the patient and review the plan of care at least every 60 days (unless the physician documents reasons why that frequency is not necessary).

State Medicaid programs may limit both inpatient and out-patient physician services. At present, 43 states have some limitation on physician services; for example, in Nevada, physician services may not exceed two office or nursing facility visits and two therapeutic injections per patient per month for treatment of illness, while emergency treatment and inpatient hospital care are not limited.

Home health care provided through Medicaid includes nursing services, home health aide services, and medical supplies, equipment, and appliances. At state option, physical, speech, and occupational therapy and audiological services can also be provided. Care must be provided by a Medicaid-certified HHA, and the beneficiary must be eligible for skilled nursing home care.

Personal care services in the home must be prescribed by a physician in accordance with a plan of treatment and must be provided by an individual who is qualified, supervised by a registered nurse, and not a member of the patient's family.

Prior to the enactment of Medicaid, medical care for the poor was provided by local governments and those hospitals and physicians offering free care. Medicaid shifted this responsibility to federal and state governments, and during the early years of the program, most states expanded their programs and benefits. Since the late 1970s, attention has switched to cost-effectiveness, and states have been given increased flexibility in service coverage, utilization control, and reimbursement. Newcomer and Bogaert-Tullis (1985) have reviewed state efforts to control expenditures by regulating benefits and reimbursement and by contracting with prepaid health providers.

Alternatives to Current Financing

The majority of the elderly assessed as dependent and requiring LTC services do receive some service. However, third-party financial support of the present system is biased toward institutional care and medically oriented noninstitutional care. Furthermore, the availability of services in both settings in unequal. Thus, while the current system is functional, the question is whether the current system is the best that can be expected for the increasing amounts of money that are expended on long term care. Most suggestions to change the current system have as a common goal at least some degree of cost containment and the encouragement of the use of presumably less expensive noninstitutional services.

A discussion of proposed changes follows with specific references noted. General discussions of alternative proposals can be found in Eustis, Greenberg, and Patten (1984, 169-206); Jazwiecki (1986); Knickman and McCall (1986); Lave (1985); Leutz (1986); and Wiener (1986).

Filial Financial Responsibility Laws

In 1983, the federal government allowed the states to reestablish filial financial responsibility laws. State Medicaid directors were given the option to require relatives of institutionalized elderly beneficiaries to contribute to the support of their care. Thus, additional funds would be raised, while acting as a deterrent to nursing home placement. This approach is based on several unfounded assumptions: that nursing home residents have families (in fact, not having relatives is a risk factor for nursing home placement, and kinless elderly are overrepresented in nursing home populations); that these families would be a ready source of financial support (since the average age of nursing home residents is over 80 years, the typical adult child is, or will soon be, dependent on retirement income); and that informal caregivers are capable of providing more care than they are already providing (although it is known that families already regard nursing homes as a last resort).

Furthermore, the cost of administrating and enforcing such a program is estimated to consume 75% of any revenues generated. Questions regarding the definition of responsible relatives, the measurement of income and assets of relatives against competing demands (e.g., family size) to identify those who could and should contribute, and the difficulty of enforcement when relatives live in different states complicate the administration of the program (Day 1985, 12-13; Horowitz 1985, 230-31). A similar program instituted in the 1950s did not lead to financial savings.

Cash Grants and Tax Credits

The payment of cash grants and the establishment of tax credits to family caregivers assumes that economic constraints on families are the key factors prohibiting continued provision of informal care, an assumption not supported by research. The dollar amounts would have to be significant in order to cover the costs of such care, which is currently being provided without charge. These programs have been shown to be administratively complicated, and make no difference in the rate of institutionalization (Day 1985, 12; Horowitz 1985, 232-33).

Long-Term Care Individual Retirement Accounts

Long-term care individual retirement accounts have been proposed as a method of encouraging saving for the cost of future health needs. It assumes a willingness to save consistently for a single uncertain goal. It is unclear whether enough can be saved to cover the potential costs of long-term care.

Home Equity Conversion

Home equity conversion relies on the fact that 75% of the elderly own their own homes, with 80% being mortgage-free. Essentially, the owner sells the paid-up home to a bank or other lending institution in return for lifelong annuity payments and the right to live in the house. Whether sufficient funds for LTC expenses could be generated is not clear. For example, only half of elderly homeowners could pay the premium for a prototype LTC insurance policy with their converted home equity payment. This program has not yet found a wide market, primarily because of the reluctance of the elderly to part with their largest financial asset (Scholen 1983; Wessel 1985).

Long-Term Care Insurance

Misconceptions by the elderly regarding their potential need for long-term care and the financial coverage available to them have limited pooled-risk (insurance) approaches. In a survey by the American Association of Retired Persons (1984), 79% of members age 65 and over polled believed that Medicare would cover all or most of the cost of an extended confinement in a nursing facility. Likewise, in a survey by Pepper (1986, 146) nearly 90% of elders believed Medicare and supplemental insurance would cover long-term care in a nursing home or at home. Medicare and private health insurance together currently pay only 2.5% of the cost of nursing home care. Half of all Medicaid spending in nursing homes goes to those who entered with some financial resources, which were depleted as a result of chronic illness. Yet, it has been shown that the elderly and near-elderly make virtually no contingency plans or preparations for potential LTC needs (Beverly Foundation 1986, 6).

When the Prudential Insurance Company offered its first policy to members of the American Association of Retired Persons in six states, only 1,200 of 215,000 members joined (a little over one-half of 1%).

Other major problems facing insurance companies developing LTC policies are adverse selection and induced need. Adverse selection results when only those who perceive (correctly) that they will need the insured services purchase the policy. Consequently, premiums cannot cover claims because too many policyholders are of higher than average risk. Adverse selection can be averted by increasing the buying base and by attracting the young and the healthy elderly, neither of whom perceive the need for such insurance. Unless this can be accomplished, companies protect their policies by increasing premiums significantly with age at purchase, screening applicants, and excluding coverage of preexisting conditions. Induced demand means that the consumption of services increases, not as a result of a change in need, but because covered services are less expensive. Induced need can be avoided by increased deductibles and copayments, elimination periods before payment begins, requirements for preceding acute hospitalization, and lifetime caps on benefits.

At present, about 75 insurance carriers sell or are developing LTC insurance policies. The number of the insured has doubled to

200,000 over the past year. There is considerable variability among policies currently being offered. Some offer only nursing home care, while others also include home health care. Premiums increase with age at sign-up, benefits are usually paid in fixed amounts for a fixed period of time or with a lifetime cap, there are elimination periods before payments begin, and there are frequently qualifying acute care stay requirements. In no case do the benefits completely cover the costs of long-term care.

In an attempt to spread the risk among a larger and healthier applicant pool, Travelers Insurance Company will be the first carrier to try to move LTC insurance into the employee benefit market. For workers in their early thirties, premiums will be $5 per month. Workers will be able to enroll their parents, but at higher premiums ($150 per month at age 75 years).

To examine the affordability of LTC insurance, a prototype individual policy which provided a benefit of $50 per day for four years after a 100-day elimination period was considered. Premiums ranged from $450 per year for issue ages 65 to 69 to $900 per year for issue ages 80 and over. Two standards of affordability were considered. Approximately 80% of the elderly age 65 to 69 could afford to buy the insurance for less than 10% of their income, but only 27% of those 80 and over could afford it. For less than 5% of their income, 47% of those age 65 to 69 could afford insurance, while only 9% of those 80 and over could buy. This decline with age occurs because the premiums increase with age, while the average income of the elderly declines with age. The percentage of elderly able to purchase insurance would be higher if they started purchasing the insurance at age 65; for example, the percentage of elderly age 75 to 79 able to buy insurance for less than 5% of their income would more than double if they had started purchasing their policies at age 65 to 69. This occurs because premiums are established by the age at which the policy is purchased. If premiums were reduced by 20%, the percentage of families able to afford coverage would increase by about 20% (Kennell 1985).

Continuing Care Retirement Communities (CCRCs)

Continuing care retirement communities provide housing and services, including health care, to persons of retirement age. The median number of residents in a CCRC as of December 31, 1981 was 218. CCRCs protect against the high risk of such a small pool of members by screening applicants, charging relatively high entrance and monthly fees, and maintaining control over decisions regarding health care utilization. Only half of CCRCs offer an extensive health care guarantee (where residents continue to pay the same monthly fee for nursing home care that they paid when living independently), while the rest have limited contracts (where residents receiving nursing home care pay the full per diem charge after a specified length of stay, ranging from 10 to 180 days). Medical or medically-related services (e.g., community's or resident's physician, referred specialist, treatment for preexisting conditions, and special duty nurses) are less likely to be included in contracts and fees offered by newer communities (Winklevoss and Powell 1984). The small number of CCRCs with complete coverage represent the only current example of full LTC insurance. However, the majority of CCRCs offer less than total coverage, and as a result, resemble expensive retirement housing with standard LTC insurance coverage.

Social Health Maintenance Organizations (S/HMOs)

In an attempt to develop a comprehensive and integrated system of health care delivery and long-term care, HCFA is sponsoring four national S/HMO demonstration projects. Extending the prepaid model to include LTC insurance should reduce the fragmentation of service delivery and funding sources. The case management approach will, hopefully, improve the efficiency of the system and decrease costs by eliminating the inappropriate use of LTC services. Of special importance, these projects represent a merging in the delivery of acute and long-term care, where cost savings generated in one system may be appropriately used in the other setting.

Medicare beneficiaries may voluntarily enroll in a S/HMO, which will provide all current Medicare benefits as well as certain LTC coverage. To protect against adverse selection, each S/HMO has established, under Medicare waiver, a quota of severely and moderately impaired elderly who can join.

Medicare reimburses the S/HMO at 100% of the AAPCC per beneficiary (an additional amount is paid if the enrollee is determined to be at increased risk of institutionalization). The enrollee also pays a premium.

Premiums and coverage for LTC benefits vary among the demonstration sites. The coverage is comprehensive (i.e., all sites cover institutional, home, and community-based care), but the depth of coverage varies. Three of the sites have a maximum annual benefit depending on the site of care, as well as a total annual maximum. The fourth site has an annual maximum for home and community-based care, a 100-day maximum for nursing home care, and a total annual maximum.

Changing Institutional Reimbursement

Reimbursement to nursing facilities can be classified as either facility-related or facility-independent.

Payments are facility-related if they depend on past, present, or projected future costs of a particular facility. Within this category, payments can be either retrospective (a facility is paid an interim rate to approximate anticipated allowable costs, with a rate adjustment made at the end of the accounting period) or prospective (the final rate of payment is determined before the accounting period begins and any surplus or deficit accrues to the facility). Facility-related retrospective payment systems do not provide an incentive for efficiency, as higher facility costs are reimbursed. However, to the extent that higher quality of care can be purchased, this system of reimbursement allows facilities to spend more to improve quality. This system may also encourage questionable accounting and inflated cost reporting.

With facility-independent reimbursement, payments are determined with reference to the costs of a certain group of, or all, facilities, rather than of a particular facility. Payments may be at a flat rate, paid identically to all facilities, or may be adjusted according to facility size, location, and patient mix. Prospective payment and facility-independent reimbursement provide incentives for efficiency, as profits are maximized by providing care at the least possible cost. However, quality of care may suffer in an attempt to maximize profits. There is also little incentive for deceptive accounting.

Presently, Medicare reimburses SNFs by the facility-related, retrospective method based on reasonable allowable costs, subject to limits applied to routine operating costs (112% of the average costs of urban and of rural facilities), and possible retroactive denial of claims. Ancillary costs, such as physical therapy, drugs, and capital expenditures, are not included in the cost limits. Hospital-based SNFs are reimbursed at a higher rate.

Prospective payment systems (PPSs) are increasingly replacing retrospective, cost-based reimbursement methodologies, because these latter methods do not reward cost-containing behavior, and therefore do not encourage efficiency. Medicare has already implemented PPSs for acute care hospitals, renal dialysis facilities, hospices, and freestanding ambulatory surgical centers. The interest in expanding this system to SNFs has been reflected in the recently enacted PPS for low-volume SNFs (SNFs that record less than 1,500 Medicare bed-days per year, equal to three or four beds occupied by Medicare patients throughout the year). It is also expected that this greater financial incentive will encourage facilities to accept more Medicare beneficiaries (as opposed to private-pay patients, who typically pay higher than publicly reimbursed rates). The plan allows low-volume SNFs the option to be paid 105% of mean operating and capital costs of all (both freestanding and hospital-based) SNFs, with separate rates calculated for urban and rural facilities. Ancillary services will be excluded and continue to be reimbursed on a cost basis. The amount of per diem reimbursement that a facility can receive will be limited to the maximum amount it charges a private-pay patient (Rudensky 1986).

The change to a PPS must incorporate case-mix adjustments for different patient needs to ensure equitable payment to providers and access for severely ill patients. Without case-mix adjustments, providers could profit by "skimming" potential admissions and admitting only patients with the lowest resource needs, thereby limiting access for more disabled patients while increasing profits. It has yet to be determined whether case-mix for nursing homes is most appropriately based on diagnoses or nursing care needs and functional status (Schieber et al. 1986).

Case-mix reimbursement, however, may provide an incentive to provide less than optimal care. If patients are maintained at lower functional levels, requiring more intensive care, the facility will receive higher payments (Chapman-Cliburn 1986, 143). One alternative is to reimburse facilities for achieving desired outcomes (see Chapter 6). Patient prognosis would be determined on admission and at regular intervals. Reimbursement would be at a base rate assigned at the time of admission, determined by the patient's estimated care needs. When follow-up assessment indicates that the patient's status matches the prognosis, the facility would be paid the base rate. If the patient does better than his/her prognosis, the facility receives the base rate adjusted upwards by an improvement factor. Conversely, if the patient does worse than the prognosis indicates, the nursing home's base rate is adjusted downwards. In this way, by comparing a patient's outcome with his/her individual prognosis, a facility is not penalized for taking seriously ill patients with poor prognoses (Kane 1976).

Within federal regulations, state Medicaid programs have considerable discretion in establishing reimbursement policies for nursing homes. In 1982, 12 states set facility-related retrospective rates for SNFs, 25 set facility-related prospective rates, 5 set facility-independent rates, and 7 used a combination of these methods. For ICFs, the respective figures were 9, 28, 5, and 8. The pattern of state Medicaid reimbursement methods have changed gradually between 1978 and 1982, with a decrease of one-third in the number of states with retrospective reimbursement systems for SNFs and a decrease of two-fifths in states with retrospective systems for ICFs (Harrington and Swan 1984, 42).

Summary

Business Approach to Long-Term Care

The LTC system for the elderly has grown rapidly since the enactment of Medicare and Medicaid in the mid 1960s. The first decade of these programs saw dramatic expansions in the number of people served and services made available. Over the past decade, the concern has centered on cost containment with more selective expansion of the system. Any discussion of the financing of long-term care for the elderly assumes that there is some agreement on what that system should accomplish. Lacking such agreement, we cannot know which services should be financed or what outcomes should be expected, or whether the system is working, much less working efficiently.

Let us look at the "business of long-term care," to identify what questions still need to be answered and to examine how the current alternatives being implemented and suggested will affect the system.

The development of any new product or service requires the identification of that product or service, and its potential market. The "demographic imperative" reveals that the number of elderly, especially those most likely to require supportive services, is increasing. Thus, the primary market is the expanding older age group, though the precise product may be less clear than the desired client goals of maximum functional independence, humane care, prolonged longevity, and the prevention of avoidable medical and social problems (Callahan 1981, 221).

The next step in planning is to develop a specific product to test, or a market survey of consumers to see what they prefer (i.e., what product or service they would be willing to purchase). The elderly prefer to remain in their homes and prefer to receive services in that setting.

The financial feasibility of the product or service must then be analyzed for its desirability, and the likelihood that the cost will not be excessive.

Two factors distinguish our LTC system, with a significant part of the expenditures being paid by the government, from more straightforward supply and demand principles: The consumers are frequently not paying for the product and the program developers/providers (the government) must answer to an enormous number of investors (taxpayers), who are also the payors. Thus, since the provider/payors cannot make a profit from this venture, they concentrate their interests on getting the most for any money they choose to invest.

In light of these unique characteristics, several important decisions must be made. First, who decides what services will be provided – the consumers or the provider/payors? If all persons cannot get all the services they want, we must then try to determine objectively what each person needs, and accordingly, their eligibility for services.

Second, does an individual's functional status alone determine need, or should needs assessment also take into account that person's environment (thereby potentially penalizing the person who has a strong support system or the money to purchase what is wanted)?

Third, must the services to be provided be proven beneficial? This, in turn, requires that we decide the meaning of "beneficial." Is it with regard to the health and function of the patient or client, or beneficial to that person, but balanced by the price to the provider/payor?

Finally, how much are we willing to pay to provide this product? If we turn to our current LTC system and assume that either too much money is already being spent or that there is a need to control future spending, then the current system must be made more efficient or smaller.

Attempts to make the system more efficient include incentives for more efficient service delivery (such as by changing reimbursement mechanisms) and encouraging alternate methods of service delivery (HMOs, S/HMOs).

The system can be made smaller by decreasing the number of services and consumers and by eliminating the most expensive services and consumers. Certificate-of-need requirements limit the number of nursing home beds (a service that is considered to be both undesirable and too expensive). Reducing the number of consumers can be accomplished by making more consumers directly able to afford care (LTC individual retirement accounts, home equity conversion), by encouraging consumers to turn to other third-party payors (Medigap, LTC insurance, CCRCs), or by simply changing government programs (increasing premiums, deductibles, or copayments; increasing the uncovered gaps in the programs; making eligibility criteria more stringent). The last method is to reduce or eliminate services to consumers who are too costly (those 85 and over and those in the last year of their lives).

Physician Responsibilities

Though physicians may not see their role in shaping major changes in the LTC system, they have clear input into at least the last of these alternatives. At present the only person who can limit services is the individual patient, through instruments like the living will. If the preferences of this person cannot be known, then limits on services can be determined on an individual basis in court or between the physician and family. Cost containment concerns have no place in influencing these individual decisions.

The physician's responsibilities regarding the financial aspects for long-term care include:

- determining the optimal match between the patient's functional abilities and existing resources

- knowing what services are available in their areas and recognizing patients who may require services (see Chapter 2)

- inquiring about the architectural features of patients' homes and what family members may be available and willing to provide informal care

- when indicated, beginning planning for these support services as early as possible (at the time of admission to an acute hospital or a nursing home, or soon after a need is identified in the office setting)

- enlisting the services of those who are knowledgeable about eligibility criteria for financing and reliable providers of service (hospital discharge planning teams, social workers, case managers)

- for patients who require institutionalization, completing forms for the determination of levels of care, and admission assessments prior to or at the time of admission to allow for review

- for home care services, developing plans of care

- providing admission orders for ADC centers, particularly when medications are to be administered

- certifying the least number of services that a patient may require, not out of a desire for cost containment, but because fostering dependence by the provision of unnecessary services is as detrimental to a patient as inadequate services.

It is easier to add services than to take them away after a patient has become dependent on them. Indeed, the system that best serves the patient is one which includes all of the necessary options for care, but is run cost-efficiently, thus eliminating the possibility of excessive services accelerating the patient's dependency.

References

American Association of Retired Persons. 1984. *Long-term care research study.* Washington, DC: American Association of Retired Persons. Photocopy.

Beverly Foundation. 1986. *Public attitudes about contingency planning for long-term care needs.* Pasadena, CA: Beverly Foundation. Photocopy.

Brody, S. J., S. W. Poulshock, and C. F. Masciocchi. 1978. The family caring unit: A major consideration in the long-term support system. *The Gerontologist* 18:556-61.

Callahan, J. J. 1981. A systems approach to long-term care. In *Reforming the long-term-care system: Financial and organizational options,* edited by J. J. Callahan and S. S. Wallack, 219-35. Lexington, MA: Heath.

Chapman-Cliburn, G. 1986. Reimbursement policy for long term care. *Quality Review Bulletin* 12:142-43.

Clark, R. L., and J. J. Spengler. 1978. Changing demography and dependency costs: The implications of future dependency ratios and their composition. In *Aging and income,* edited by B. R. Herzog, 55-89. New York: Human Sciences Press.

Day, A. T. 1985. *Who cares? Demographic trends challenge family care for the elderly.* Population trends and public policy, edited by P. M. Scommegna, no. 9. Washington, DC: Population Reference Bureau.

Eustis, N. N., J. N. Greenberg, and S. K. Patten. 1984. *Long-term care for older persons: A policy perspective.* Monterey, CA: Brooks/Cole.

Garibaldi, R. A., S. Brodine, and S. Matsumiya. 1981. Infections among patients in nursing homes: Policies, prevalence, and problems. *The New England Journal of Medicine* 305:731-35.

Harrington, C., and J. H. Swan. 1984. Medicaid nursing home reimbursement policies, rates, and expenditures. *Health Care Financing Review* 6(1):39-49.

Health Care Financing Administration. 1983. *The Medicare and Medicaid data book, 1983.* Washington, DC: Health Care Financing Administration, pub. no. 03156.

Horowitz, A. 1985. Family caregiving to the frail elderly. In *Annual review of gerontology and geriatrics,* vol. 5, edited by C. Eisdorfer, M. P. Lawton, and G. L. Maddox, 194-246. New York: Springer.

Jazwiecki, T. 1986. Financing options for long-term care services. *Business and Health* 3(5):18-19, 22-24.

Kane, R. L. 1976. Paying nursing homes for better care. *Journal of Community Health* 2:1-4.

Kane, R. L. 1984. Long-term care: Policy and reimbursement. In *Geriatric medicine, vol. 1: Medical, psychiatric, and pharmacological topics,* edited by C. K. Cassel and J. R. Walsh, 380-96. New York: Springer-Verlag.

Kane, R. L., D. Hammer, and N. Byrnes. 1977. Getting care to nursing-home patients: A problem and a proposal. *Medical Care* 15:174-80.

Kennell, D. L. 1985. Can the elderly afford long term care insurance? *American Health Care Association Journal* 11(6):6-8.

Knickman, J. R., and N. McCall. 1986. A prepaid managed approach to long-term care. *Health Affairs* 5(1):90-104.

Langwell, K. M., and J. P. Hadley. 1986. Capitation and the Medicare program: History, issues, and evidence. *Health Care Financing Review* (annual supplement):9-20.

Lave, J. R. 1985. Cost containment policies in long-term care. *Inquiry* 22:7-23.

Lawton, M. P. 1980. *Environment and aging.* Monterey, CA: Brooks/Cole.

Leutz, W. 1986. Long-term care for the elderly: Public dreams and private realities. *Inquiry* 23:134-40.

Liu, K., K. G. Manton, and B. M. Liu. 1985. Home care expenses for the disabled elderly. *Health Care Financing Review* 7(2):51-58.

Lloyd, S., and N. T. Greenspan. 1985. Nursing homes, home health services, and adult day care. In *Long-term care: Perspectives from research and demonstrations,* edited by R. J. Vogel and H. C. Palmer, 133-66. Rockville, MD: Aspen.

Manning, W. G., A. Leibowitz, G. A. Goldberg, et al. 1984. A controlled trial of the effect of a prepaid group practice on use of services. *The New England Journal of Medicine* 310:1505-10.

McCoy, J. L., and B. E. Edwards. 1981. Contextual and sociodemographic antecedents of institutionalization among aged welfare recipients. *Medical Care* 19:907-21.

National Center for Health Statistics. 1977. *Characteristics, social contacts, and activities of nursing home residents, United States, 1973-74 National Nursing Home Survey*. Washington, DC: Government Printing Office, pub. no. HRA 77-1778.

National Center for Health Statistics. 1986a. *Americans needing home care, United States*. Washington, DC: Government Printing Office, pub. no. PHS 86-1581.

National Center for Health Statistics. 1986b. *Nursing and related care homes as reported from the 1982 National Master Facility Inventory Survey*. Washington, DC: Government Printing Office, pub. no. PHS 86-1827.

Newcomer, R. J., and M. P. Bogaert-Tullis. 1985. Medicaid cost containment trials and innovations. In *Long term care of the elderly: Public policy issues*, edited by C. Harrington, R. J. Newcomer, C. L. Estes, et al., 105-23. Beverly Hills: Sage.

Palmer, H. C. 1985a. Home care. In *Long-term care: Perspectives from research and demonstrations*, edited by R. J. Vogel and H. C. Palmer, 337-90. Rockville, MD: Aspen.

Palmer, H. C. 1985b. Adult day care. In *Long-term care: Perspectives from research and demonstrations*, edited by R. J. Vogel and H. C. Palmer, 415-36. Rockville, MD: Aspen.

Palmore, E. 1976. Total chance of institutionalization among the aged. *The Gerontologist* 16:504-7.

Pawlson, L. G., and R. A. Berenson. 1986. Financing and delivery of health care services: Changes and more changes. In *Geriatric medicine annual, 1986*, edited by R. J. Ham, 260-68. Oradell, NJ: Medical Economics.

Pepper, C. 1986. Catastrophic health insurance: "Medigap" crisis, introduction and executive summary. In U.S. Congress, House Subcommittee on health and long-term care of the Select Committee on Aging. *Catastrophic health insurance: The medigap crisis*, 140-50, 99th

Cong., 2d sess., June 25. Washington, DC: Government Printing Office, comm. pub. no. 99-587.

Preadmission screening survey. 1986. *Nursing Home Care & Management* 1(2):5-6.

Rango, N. 1982. Nursing-home care in the United States: Prevailing conditions and policy implications. *The New England Journal of Medicine* 307:883-89.

Ray, W. A., C. F. Federspiel, and W. Schaffner. 1980. A study of antipsychotic drug use in nursing homes: Epidemiologic evidence suggesting misuse. *American Journal of Public Health* 70:485-91.

Rubenstein, L. Z., K. R. Josephson, G. D. Wieland, et al. 1984. Effectiveness of a geriatric evaluation unit: A randomized clinical trial. *The New England Journal of Medicine* 311:1664-70.

Ruchlin, H. S., J. N. Morris, and G. M. Eggert. 1982. Management and financing of long-term-care services: A new approach to a chronic problem. *The New England Journal of Medicine* 306:101-6.

Rudensky, M. 1986. Skilled nursing facilities offered prospective pricing system option. *Modern Healthcare* 16(20):114.

Schieber, G., J. Wiener, K. Liu, et al. 1986. Prospective payment for Medicare skilled nursing facilities: Background and issues. *Health Care Financing Review* 8(1):79-85.

Scholen, K. 1983. Financing home care with home equity. *Pride Institute Journal of Long-Term Home Health Care* 2(2):43-45.

Senate Special Committee on Aging. 1986. *Aging America: Trends and projections*. 1985-86 ed. Washington, DC: Department of Health and Human Services.

Smith, K. F., and V. L. Bengtson. 1979. Positive consequences of institutionalization: Solidarity between elderly parents and their middle-aged children. *The Gerontologist* 19:438-47.

Solon, J. A., and L. F. Greenawalt. 1974. Physicians' participation in nursing homes. *Medical Care* 12:486-97.

Vicente, L., J. A. Wiley, and R. A. Carrington. 1979. The risk of institutionalization before death. *The Gerontologist* 19:361-67.

Vladeck, B. C. 1984. Medicare hospital payment by diagnosis-related groups. *Annals of Internal Medicine* 100:576-91.

Wachtel, T. J., C. Derby, and J. P. Fulton. 1984. Predicting the outcome of hospitalization for elderly persons: Home versus nursing home. *Southern Medical Journal* 77:1283-85, 1290.

Waldo, D. R., and H. C. Lazenby. 1984. Demographic characteristics and health care use and expenditures by the aged in the United States: 1977-1984. *Health Care Financing Review* 6(1):1-29.

Waldo, D. R., K. R. Levit, and H. Lazenby. 1986. National health expenditures, 1985. *Health Care Financing Review* 8(1):1-21.

Weissert, W., T. Wan, B. Livieratos, et al. 1980. Effects and costs of day-care services for the chronically ill: A randomized experiment. *Medical Care* 18:567-84.

Wessel, P. 1985. IRMA: A long-term home-equity conversion program. *Pride Institute Journal of Long-Term Home Health Care* 4(2):29-31.

Wiener, J. M. 1986. Financing and organizational options for long-term-care reform: Background and issues. *Bulletin of the New York Academy of Medicine* 62:75-86.

Willemain, T. R., and R. B. Mark. 1980. The distribution of intervals between visits as a basis for assessing and regulating physician services in nursing homes. *Medical Care* 18:427-41.

Winklevoss, H. E., and A. V. Powell. 1984. *Continuing care retirement communities: An empirical, financial, and legal analysis.* Homewood, IL: Irwin.

For Further Reading

Aging America: Trends and Projections. 1985-86 edition. Best single source of data regarding status of aging in the United States. Prepared by the U.S. Senate Special Committee on Aging in conjunction with the American Association of Retired Persons, the Federal Council on the Aging, and the Administration on Aging. Out of print, but limited number of copies available without charge from the American Association of Retired Persons, 1909 K St., N.W., Washington, DC 20049, Attn: Federal Legislation.

Health Care Financing Review. Original and review articles concerning health care delivery to the elderly. PUblished quarterly (plus an annual supplement) by the Health Care Financing Administration's Office of Research and Demonstrations. Available ($18 per year, $4.25 per single issue) from the Superintendent of Documents, U.S. Government Printing Office, Washington, DC 20402, Stock no. 717-011-00000-7.

The Medicare and Medicaid Data Book. 1983 edition. Descriptive reports and statistics on the Medicare and Medicaid programs. Available from the Superintendent of Documents, U.S. Government Printing Office, Washington, DC 20402. Next edition (containing data as of 1985) will be available August 1987.

Medicare and Medicare Guide. Comprehensive reference regarding Medicare and Medicaid programs. Subscription ($630 per year) includes four looseleaf volumes and biweekly updates. Available from Commerce Clearing House, Inc., 4025 W. Peterson Ave., Chicago, IL 60646.

Chapter Nine

Information, Computers, and Medical Care

Steven A. Levenson, M.D.

Chapter Objectives

This chapter will:

- Consider the importance of compiling accurate information in LTC

- Describe the data needs of the physician practicing LTC medicine

- Consider the possibilities for information management in the LTC system of the future

- Propose a physician role in LTC information system design and implementation

- Discuss the prospects for computers in these information systems.

The Importance of Information

The long-term care system of the future will rival or exceed the acute medical care system in size, patient load, and overall importance. It will cover many sources and sites of care, and track patients with multiple problems over many years. That is, its emphasis will shift from service *sites* (hospital, nursing home, clinic, etc.) to service *needs*. An older person is not just a nursing home or a hospital patient, but one who will have needs met by services at several different sites, delivered by many different individuals over many months or years. Since accurate and complete information is the basis for adequate diagnosis, treatment, and placement, many of the deficiencies in patient care of the elderly can almost certainly be traced to inadequate and poorly functioning information systems.

There are well over a million older people at any one time in American nursing homes. Almost all of them, like many of the ambulatory elderly, also receive care from other parts of the system. The nursing home (NH) must be brought in line with the other parts of the health care system. Quality care depends on accurate, complete information, which can be located quickly and be readily passed on, as needed, to other providers in other parts of the health care system.

The health care system is just beginning to recognize the value of good information management to quality and cost-effective patient care. Handwritten, people-dependent systems are unreliable, often inaccurate and illegible, and sometimes unavailable when needed. In addition, they offer hinder health care professionals attempting to care for patients, especially the elderly. "Such records impede efficient health care, make careful and timely audit impossible, and create barriers to clinical research" (Levinson 1983, 607).

Information and Truth

From reading the newspapers or watching television, we know instinctively that there is a critical difference between information and truth. Information is all around us, but *truth* depends on the manner in which that information is arranged, presented, and interpreted in relation to other information. When we base a conclusion on inaccurate or incomplete information, we are less likely to reach a desirable goal or conclusion because we are less likely to be acting on truth. Such has been the unfortunate lot of LTC in the past.

Providing proper medical care depends on having the most accurate, current, and complete information possible. But since much of the information pertaining to a LTC patient is either inaccurate, incomplete, or missing entirely, care and treatment are likely to be inadequate or inappropriate. In addition, standardized terminology and criteria are essential to provide a consistent basis for evaluating, comparing changes in condition, and proving the value of various treatments or services. Only by reproducible, objective data do we stand a good chance of finding those things that can truly help the elderly at a reasonable cost. Good information management is thus central to improving quality of care in LTC.

Most quality assurance in LTC depends not so much on observing patients, but on analyzing information related to those patients. An equally important part of quality assurance, however, is the evaluation of the *quality of the information itself,* and the design of policies and procedures to monitor and improve on the information process.

The long-term care system requires three essential areas of information:

- recording, retrieval, and transfer of basic patient information

- search and retrieval of medical and other factual data bases to assist in diagnosis and treatment

- education of patients and other nonmedical staff, on such topics as understanding of illnesses, medications, prevention, risk factors, etc.

Good information management should thus stress developing data that are accurate and complete, consistent from one person to the next, and include valid definitions, criteria, and standards for individual data items.

Information Flow

Information in the LTC continuum flows in several major directions, as seen in Figure 9-1:

- physician to physician

- physician to other health professionals, and vice versa

- physician to hospital, and vice versa

- hospital to NH, and vice versa

- physician to NH, and vice versa

- physician to outpatient or home service provider, and vice versa

- third-party payor to physician, and vice versa

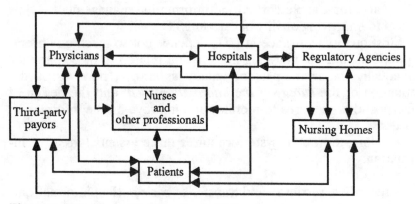

Figure 9-1 The Flow of information in LTC

- third-party payor to institution, and vice versa

- regulatory agency to physician, and vice versa

- regulatory agency to institution, and vice versa

- physician to patient, and vice-versa.

The ultimate goal in LTC, a formidable, but achievable task, should be the consistency and interchangeability of information among *all* these originators and recipients. *Each piece of information should be recorded only once, and then be readily available to all who need it, as needed.*

LTC and the Clinical Information System

A central concept is that of the "clinical information system," defined herein as a coordinated approach at any and all levels (programmatic, institutional, community, state, or national) to the systematic collection, storage, analysis, retrieval, transfer, and use of information concerning patients, their health and illnesses, and any associated needs or problems.

The *computerized* information system, considered below, simply refers to the use of computers as the key tool for the aforementioned processes of collection, storage, etc.

All medical personnel and information systems process three items (Blum 1986): *data*, the uninterpreted items; *information*, interpreted sets of data; and *knowledge*, the rules, relationships, and experience by which data become information.

Examples of data are a patient's vital signs and laboratory test results, or observations of behavior and Activities of Daily Living (ADL) function. Examples of information are the facts about medical illness given in medical textbooks. Examples of knowledge are the rules about diagnostic probability that underlie medical practice.

In contrast to biomedical engineering applications, such as the CAT Scan, which process limited amounts of data and do not maintain long-term data bases, information applications require a long-term data base.

Handling information is costly and time-consuming. Blum (1986) notes that Jydstrup and Gross found that about 25% of hospital operating costs was spent on information handling, and that a small minority of documents accounts for about half the total costs. Nursing staff spent about 30% of their time in information handling, representing 25% of their paid time. In reality, the cost of information handling as a percentage of total operating costs in hospitals is greater for the clinical staff than for the administrative departments (Blum 1986, 219). The same is almost certainly true in LTC.

The LTC Medical Record

Today, the written medical record is the major tool of LTC information. "The medical record plays a key role in today's medical practice. It is a medium for communication among providers, an informative source for follow-up, a resource for research, a legal record, and more. . . . There are many styles and forms for medical records; the problem-oriented medical record (POMR) is one example. All records contain some textual information (name and address) and some coded information (race and sex). The medical data may include text or codes for complaints, diagnosis, and therapies. Test results are incorporated into the record; they may be in the form of individual reports, flow sheets, or graphs. It is assumed that patient care is better when medical records are available than when they are not. However, the contents and structure of in-

dividual records are subject to personal preferences and local standards." (Blum 1986, 255)

Ultimately, a medical record should follow an elderly individual
throughout all parts of the health care system, quickly provide accurate and complete information, protect patient privacy, be updated conveniently and quickly, and provide the data for any necessary reports and to assist with actual care decisions. The current
reality, however, is very different, since the LTC medical record
often cannot support extensive information needs.

Information needs in various settings

Two major reasons for clinical information systems (CIS) include communication and the organization of data to facilitate
decision making. In acute care, "the primary reason for information
handling is communications" (Blum 1986, 221), and the primary
function of a CIS is to *support* such communications. These include
such items as intershift communications, orders from physicians to
nurses, vital signs, and medication and test orders, and charges post-
ing.

By contrast, the encounters in ambulatory care are brief and
sporadic, with more patients and less information, having a necessary link between visits, and no great need for timely communication between services. "Since an ambulatory care system does not
focus on the communication functions, its primary impact on patient
care is through the contents and availability of the medical record
used by the providers and ancillary services." (Blum 1986, 253)

Having features of both acute and ambulatory care, the NH requires a CIS that offers some of both worlds: multiple systems and
professional services that need to communicate with one another
regularly, and sporadic brief medical encounters that must be linked
together over a potentially long time span. There are far fewer admissions per annum than in the hospital, but the record of each individual is long, often complex, and contains much hard-to-find
documentation, some of which is pertinent to current care. The
proper CIS must therefore be a hybrid of the two systems.

Home-based care, another part of the LTC continuum, also
presents some special information needs. Hospital care is usually
episodic, and the outcome is for the individual to leave the system.
Each admission or readmission is a new episode, and starts a new

recording and set of data. In the NH, however, care is continuous over time. Home care, on the other hand, is somewhere between the two: it is neither episodic, as in the hospital, nor continuous, as in the NH. Current reimbursement requirements are for services to be rendered within a definitive time span at predetermined frequencies, and to result in some specific changes in the individual's condition and function. Whereas in both acute care and the NH, each individual service is provided in the context of the *overall* care, in home health care, each individual service must account for its continued need. Therefore, the main measure of quality is the *individual visit*, which must be adequately documented and justified.

The Medicare treatment plan report requires an initial treatment plan submitted with the first claim for a home health episode, and then recertified treatment plans with subsequent claims at 60-day intervals thereafter. This requires both coded data and free-form narrative text.

Information and the LTC Physician

The LTC physician has four major information-related roles: recipient, provider, reviewer, and systems designer.

To be effective in all of these roles, the physician must:

- collect accurate data
- help standardize terminology and improve data collection accuracy
- provide and review the rules by which data are interpreted
- review the format, accuracy and applicability of the information generated by such systems.

In each role, the physician needs or conveys information about patients, geriatrics, matters related to medical practice and LTC, resources, and other professionals.

Patient-related information includes past medical history, reports of recent hospitalizations, changes in condition, response to treatments, patient wishes, and the results of tests and consultations by others.

Geriatrics-related information includes knowledge of the biology of aging, syndromes and illnesses accompanying aging, management of chronic illness and pain, guidelines for approaching both clinical and ethical issues, therapeutics, opportunities for personal education, and the work and efforts of others in the field (See Chapter 10).

Medical practice and LTC-related information includes reimbursement, liability, regulations, and laws pertinent to LTC (See Chapters 8 and 11).

Resource-related information includes referral and consultative sources, and available LTC programs and facilities (See Chapter 2).

Professional-related information refers to other fields related to the elderly, such as social, psychological, biological, administrative, and nursing (See Chapter 7).

The Patient Data Base

A data base is defined as a collection of information. Thus, both a patient medical history and medications list, and the list of books about geriatrics in a medical library, are considered data bases. But whereas the latter is provided *to* or *for* the physician by others, the patient data base is created *by* the physician along with other health professionals. Therefore, while the physician is concerned with accessing outside data bases, he must also be concerned with the design and validation of patient data bases.

The physician provides a large portion of the LTC *patient data base*, the collection of information about an individual elderly patient at specific times. This information is in two categories: known facts, or information obtained from objective testing and evaluation, and conclusions or opinions based on that known information and other new information. Information based on known facts or on testing and evaluation may include:

- current diagnoses, symptoms, and complaints
- hospital course
- past history and surgeries
- physical examination
- laboratory data

- allergies
- immunizations
- treatment and therapies – currently received
- activities of daily living and functional capacity
- sensory impairments
- dentition
- psychological assessment
- social data
- physician lists.

Let us address some of these individually.

Diagnoses. Nothing in geriatric medicine is more important than accurate diagnosis and recording of diagnoses, as the foundation for interdisciplinary communication, initiation of proper treatment, accurate prognosis, presentation of appropriate treatment options to patients and families, and appropriate testing and follow-up. Unfortunately, this remains one of medicine's weakest areas. Diagnoses are often incomplete, inaccurate, or use personalized styles or abbreviations, or are missing entirely.

One possible solution is to require each physician, on admission or entry of an individual into the LTC system, to complete a problem list, using standardized terminology, and to supplement this with additional diagnoses. Using a preprinted checklist takes little time, ensures standardized terminology, and bypasses the legibility problem (See Appendix 9-A).

A related quality assurance activity would be a review of the record to see if it contains information to adequately and appropriately support the diagnostic conclusion (e.g., are there some objective test results to confirm a diagnosis of "dementia?").

Hospital course. Relevant results of previous institutional stays are often unavailable or incomplete. Tests may be repeated because no one has bothered to notice when they were last done.

A possible solution is for each LTC facility to adopt, with the assistance of the medical staff, a policy requiring certain information of acute hospitals prior to accepting a transfer for admission. Each home-based or outpatient program should establish a required set of information before accepting a new patient into a program. The medical staff of each NH should work with the appropriate committees of its local hospitals to improve the quality and consistency of the records sent on patient transfer and the information they contain.

Past history. An older patient is likely to have an extensive past history. This should not have to be elicited and rewritten repeatedly upon each new hospital or NH admission, or when seen by another physician or consultant. Each time this is redone, the possibility of inaccuracies or incomplete information becomes greater. The past history should be done once, updated as appropriate, and available for all who need it.

Laboratory data. Baseline laboratory data are extremely helpful in the event of subsequent changes in condition. These can be obtained from physicians' offices or the acute hospital record, or can be drawn after admission to a NH. At a minimum, they should include: hemoglobin and hematocrit, BUN (blood urea nitrogen), creatinine, and an EKG (electrocardiogram). A chemistry profile is helpful in certain specific cases, such as undernutrition, decubitus ulcers, edema, or weight loss. There should also be pertinent laboratory tests to follow specific individuals on particular medications (for example, prothrombin time for those on Coumadin; BUN and creatinine for those on diuretics).

Allergies. An accurate and complete listing of medication, food, and other allergies is extremely important, especially in avoiding potential complications of subsequent medications ordered to which the patient might be allergic.

Immunizations. It is important to know if the individual received flu vaccine previously, and if he or she had any reactions. It is even more important to know whether the patient received Pneumococcal vaccine, since this should not be repeated.

Treatments and therapies. A description of currently and previously received treatments and therapies can help staff decide what to try again, what did not work, and what new measures might be worthwhile.

Activities of daily living and functional capacity. As mentioned previously, function is a major issue in the LTC patient. Since illness may or may not affect function significantly, it is important to clarify functional capacities. For instance, to what extent can the individual dress, bathe, feed, or groom himself? How much assistance is needed?

Psychological assessment. In a LTC population with increasing mental and behavioral dysfunctions, a thorough psychological assessment is essential. This should include at least a test of cognitive function (such as the mini mental status exam), and where indicated, tests for depression, personality, perception, and anxiety.

Physician lists. Lists of physicians who have attended or consulted on a patient are extremely helpful for staff who must contact them. It also helps to know when there is no physician, so that other medical care sources can be contacted in the event of an emergency.

Appendix 9-B is an example of how much of the above information can be arranged in a computerized data base for further analysis and retrieval.

As such information is collected, it is used to support additional conclusions about the patient's needs and care plan, including:

- prognosis
- rehabilitation potential
- objectives and goals for the individual
- orders for care
- required level of care, and the reasons why continued care is needed at that level
- competency assessment
- discharge plans and follow-up arrangements, where applicable.

Prognosis. Prognosis can be designated as *excellent, good, fair, poor,* or *terminal.* As always, exactly *what* these terms mean depends on how they are defined at the outset.

Rehabilitation potential. This refers to the individual's capacity to benefit from some therapeutic modality, such as physical or occupational therapy, to at least maintain and possibly improve overall or partial function. This, too, may be designated by *excellent, good, fair, poor,* or *none.*

Objectives and goals. Again, since what we choose to do for LTC patients depends on the goals and prognosis, establishing such aims should precede choices of treatment.

Goals should be both short-term (for example, stabilize cardiac condition, or adjust to environment) and long-term (improve ambulation, reduce number of medications, encourage self-care). These should be documented, and are a very useful basis for considering quality of care, by subsequently comparing results with expectations or objectives. Progress notes should periodically indicate the extent to which goals have been achieved, and the prospects for further efforts.

Orders for care. These should include both drug and nondrug orders, such as medications, treatments, restorative and rehabilitative services, activities, therapies, social services, diet, and special procedures recommended for the patient's health and safety (see Chapter 4). They should be written according to established protocols, so that those who must carry out the orders know *exactly* what the terms mean. For instance, does a "low sodium diet" mean "no added salt on the tray," "4-6 grams," or "40-60 milliequivalents"? Only by defining things first can we check for accuracy of orders and consistency of care.

Level of care, and its rationale. Level of care (e.g., domiciliary or intermediate) designations are often required to justify payment. They are also important indicators for quality of care and utilization reviews. The services and therapies ordered for an individual should be consistent with needs, and they should be at the level of care appropriate for those needed services (see Chapter 6). For instance, the person who needs constant nursing monitoring and medical evaluation for repeatedly unstable problems does not belong at the domiciliary level of care until those problems are evaluated or stabilized by treatment. On the other hand, the individual in a skilled NH who can take care of all his daily needs, and is mentally intact and physically stable may be able to be transferred to the less costly and less intensive domiciliary setting, or even discharged to the community and followed in a day care program. The physician should periodically reconsider and document a person's need to remain at a particular level of care.

Competence assessment. A competence assessment should consider the person's potential to function in various settings or roles. Such evaluations clearly depend on first gathering appropriate and accurate factual information about an older patient (see Chapter 12).

Discharge and follow-up plans. The record should indicate how and by whom the individual will be followed, outline the plan of care, and list appropriate medications. Discharges to other facilities, such as hospitals, should also include pertinent information about past history, clinical course while in a NH, and the results of pertinent tests and consultations.

The Transfer of Information

As individuals move through the LTC system, information moves with them. Common situations are hospital to NH, NH to hospital, and physician to physician or clinic. Physicians should be just as concerned with the information that moves as with the patients themselves. Such information should be, but often is not, accurate, complete, up-to-date, and understandable.

Physicians should help acute and LTC institutions adopt protocols and checklists to remind people of the information that should accompany patients from one place or professional to another. For example, individuals transferred from NH to hospital should have documentation of a reason for transfer, current medications, progress notes pertinent to the current situation, recent laboratory test results, and statements related to patients' wishes, such as a living will. Physicians transferring patients to nursing homes should provide, among other things, current medication lists, test results, lists of diagnoses, and pertinent summaries of recent assessments and care.

Improving LTC Information

Physicians, working with other health professionals, can do many things to help establish quality information systems in LTC, especially by assisting in the standardization, verification, and planning of such systems.

Plans must be made for recording information in a standard form. Coding must be consistent so that different people will enter the same information identically. The criteria for describing someone as "severely agitated," "confused," or "lethargic" should be the same for physicians, nurses, aides, and social workers, even if some of these people might be better qualified to judge than others. Consider this observation:

> Before you decide what you want to store in the medical record, consider each kind of data and how it can be obtained. There are many sources of clinical data: physicians' notes, nursing notes, and laboratory results; and each kind of data may come from many different sources. For example, inpatient laboratory data might come from three different hospitals you visit. . . . A diagnosis can come from the physician's progress notes, but it may also come from a billing system – often more easily (McDonald 1987, 7).

Therefore, decisions must be made about who will *enter* each piece of information, who will *verify* each piece, and who will be allowed to *access* data. For example, should changes in mental status or level of consciousness be recorded by the nurse, a psychiatrist, the attending physician, the aide, or all the above? If the answer is "all the above," then they all need to use the same definitions and criteria. We must also decide which pieces of information are needed for various reports, and where those data should be stored so we may best find and use them.

Several broad attempts to standardize, code, and verify LTC information have been made, and are available to use intact or to modify for applications. Two of these are the OARS (Older

Americans Resources and Services) Assessment Methodology, developed at Duke University (Duke University 1978), and the Cornell University Long-Term Care Information System (LTCIS) (Falcone 1982; 1983).

The Role of Computers in LTC Information Systems

Computers may be used in LTC either alone–to accomplish specific tasks for individuals or small groups–or as part of a coordinated clinical information system. As practitioners, LTC physicians can be aided in patient assessment, diagnosis, and therapy, as well as in receiving payment for their services (see below). As participants in a LTC *system*, they can benefit themselves and patients by using computers intelligently as part of a CIS.

Evaluation, organization, and rearrangement of clinical information systems must be done regardless of any computerization, and are essential for the ultimate success and value of any such computerization. The computer can be enormously helpful in data storage, analysis, reporting, and retrieval. But professionals must still help plan and execute the *input* and *design*.

A computer will do only as it is told to, and will not salvage a poorly designed clinical information system. Therefore, it is not computerization itself, but a *well thought-out*, intelligently designed information system using computer support, that will benefit users and patients. Neither will a computer take the place of good communication between staff. A well-designed medical system will enhance and facilitate good communication, but a poorly designed or implemented system will frustrate people, risk loss of data, and waste time and money (McLean and Kapkin 1983).

A computer system will give us information, either analyzed or unanalyzed, but will not guarantee us absolute truth. Reliable information is highly dependent on the accuracy of what is entered, and the way the program is set up to process that information (garbage in; garbage out"). Both input and programming are subject to human error and individual interpretation. Therefore, a well-designed computer system must include built-in error-checking protocols for data entry. A parallel system should be run in the beginning to double-check for accuracy.

What information we collect and how we arrange it is largely determined by what we feel is important and how we intend to use it at the time we first collect it. Proper use of the computer therefore requires preliminary planning: What data do we want to collect about patients, how might we want to use these now and in the future, and how shall we arrange it for easy storage and retrieval?

Nevertheless, the computer has enormous potential as a revolutionary tool for LTC professionals, including physicians. In 1970, a physician wrote:

> Many discussions during the past decade have considered the use of computers as an adjunct to medicine. Few, however, have fully explored the possibility that the computer as an intellectual tool can reshape the present system of health care, fundamentally alter the role of the physician, and profoundly change the nature of medical manpower recruitment and medical education – in short, the possibility that the healthcare system by the year 2000 will be basically different from what it is today (Schwartz 1970, 1257).

Because of its needs for manpower and for information, the LTC system is the vanguard of those substantial changes in future health care. The new technologies, especially computers, have a critical role in facilitating comprehensive, efficient and cost-effective health care systems. Without them, substantial improvements in the quality of LTC will be largely unattainable. With them, the possibilities for such improvement are endless.

Intelligent computerization could help tremendously with problems unique to the elderly. Older people often carry multiple diagnoses and receive many medications, have extensive medical records, and are treated by many different parts of the health care system. They often have limited memory, attention span, and sensory capabilities. It often takes longer to take their history, examine them, and explain their diagnoses and medications to them. Since for many physicians, the elderly comprise the predominant patient population, computerization can help to identify these problems efficiently and accurately.

Ultimately, the computer-stored medical record can present all information legibly, and allow users to organize and report the same information in various formats to suit their needs. It eliminates the problem of unavailable charts after discharge or when being used by others. But "most important, the computer record can assure quality care. It can detect clinical problems or trends reflected in the record and call them to physicians' attention. It can statistically summarize a practice's experience with a particular disease or therapy. Physicians can use these features to guide future clinical practices and policies" (McDonald 1987, 7).

The effective use of computers will force us to rethink the true purpose of medicine, which is not to memorize information, but to apply information:

> The physician is an information manager who acquires, processes, stores, retrieves, and applies information related to 1) individual patient history and clinical course, 2) diagnostic and therapeutic protocols, 3) disease patterns in patient populations, 4) functioning of the health care system, and, 5) the vast store of published knowledge. Little occurs in the clinical encounter that is not in some way related to obtaining, processing, or applying information (Levinson 1983, 607).

Figure 9-2 shows that the patient data base is the centerpiece of a computer-based medical information system, just as personnel and financial data bases are central to the operations of hospitals.

Data-gathering and organizing programs (Fig. 9-3) facilitate the *collection and arrangement* of all aspects of information about the patients, their problems, illnesses, and needs. These include the ways in which physicians gain access to information, as well as the information itself.

Diagnosis and treatment programs (Fig. 9-4) are all those which facilitate the physician's ability to *translate raw data* into diagnoses, to choose the most appropriate treatments based on those diagnoses, and to help the patient find the best combination of placement and service to meet their needs once the diagnoses and treatments are established.

Lastly, *output* programs (Fig. 9-5) are those which facilitate the production of reports, patient care analyses, and instructional and educational materials based on patient information and on diagnosis and treatment data.

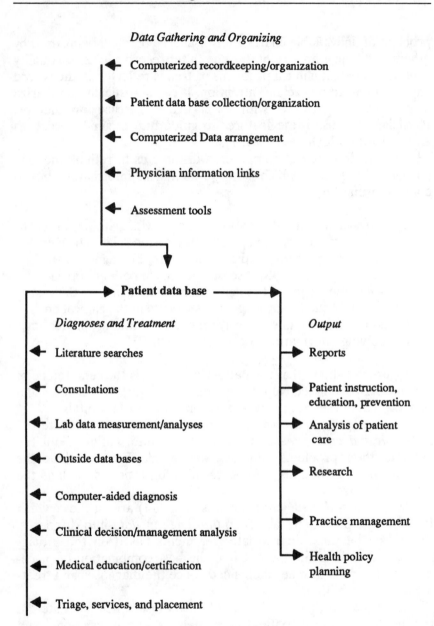

Data Gathering and Organizing

◄ Computerized recordkeeping/organization

◄ Patient data base collection/organization

◄ Computerized Data arrangement

◄ Physician information links

◄ Assessment tools

Patient data base

Diagnoses and Treatment

◄ Literature searches

◄ Consultations

◄ Lab data measurement/analyses

◄ Outside data bases

◄ Computer-aided diagnosis

◄ Clinical decision/management analysis

◄ Medical education/certification

◄ Triage, services, and placement

Output

► Reports

► Patient instruction, education, prevention

► Analysis of patient care

► Research

► Practice management

► Health policy planning

Figure 9-2 The computer-based information system

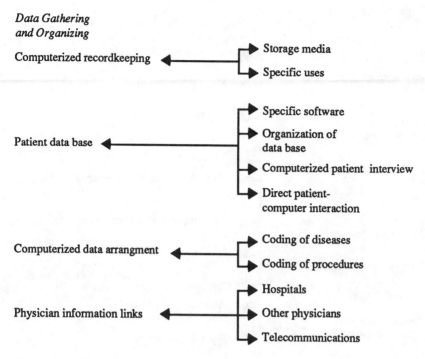

*Data Gathering
and Organizing*

Computerized recordkeeping
- Storage media
- Specific uses

Patient data base
- Specific software
- Organization of data base
- Computerized patient interview
- Direct patient-computer interaction

Computerized data arrangment
- Coding of diseases
- Coding of procedures

Physician information links
- Hospitals
- Other physicians
- Telecommunications

Figure 9-3 Data gathering and organizing programs

To summarize, a comprehensive LTC computer-based clinical information system concerns the *input, processing,* and *output* of information, with the patient data base at its core.

Unfortunately, for the most part, only expensive mainframe, hospital-based computer systems have been available, often requiring extensive costly custom programming. This has limited their usefulness and availability for thousands of small-to-medium-sized health care facilities, such as nursing homes, in the U.S. and abroad, and for such individual users as physicians. Both physicians and facilities still use computers predominantly for financial and administrative matters, including hospital admissions, census, billing and finances, and medical records functions, and are only beginning to consider their potential for enhancing patient care.

The computer has applications in *all* aspects of LTC, as mentioned previously. Some of these are described below.

Diagnosis and Treatment

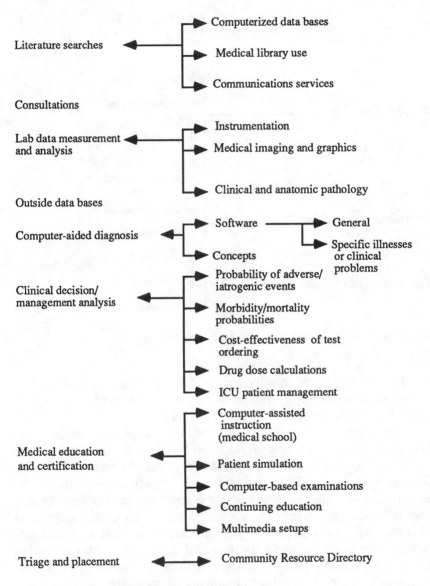

Figure 9-4 Diagnosis and treatment programs

Output

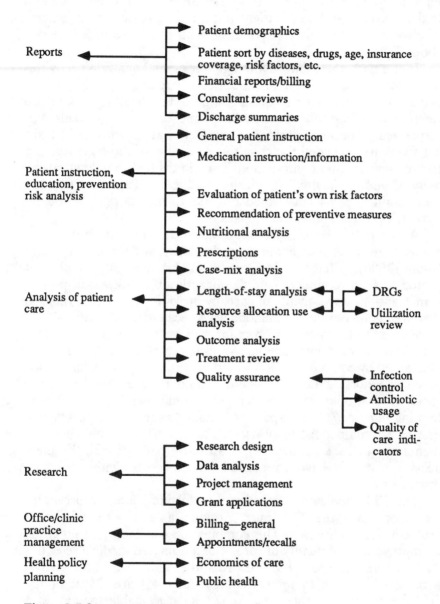

Figure 9-5 Output programs

Patient management and quality assurance. Besides recording and finding current and past patient information, patient management involves correlating that information with our store of knowledge about disease.

In the past, these information gathering and analyzing activities were done mainly by hand and foot, searching medical records departments and patient files, going to the library, looking up references, calling colleagues on the phone, or reading journals. Not surprisingly, "optimal performance of clinical informational tasks has for years exceeded the cognitive capability of the human mind; the physician-patient interaction is an individual, handcrafted activity of uneven quality" (Levinson 1983, 607). To minimize these shortcomings, physicians would be wise to incorporate computers into their patient management tasks.

A computerized clinical information system can speed communications, reduce or eliminate redundancy, and lower error rates (Blum 1986). Clement McDonald (1976) has suggested that protocol-based reminders can significantly affect physician performance and improve quality of care, by providing timely information that even good physicians cannot always recall when needed.

For example, computer programs can warn physicians of potentially harmful drug interactions. An example of a quality assurance item aided by computerization would be a rule that every known hypertensive nursing home resident should have a blood pressure check at least quarterly. The computer could then be programmed to print all names of those patients with a diagnosis of hypertension, first as a reminder list to physicians to order this monitoring, and then as a quality assurance list of all those patients with the diagnosis who do not have a recorded blood pressure within the past three months.

The LTC medical record must therefore provide the current information, and the CIS must provide a link with rule-based protocols for quality care. This combination has enormous potential to improve overall quality of care. The automated medical record is " . . . superior to the written record and . . . automated record systems provide tools to improve the quality of care. Most of the evidence to support these claims has been available for almost a decade" (Blum 1986, 290). Major factors holding back widespread use of such systems have been cost and lack of software. Cost is no longer a constraint with the newer microcomputers, and software development is rapidly expanding.

Home- and office-based computers can unite physicians, hospitals, and LTC facilities, providing rapid access to critical patient information, and enabling more accurate and timely advice and assistance.

> The office computer has the potential to rapidly expand our currently narrow base of information on common disorders. It will cause an explosive growth in the dimensions and detail of our knowledge about wellness, minor and major illnesses, and prognosis. It will bring thousands of new clinical syndromes to our attention. It will describe the natural history or a variety of minor and chronic illnesses. In the end, hitherto unsuspected prodromes to chronic illnesses will be identified (Reid 1984, 66).

Data input. Computers can contribute greatly to better data collection and input, especially by offering assistance to those with sensory impairments, and having patience for those who are slow or who do not at first understand. Fears that such uses of computers dehumanize the doctor-patient relationship are baseless. One physician who has spent twenty years working on patient/computer dialogues claims that, "In our experience, concern about the computer as a depersonalizing influence in dialogue with patients—a concern expressed mostly by professionals—has been unfounded. Computer interaction thus far has been pleasant and interesting for most patients, and has been effective in helping them to communicate information about their medical problems" (Slack 1984, 59).

Medical information data bases. Computerized data bases provide access to information when we need it. They are more up to date than journals and standard textbooks, generally having the most current information on line within days to weeks, not months or years. Search time is in seconds to minutes, rather than the hours or days it would take to go through a library or volumes of *Index Medicus*. In addition, computers can locate and crossmatch information far more thoroughly and rapidly. By interacting directly with the service, the physician has the opportunity to see the results of his search instantaneously, and to try various modifications.

Within a few years physicians will obtain most, if not all, of their current medical information through one or more of these sources. The coming use of optical disk mass storage will enable physicians to retrieve, print out, and store large amounts of information for ready access. Entire medical reference libraries will be available for individual use on a few inexpensive laser disks, easily replaced by updates.

Successfully implemented on-line networks include AMANet, launched in 1982 by the AMA in collaboration with GTE Telenet. The contents include drug and diagnostic information, disease classification and terminologies, medical procedure coding, legislative updates, socioeconomic statistics, and an AMA bulletin board. Other facets of this service include computer-assisted self-assessment teaching programs in such areas as arrhythmias, basic life support, and hypertension management, and EMPIRES (Excerpta Medica Physicians Information Retrieval and Education Service), which provides physicians with 50,000 new citations a year, mostly accompanied by bibliographies and abstracts (Morse 1984; Swerdlow 1984; and Wright 1984).

Other services, like Bibliographic Retrieval Service's BRS/Colleague and Lockheed's DIALOG, provide capabilities for retrieving texts of journals and textbooks, and scanning bibliographies in a wide array of business, science, engineering, general knowledge, and medical subjects. Using such data bases, the physician could, for instance, search for articles about the future of care for the elderly in the popular press, major daily newspapers, and in the medical, psychological, and sociological literature (Wright 1984). PaperChase is a bibliographic retrieval program developed at Beth Israel Hospital in Boston, and has facilitated access to hundreds of thousands of articles from the medical literature. It is generally updated even more quickly than *Index Medicus* (Mula 1984) and has gained popularity with its physician users.

These services are usually offered on a subscription basis, with either an initial or annual fee, or both, plus a charge for on-line time. Most include a certain amount of free use time, and some allow the user to place orders directly for reprints of the articles themselves. Presently, the main drawback for some individual users is cost, but eventually, with more users, costs will probably drop while ease of use and compatibility increase. Some of these services will also become available on optical disk.

Diagnosis and treatment assistance. Geriatrics is a particularly appropriate area for computerized diagnostic assistance, because of the multiple complex coexisting problems and syndromes of the typical geriatric patient, and the often nonspecific presentation of illnesses in this population. In addition, the computer can quickly provide answers to important questions in an increasingly cost-conscious era: Which laboratory test(s) are most likely to provide useful information? What is the probability that a given set of results implies or confirms a particular diagnosis? What is the likelihood that a given patient can be safely observed rather than immediately undergoing a procedure or an extensive workup? "Evidence now exists . . . to show that a consistently applied clinical decision-making strategy can be directly translated into better patient outcomes" (Jenkin et al. 1978, 218).

Both community- and institution-based practitioners desire practical, readily accessible diagnostic assistance. Thus far, the use of the computer as a diagnostic tool has been somewhat limited by cost, by the need for large computers with massive data storage capabilities, and by the difficulty of writing programs that can reason and consider relevant information in the same manner as a skilled physician. But the farsighted predict that the successful evolution of computer-based diagnostic systems will result in faster and more accurate diagnoses, and decreased patient stays (Reid 1984).

There is a growing body of diagnostic applications. For instance, the Problem-Knowledge Coupler is a problem-oriented diagnostic program developed for a microcomputer. MYCIN is a program for consulting on infections. Both of these depend on having rules, each of which uses certain facts from which subsequent premises can be deduced. If the facts establish a premise as true, then that premise serves as the basis to deduce another one (Batson 1984; Yu, et al. 1979).

Probably the most comprehensive of these programs is the *Quick Medical Reference*, known in other versions as *Caduceus* and *Internist*. Developed over more than a decade, its goal is to assist with the diagnosis of all important diseases in internal medicine. Using this program, a physician can obtain a disease profile in less than a minute, and learn of interrelationships with other illnesses that would otherwise take many days to locate (Bruer 1984). Copies for actual use should be available by late 1987.

The potential for such software to assist in clinical decision-making for complex elderly patients, many in nursing homes, and many unable to provide significant clinical histories, is very great. These programs will not replace physician data gathering and data analysis, but should greatly aid in the more timely and accurate handling of acute and progressive chronic problems, and in reminding physicians to consider diagnoses and confirmatory tests that they might otherwise have forgotten.

The importance of the computer in assisting our management of some difficult ethical issues concerning the elderly should not be underestimated. To offer elderly patients the chance to make choices on their own behalf, the physician must present them with realistic options. " 'The proliferation of medical technology and interventions force choices about what should be done for a patient. Pathophysiology and detailed knowledge of disease mechanisms do not dictate these choices. There is relatively little in medical education to impart systematic skills for dealing with choices, risks, benefits, uncertainties, and values' " (Bruer 1984, 31). (Further discussion of ethical issues can be found in Chapter 12.)

The computer can provide much more detailed analyses to help establish prognoses and choose options: How likely is this treatment to help? What is this person's likely prognosis with or without a given treatment? How likely is this test to provide useful information? Armed with such details, both physician and patient have a more substantial basis for making critical choices.

Information Output. The third major area of computer use (besides information input and analysis) is information output.

Computers can be used to educate older patients and those who care for them. For instance, drug dosage schedules could be printed out by medication and time of day, and patient weights or blood pressures over time could be plotted. The older patient can obtain information about his condition and medications at his own pace, without extensive staff and physician time. Not only are the advantages of visual presentation apparent for those many elderly with partial or total hearing impairment, but improvements in computer voice recognition technology will allow for better access by the visually impaired, as well.

Other software has included interactive instruction in cardiac risk factors (Chen et al. 1984) and weight control (Ellis and Raines

1981). The "Health Hazard Appraisal" identifies risk factors associated with increased morbidity and mortality at a given age, and is especially adaptable to computerization (Reid 1984).

Patient care analyses, quality assurance, and policy and planning. Data required for developing and analyzing case management systems come from medical records, patient bills, and the general ledger. Microcomputer-based programs are being integrated with hospital-wide information management systems, to facilitate interaction between individual practitioners and the institution, to help gather and analyze data, and as a teaching device. A properly designed system should increase the accuracy and completeness of diagnoses and recordkeeping, in addition to providing invaluable information for research and program planning. These same systems are also applicable in the NH and in other LTC programs.

The computer also has value in assisting public policy and health-planning decision making. For example, microcomputer-based software has been developed to project demographic trends among the elderly (Davis 1983).

LTC Information Systems of the Future

Future information systems must move as quickly as possible to fully utilize computers. Previous reasons for not computerizing are becoming invalid as certain obstacles have been, or are being, gradually diminished. Fairly comprehensive systems can be purchased at reasonable costs even by one or several individuals. Rapidly retrievable inexpensive mass storage on hard disks or optical disks is possible. Problems of moving information from one computer system to another are being addressed.

At this time, there are no truly comprehensive, easy to use, flexible, readily modifiable computerized clinical information systems for LTC. Much of what is now being marketed provides specific solutions to limited problems for individual users, and much of what is now being accomplished is by individual or small groups of users.

Nevertheless, there are clearly many opportunities for individuals to use currently available tools to help solve certain problems. Furthermore, physicians should already be finding more ways for computers to help with medical care in LTC, because "Medical record systems are coming, and will unleash a host of 'intelligent' clinical support systems. It is not too early to be thinking about how to capture the various kinds of information you'll want to store in the system. Indeed, such considerations should influence current decisions about computer systems for order entry, billing systems, and so on, within an institution" (McDonald 1987, 8).

In just a matter of time, the encounter with the older patient and the use of the information derived from these encounters will be assisted at each step by computers.

Information Gathering

The patient will interact directly with the computer, not only by typing in answers at a keyboard, but also by touching the screen, pointing with a mouse, or talking directly to a computer with voice-recognition capabilities.

The physician will enter information directly from his history and physical examination into the computer. The computer will prompt him to use standard terminology, and will eliminate the use of confusing personal abbreviations, acronyms, and symbols. It will automatically code and organize patient problems and physician procedures for later production of a variety of reports. Through either direct links to other community facilities, or by the use of special laser-based recordings carried by patients, or both, physicians will have rapid access to any relevant information, past or present, on any patient from every source of care in the health care system.

Many objective data measurements now done manually will be obtained and analyzed automatically with instruments directly connected to computer input terminals; among them, blood pressure, pulse, temperature measurements, and electrocardiograms.

Patient Diagnosis and Treatment

Every aspect of patient diagnosis and treatment will also be assisted by the computer, which will suggest to the physician probable diagnoses for a given set of signs and symptoms, and the least costly tests most likely to help confirm diagnoses. Lab test results will be made immediately available to the physician via electronic mail. They will be filed in the patient's record, either automatically or after the physician has seen them, depending on physician choice. Abnormal test results will be automatically flagged until the physician reviews them, at which time they will be filed. The doctor will be able to have test results over a period of time plotted in a variety of graphs and charts that will make trends readily apparent.

If a physician wishes a consultation, both the request and the relevant patient information will be transmitted electronically. The consultant's report will be returned to the initiating physician by the same route.

Those desiring to search for information on their own will be able to do so without leaving their home, office, or clinic. Each physician will have access to the full range of medical literature and information sources. Current journals and many comprehensive medical and nonmedical data bases will be available by telecommunications. Many textbooks and journals will be available on (optical) laser disks, and will be updated easily for a fraction of the cost of printing new editions. In a matter of minutes, relevant material will be tracked and printed out.

Actual patient management will be facilitated in several ways. Iatrogenic events will be reduced as physicians are able to receive instant analysis of the probability of complications and adverse reactions to drugs, treatments, tests, or procedures. Management of a variety of specific problems, from renal failure to shock to arrhythmias, will be supported and enhanced by computer-based protocols and calculations.

The computer will usher in a whole new era in education and re-education. These will be self-paced, ongoing rather than intermittent, convenient, timely, and cost- and time-effective.

Triage and placement of the patient will be greatly facilitated by a system wherein the patient's needs can be entered into the computer and quickly matched with available community resources.

Output

Financial and business management of all kinds of medical practices will be facilitated by computer. Billing will be achieved quickly and accurately without the need to exchange paper forms. Electronic claims entry systems facilitate electronic transmission of Medicare Part B claims to Blue Cross and Blue Shield offices. Claims can be acknowledged within a short time, and payments made or denied within much less time. Predictions are that, within the next five years, most claims will be electronically processed.

It will be possible to easily sort any collection of patients into categories according to any desired characteristic, such as age, medications, risk factors, or diagnoses. Reporting of patient care, hospital utilization, outcome of treatment, and quality of care measures will all be readily attainable.

Patient appointments and recalls will also be facilitated. For example, if a physician needs to recall all those patients taking a certain drug, he can quickly bring up a list of all such patients, and generate a personalized form letter at the same time, in addition to having all the envelopes addressed, as well.

Prescriptions, medication directions, instructions on self-care, and education on medical problems can all be produced to benefit patients. These will be personalized and will offer the patient the kind of information that the physician, with his limited time, simply cannot provide. This may be in the form of text, charts, graphs, or a variety of entertaining and educational formats. In addition, the computer can assist in assessment of risk factors and recommendation of preventive measures.

In conclusion, clinical information management—largely ignored by physicians in the past in favor of other things considered to be more important to patient management—is fundamental to providing quality long-term care. And despite fears of potential dehumanization, computers actually offer the proven potential to unleash creativity, essentially by giving us the tools to turn ideas into reality. Much of this great potential is as an interactive tool to help us use information to care for patients most efficiently. By handling critical areas of information retrieval, storage, and analysis, computers allow the practitioner to spend more time interacting with the patient.

Physicians will have a key role in the design, use, and quality control of such systems, and must be involved in their testing and implementation. Without effective clinical information management, many goals in improving quality of care in the LTC system, especially in the NH, would be largely unattainable. With such systems, the possibilities will be limited only by our imagination.

Guidelines for Physician Input

Below are some suggested ways for physicians to create or refine LTC clinical information systems. Many LTC physicians will wish to be involved only as end users, rather than as participants in the design or implementation of such systems. Nevertheless, certain general principles apply in any setting, from the doctor's office to the nursing home:

- Review the strengths, weaknesses, and scope of the current information system, whether paper-oriented or computer-oriented, and the uses for that information.

- Analyze what is to be accomplished with changes or additions.

- Start with the *endpoint.*

- Decide which data are needed to produce reports.

- If computerized, consider the setting in which the computer is to be used.

- If computerized, review and select software appropriate for the desired tasks.

- If computerized, choose the hardware that will run that software.

- Design the information system manually.

- Test the design for accuracy and ease of use.

- Make necessary modifications.

- Be sure full, complete, and clear instructions for use exist for all levels of user.

Current system review. Because common practices are so habitual, it is often difficult to realize their strengths and weaknesses without stopping to assess them. Such appraisals should include, among other things, who collects and enters data; how the data are stored and retrieved; how much duplication of entry of identical information exists; how information is analyzed, retrieved, and verified; how and when information is transmitted to, and received from, others; and what kinds of backups and security exist to protect information,

or limit access. If computerized, is current storage capacity sufficient? How easy is the system to use? How dependable is the system? How flexible is it, and how easy is it to change data bases,
reports, or user entry screens? How well can the data be protected?
How often is the system out of commission?

Goals and objectives. Design of any information system starts with
paper and pencil, and a number of questions about what *must* be accomplished (billing, appointments, reports to health department,
quality assurance, etc.) and what one would *like* to accomplish (of-
fice-nursing home link, diagnostic assistance, patient education).

Working backwards from the endpoint. Unless we are just collecting
information for its own sake, we must first understand what we want
in the final analysis before we can detail what information needs to
be input initially. For example, if we want to know what information
we should collect about patient falls in a NH, we must first know
what we would like to see in the end report (breakdown by shift, by
unit, by patient, by medications in use, by nursing staff, etc.). We
also want to be able to modify our input or report forms easily, in
case we later decide to look at some other factors (incontinence,
mental status, or distance from bathroom). Similarly, if we want to
print out prescriptions after a patient visit, we must be sure to first
include all the necessary information in the data file as we record it.
The same is true for everything from billing to quality assurance.

Software review and selection. In most cases, one may choose from
two broad categories of software: those designed for a specific application (diagnostic assistance, patient and insurance billing,
patient appointments), and generic software that can be adapted for
specific needs (spreadsheets, data bases, and word processing
software). The choice depends on cost (specifically designed
software usually costs much more); time (generic software must be
set up from scratch to meet the specific need, and may or may not
be flexible enough to make the task comparatively easy); interest
(not all physicians would want to be involved in the setup); and applications (what will it all be used for); and ease of integration (how
readily the data from one program can be combined with the data
from others).

Choosing hardware. Hardware choices depend on software (can it run what one wants to use); cost of computer and such peripherals as printers and modems; capacity and speed (what may easily sort and search a list of 100 patients could bog down the system when the list grows to 2,000); ease of modification or repair; and quality and reliability. Unlike in the past, it is almost always possible to select a computer system that can be used for more than just specifically dedicated software.

System design. A system must blend together users and uses, and ensure accurate, reliable and complete entry, retrieval, and analysis of information. Technical understandings leading to successful design and implementation are beyond the scope of most physicians' knowledge base, and require consultative assistance.

Testing, verification, and implementation. This part can be more time-consuming than actual design, but is critical if accuracy, dependability, and ease of use are to be assured. Without these three things, an information system can become more of a liability than an asset.

Further information on clinical information system design, and computerization for physicians, is available in the sources listed below.

Appendix 9-A Sample Preprinted Information Form for
Use in the Nursing Home

PHYSICIAN PROBLEM LIST

Directions: Circle the appropriate diagnoses. Write additional clarifying information, where indicated, to the right of the diagnosis. Indicate, where possible, dates of onset or resolution.

DIAGNOSES	ICDA	ONSET DATE	RESOLVED DATE
Allergies, to:			
Alzheimer's Disease	331.0		
Amputation, site:			
Anemia, iron deficiency	280.9		
Anemia, unspecified type	285.9		
Angina pectoris	413.9		
Arrhythmia, cardiac, specifically:			
Arteriosclerotic cardiovascular			
disease	429.2		
Arthritis, rheumatoid	714.0		
Bronchitis, acute	466.0		
Cancer, breast	174.9		
Cancer, colon	153.9		
Cancer, esophagus	150.9		
Cancer, lung	162.9		
Cancer, pancreas	157.9		
Cancer, prostate	185		
Cancer, renal cell	189.0		
Cardiac arrest	427.5		
Cataract Surgery	13.69		
Cellulitis, site:	682.9		
Cerebrovascular accident/CVA/			
Stroke, acute	436		
Cerebrovascular accident/CVA/			
Stroke, old, with residua	438		
Chronic obstructive pulmonary			
disease	496		
Confusion	298.9		
Congestive heart failure	428.0		
Constipation	564.0		
Cystostomy	57.21		

DIAGNOSES	ICDA	ONSET DATE	RESOLVED DATE
Debility, generalized	799.3		
Decubitus ulcers, site(s):	707.0		
Degenerative joint disease (osteoarthritis), site:	715.9		
Dehydration	276.5		
Dementia, multi-infarct	290.4		
Dementia/Organic brain syndrome/ Chronic brain syndrome	290.0		
Depression, major, with psychotic features	296.2		
Diabetes mellitus, insulin dependent	250.00		
Diabetes mellitus, non-insulin dependent	250.01		
Diabetic neuropathy	250.6		
Diverticulitis	562.1		
Diverticulosis	562.10		
Edema, peripheral	782.3		
Fracture, femur, neck, closed	820.8		
Fracture, femur, other than neck, closed	821.0		
Gangrene, site:	785.4		
Gastrointestinal bleeding, site:	578.9		
Heart block, complete	426.9		
Hemorrhoids	455.6		
Hepatic failure	570		
Herpes Zoster	053.9		
Hypertension/HBP/High blood pressure	401.9		
Hypotension	458.1		
Hypotension, orthostatic	458.0		
Incontinence, urine	788.3		
Incontinence, bowel	787.6		
Intracerebral hemorrhage	431		
Ischemic heart disease	414.9		
Lethargy	780.7		
Leukemia	208.0		
Lymphoma	202.8		
Manic depressive illness	296.80		

DIAGNOSES	ICDA	ONSET DATE	RESOLVED DATE
Myocardial infarction, acute, site:	410.9		
Myocardial infarction, old	412		
Obesity, morbid	278.0		
Osteoporosis	733.00		
Pacemaker, permanent	37.77		
Pacemaker, temporary	37.70		
Parkinsonism/Parkinson's disease	332.0		
Peptic ulcer disease	536.9		
Peripheral vascular disease	443.9		
Personality disorder, type:	301.9		
Pneumonia, aspiration	507.0		
Pneumonia, site:	486		
Polymyalgia rheumatica	725		
Prostate, transurethral resection	60.2		
Renal failure, chronic	585		
Respiratory failure	799.1		
Seizure disorder, convulsive	345.1		
Seizure disorder, nonconvulsive	345.0		
Septicemia	038.9		
Transient ischemic attack/T.I.A.	435.9		
Others:			

Appendix 9-B A sample computerized data base
for an ambulatory geriatric center

Field	Field name	Type	Width	Description
1	NAME	Character	20	PATIENT NAME
2	SSN	Character	11	SOCIAL SECURITY NO.
3	DOB	Date	8	DATE OF BIRTH
4	SEX	Character	1	SEX: Male, Female
5	RACE	Character	1	RACE: White, Black, Hisp, Asian, Other
6	CLINDT	Date	8	DATE OF CLINIC

DIAGNOSES

7	DIAG1	Character	30	PATIENT DIAGNOSES (Max of 20) CORRECTED OR MODIFIED AS NEEDED DURING CLINIC VISITS (Max of 20)
8	DIAG2	Character	30	
9	DIAG3	Character	30	
.	DIAG ...	Character	30	
.	DIAG ...	Character	30	
.	DIAG ...	Character	30	
26	DIAG20	Character	30	
27	LASTVISIT	Date	8	DATE OF LAST CLINIC VISIT
28	MED RENEW	Date	8	DATE MEDICATIONS WERE LAST RENEWED

MEDICATION

29	MED1	Character	35	MEDICATIONS, DOSE, ROUTE & FREQUENCY PRESCRIBED (Max of 10)
30	MED2	Character	35	
.	.MED ...	Character	35	
.	MED ...	Character	35	
38	MED10	Character	35	

PRIOR HOSPITALIZATIONS

39	ADMDT1	Date	8	DATE OF LAST FIVE
40	DCDT1	Date	8	HOSPITAL ADMISSIONS
41	ADMDT2	Date	8	(MOST RECENT TO

Field	Field name	Type	Width	Description
42	DCDT2	Date	8	LEAST RECENT)
43	ADMDT3	Date	8	
44	DCDT3	Date	8	
45	ADMDT4	Date	8	
46	DCDT4	Date	8	
47	ADMDT5	Date	8	
48	DCDT5	Date	8	

VITAL SIGNS FROM PRIOR CLINICS

Field	Field name	Type	Width	Description
49	VITALDT1	Date	8	VITAL SIGNS FROM LAST
50	WT1	Numeric	3	FIVE PATIENT CONTACTS
51	PULSE1	Numeric	3	(MOST RECENT TO LEAST
52	RESP1	Numeric	2	RECENT)
53	BP1	Character	7	
54	BPSTAND1	Character	7	VITALDT = DATE
55	VITALDT2	Date	8	OBTAINED
56	WT2	Numeric	3	WT = WEIGHT
57	PULSE2	Numeric	3	PULSE = PULSE RATE
58	RESP2	Numeric	2	RESP = RESPIRATION
59	BP2	Character	7	BP = SITTING BLOOD
60	BPSTAND2	Character	7	PRESSURE
.	VITALDT ..	Date	8	BPSTAND = STANDING
.	WT ..	Numeric	3	BLOOD PRESSURE
.	PULSE ..	Numeric	3	
.	RESP ..	Numeric	2	
.	BP ..	Character	7	
.	BPSTAND ..	Character	7	
73	VITALDT5	Date	8	
74	WT5	Numeric	3	
75	PULSE5	Numeric	3	
76	RESP5	Numeric	2	
77	BP5	Character	7	
78	BPSTAND5	Character	7	
79	VST INT	Character	15	INTERVAL (Days) BETWEEN VISITS (Auto-Calc'd by UPDATE.PRG)

—— —— —— ——
< Recent .. visits .. Distant >

PATIENT CARE PLAN

Field	Field name	Type	Width	Description
80	PLAN1	Character	40	PLAN FOR CURRENT
81	PLAN2	Character	40	VISIT. THIS INFORMATION

Field	Field name	Type	Width	Description
82	PLAN3	Character	40	SUMMARIZES THE CARE
83	PLAN4	Character	40	PLAN. IT MAY BE UP-
84	PLAN5	Character	40	DATED FROM THE LAST
85	PLAN6	Character	40	VISIT JUST PRIOR TO
86	PLAN7	Character	40	CLINIC DAY. IMPROVES
87	PLAN8	Character	40	CONTINUITY OF CARE
88	PLAN9	Character	40	WITHIN A TEACHING
89	PLAN10	Character	40	HOSPITAL
				(Max of 10 lines)
90	FLU	Date	8	DATE OF FLU VACCINATION
91	PNEUMONIA	Date	8	DATE OF PNEUMOVAX VACCINATION
92	RESIDENCE	Character	1	PLACE OF RESIDENCE: H = HOME N = NURSING HOME F = FOSTER HOME D = DOMICILE O = OTHER
93	EXPIRED	Date	8	DATE PATIENT EXPIRED (For longitudinal follow-up)
94	DUMMY	Numeric	1	(UTILITY VARIABLE USED FOR TEMPORARY MANIPULATION)

Total Number of Spaces in File - > 1686

Reprinted by courtesy of Thomas A. Teasdale, M.P.H., Veteran's Administration Medical Center, Houston, Texas.

References

Batson, E. 1984. Data base management systems. *Postgraduate Medicine* 75(1):301-304.

Blum, B. 1986. *Clinical information systems.* New York: Springer-Verlag.

Bruer, J. T. 1984. Can computers take the drudgery out of medical education? *MD Computing* 1(3):29-33.

Chen, M. S., T. P. Housten, and J. L. Burson. 1984. Microcomputer-based health education in the waiting room: a feasibility study. *Journal of Family Practice* 18(1):149-150.

Davis, K. 1983. Health implications of aging in America. *Proceedings of 7th Annual SCAMC*, New York:IEEE Press, 688-691.

Duke University. 1978. *Multidimensional functional assessment: The OARS methodology.* Durham: Duke University Center for the Study of Aging and Human Development.

Ellis, L. B., and J. R. Raines. 1981. Health education using microcomputers: initial acceptability. *Preventive Medicine* 10:77-84.

Falcone, A. 1982. *Long-term care information system assessment process.* New York: Cornell Long-Term Care Assessment Training Center.

Falcone, A. 1983. Comprehensive functional assessment as an administrative tool. *Journal of the American Geriatrics Society* 31:642-650.

Jenkin, M. A., L. Cheezum, V. Essick et al. 1978. Clinical patient management and the integrated health information system. *Medical Instrumentation* 12:217-221.

Levinson, D. 1983. Information, computers and clinical practice. *Journal of the American Medical Association* 249:607-609.

McDonald, C. J. 1976. Protocol-based computer remainders, the quality of care and the non-perfectability of man. *New England Journal of Medicine* 295:1351-1355.

McDonald, C. J. 1987. Computer-stored medical records: their time is nigh. *MD Computing* 4(1):7-8.

McLean, J. C., and I. A. Kapkin. 1983. Negative impact of computerized record keeping in a psychiatric department. *Canadian Journal of Psychiatry* 28:114-116.

Morse, C. F. 1984. AMA data bases—instant access to medical information. *Physicians and Computers* 1(10):10-22.

Mula, R. 1984. Making molehills out of paper mountains. *Physicians and Computers* 1(12):10-13.

Reid, R. 1984. The physician in the information age: a reflection on microcomputing and the practice of medicine. *MD Computing* 1(1):66-71.

Schwartz, W. B. 1970. Medicine and the computer—the promise and problems of change. *New England Journal of Medicine* 283:1257-1264.

Slack, W. V. 1984. A history of computerized medical interviews. *MD Computing* 1(5):52-59.

Swerdlow, R. H. 1984. Information overload? Let a computer give you a hand. *Medical Economics* January 23: 123-130.

Wright, W. 1984. Dialing for data—telecommunications in the doctor's office. *Physicians and Computers* 1(2):8-13.

Yu, V., B. Buchanan, E. H. Shortliffe, et al. 1979. Evaluating the performance of a computer-based consultant. *Computer Programs in Biomedicine* 9:95-102.

For Further Reading

Geriatric Patient Assessment

Kane, R., and R. Kane. 1981. *Assessing the Elderly*. Lexington, Mass: D.C. Heath. A comprehensive review of the many scales and measuring tools for physical, mental, social, and functional evaluations of the elderly, plus a discussion of the problems of using such tools, and recommendations for selecting the right ones.

Israel, L., D. Kozarevic, and N. Sartorius (eds.), *Source Book of Geriatric Assessment* (2 vols.), New York: S. Karger. A collection of the forms and tools used in a wide variety of geriatric assessments.

Systems Analysis

Waters, K. A., and G. F. Murphy. 1983. *Systems Analysis and Computer Applications in Health Information Management*. Rockville, Md.: Aspen Systems. An excellent reference source, with many flow diagrams, charts, tables, and worksheets, for analyzing the flow of informaton and the systems needs of a program or institution.

Clinical Information Systems.

Blum, B. 1986. *Clinical Information Systems*. New York: Springer-Verlag. A very readable, informative, and nontechnical overview of the history of computers in medical care; explanations of the various aspects and considerations in clinical information systems; and a review and analysis of a number of different available systems.

Solomon, M. 1985. *Using Computers in the Practice of Medicine*. Englewood Cliffs, N.J.: Prentice-Hall. Focuses on selection, purchasing and use of computers in practice management and patient management, including a comprehensive example of a programmed medical history questionnaire and a very extensive reference section.

Various Clinical Applications

Society for Computer Applictions in Medical Care. 1986. *Annual Proceedings of the Symposium on Computer Applications in Medical Care*. The papers of the participants in one of the world's largest regular gatherings of those interested in using computers in medicine, are published following the annual meeting of the Society for Computer Applications in Medical Care, held each October or November. Applications described cover all aspects of medical practice, administration, teaching, and research. Available from IEEE Computer Society, P.O. Box 80452, Worldway Postal Center, Los Angeles, CA 90080.

Periodicals of Interest to Clinicians and Physician Administrators

MD Computing. Springer-Verlag Publications. P. O. Box 2485, Seacaucus, N.J. 07094. Articles on concepts and principles of medical computing, as well as specific software and applications. Useful for both interested practitioners and those interested in development and implementation.

Physicians and Computers. P&C Publications, 2333 Waukegan Road, Suite S280, Bannockburn, IL 60015. Practical applications and reviews of specific applications and software packages.

Chapter Ten

Geriatric Medical Education in Long Term Care

Susan G. Scholer, M.D. and Jane F. Potter, M.D.

Chapter Objectives

This chapter will:

- highlight the physician's personal educational needs in geriatrics
- outline the physician's role in the education of others (staff, patient, families)
- discuss quality assurance assessment as an educational tool in long-term care.

Introduction

Education in the LTC setting can greatly improve physician, nursing, and social care of the aged patient. The same knowledge base long-term care physicians use to deal with the problems of aging can be used to educate other health care professionals, administrators, and the community about special concerns in long-term care. The overall goal is to improve patient care, and thereby enhance quality of life.

Educational Needs of the LTC Physician

T. Franklin Williams, Director of the National Institute on Aging, said this about physician education in geriatrics: "The rapidly changing knowledge base in geriatrics makes it difficult to keep up. Our primary job as teachers is to understand and emphasize the unity of knowledge, and all of use have a responsibility to keep up to date on the full spectrum of knowledge" (Williams 1986, 51).

In the long-term care setting, physicians play a primary role in medical care of the elderly, and establish standards for health care maintenance. The problems affecting older adults can result from cumulative effects of normal aging as well as from pathological states. The diagnosis and treatment of illness superimposed on an aging body often requires specialized medical knowledge and skills. This knowledge should not be limited to geriatricians or those physicians who limit their practice to older adults. Rather, all physicians should be educated about the normal aging process, common medical problems seen in the elderly patient, and the socioeconomic factors that may complicate their care (Swanson 1979).

Pertinent areas of physician knowledge include the physiology of aging and of functional assessment and rehabilitation; identifying and treating common problems that contribute to the functional decline of the older person, such as depression, dementia, and incontinence; and the interdependence of the medical, social, and economic needs of the older patient.

Geriatrics and Gerontology

A thorough knowledge of age-related physiological changes is fundamental to avoid mislabeling normal aging as disease. These physiologic changes also influence the presentation of disease and the response to treatment, and can predispose individuals to certain complications (Rowe and Besdine 1982).

Two concepts should be kept in mind in any review of this topic. First, variability in test performance increases with age. As people grow older, they become less like each other. This is related to a number of factors, including other disease states, different life experiences or exposure, and various physiological changes. Second, function declines with age.

Some variables, however, do not change with age. Rowe and Minaker (1985, 938) in the *Biology of Aging* stated: "Perhaps the most important type of change that occurs with aging is no change at all." Nevertheless, certain predictable age-related changes *do* occur in the major organ systems, modified by a number of factors, including environment and inheritance (Finch, 1985; Andres, 1985).

Functional Assessment and Rehabilitation

As people grow older, they develop chronic diseases which can result in physical, psychological, or mental impairments. Conservative estimates suggest that 60 percent of adults aged 85 years of age and older have some activity limitation due to physical impairment alone (Rice 1982). Accordingly, physicians must be knowledgeable about assessment and rehabilitation.

The goal of functional assessment is to provide a comprehensive evaluation of the individual's physical, mental, and social abilities, and to then orient the care plan to maximize function. Careful and appropriate use of functional assessment has resulted in more appropriate care and less use of institutions as placement for the old (Williams 1973).

To be effective, the physician must accurately assess both what the patient is *capable* of doing and what the patient does. Subsequent measurement of the patient's physical status, his ability to perform self-care activities, his emotional and mental abilities, and his social interactions will prove invaluable when intervention becomes necessary. Assessment tools can measure all aspects of the patient's function. These tools are used to evaluate the patient's current status, to document any changes, and to predict outcomes, and are flexible enough to be used for both clinical and research purposes. The problems of an older patient, which seem overwhelming when reviewed as a whole, become more understandable and treatable when separated into distinct parts. Because the loss of function can have devastating consequences for the older adult, an organized approach to those problems causing loss of function is advised.

Since most disability conditions are age-related, knowledge of rehabilitative medicine is essential to the management of chronic diseases in the elderly. The increasing incidence of peripheral and cerebrovascular disease with age finds more patients with amputations and strokes, with residual hemiplegia and aphasia (Wade 1985). People with chronic cardiopulmonary and neurologic diseases are living longer because of improved medical and surgical treatment. The incidence of hip fracture increases with advancing age, and by extremely old age, one out of every three women and one out of every six men will have had a hip fracture (Melton 1983).

In contrast to the increasing number of patients requiring rehabilitation for treatment of chronic disabilities, there is a dearth of interest in this area by the medical community. Medical schools devote little, if any, time to this subject. The physician entering the field of long-term care today often finds himself poorly prepared in the areas of assessment of musculoskeletal function, gait analysis, rehabilitation for degenerative disease of the central nervous system, and knowledge about prescribing physical and occupational therapy.

Geropsychiatry

Psychiatric disorders, a common cause of disability in the elderly patient, are often overlooked or misdiagnosed. Also, the older population tends to under-utilize psychiatric services, possibly because of the patient's inability to recognize his psychiatric symptoms or because of the stigma attached to psychiatric care. Among the important topics here are depression, dementia, anxiety disorders, parkinsonism, and stroke (Butler 1977 and Goodnick, Gershon, and Salzman 1984).

Common Medical Problems of Old Age

Certain disabling conditions, common to the older population, are seen disproportionately in long-term care facilities. Urinary incontinence afflicts as many as half of all residents, and the recognition and therapeutic approach must be understood by physicians practicing in this setting (Williams 1982; Resnick 1985; Ouslander 1982). The prevalence of dementia is striking in nursing homes, where significant cognitive impairment affects up to 50-60% of the residents (Goodnick, Gershon, and Salzman 1984), and effective treatment and coping strategies are essential to the management of these disorders.

Medications and the Elderly

More chronic diseases unfortunately mean more prescription drugs for the elderly (Lamy 1980), including nursing home residents. It has been reported that more than 85 percent of elderly ambulatory patients and 95 percent of elderly institutionalized individuals receive drugs (Laventurier and Talley 1977). Twenty-five percent of these drugs may be ineffective or unneeded (Bergman 1975). The average number of prescription drugs per patient has been variously estimated to be 5-12, and the leading category of drugs prescribed for nursing home patients are tranquilizers (Lamy 1980). Because of pharmacokinetics and pharmacodynamic changes associated with aging, the older individual is at greater risk for drug toxicity, a risk increased by each additional drug in the regimen.

Drug reviews in nursing homes are vital to ensuring appropriate quality care. The physician should taper or discontinue those medications that should be used in smaller doses or not at all. For instance, the long-term use of Digoxin in the elderly has been extensively reviewed. A study by Wilkins and Khurana (1985) looked at the usefulness of maintenance Digoxin therapy in 19 nursing home patients with a normal sinus rhythm. Eighteen of these 19 patients tolerated discontinuation of the drug without adverse effects. The authors concluded that Digoxin therapy for episodes of congestive heart failure can very likely be discontinued after the primary problem has been resolved. The only contraindication to discontinuing the drug was a history of supraventricular tachycardia or atrial fibrillation with a rapid ventricular response.

Psychosocial and Economic Aspects of LTC

The medical and social needs of the older individual are intimately intertwined. A change in social status can precipitate a physical or psychiatric illness (e.g., the death of a spouse leading to depression). Changes in physical status can lead to social problems (such as stroke resulting in institutionalization). The physician involved in long-term care must not only become adept at recognizing specific medical problems of the older individual, but also at recognizing social solutions to such problems as loneliness, withdrawal, and weight loss. Because many physicians know very little about the social support systems in their community, these services tend to be under-utilized. Given the appropriate data base, LTC physicians can help ensure that their patient's social needs are appropriately assessed and provided for. Combined with the appropriate medical care plan, this approach should achieve the best functional outcome—the ultimate goal of long-term care.

Knowledge of financing of medical care in long-term care is also quite important because the LTC physician orders treatments and services which must be paid for. This is discussed further in Chapter 8.

LTC Administration

The administrator in the long-term care setting has unique responsibilities that require a combination of technical and human skills and a good deal of foresight. In the past, the roles of the administrator and the physician were kept separate, with a minimum of interaction between the two. The different perspectives were described by K.G. Gordon and R. Stryker (1983, 14): "Health care professionals have predominantly hospital-based educations and bring practices to the nursing home that are often counterproductive to the care of residents. On the other side, many nursing home administrators and owners have never been associated with hospitals, so they are unable to clearly explicate the desired differences."

Knowledge of administrative issues is critical for medical directors and principal physicians, and should be of more than passing interest to physicians who care for LTC patients. The administrator can educate the physician about the internal organization of the nursing home, and how best to accomplish his or her goals. By working together, the physician and administrator should be able to positively influence the quality of care provided by their facility.

Ethical Concerns in LTC

The physician trained to save lives is often faced with very different situations in the nursing home, where multiple chronic illnesses are the rule rather than the exception. Relevant issues include competence determinations, consent, patient choice, living wills, terminal care, and family involvement. Physicians must have an understanding of these ethical issues to provide appropriate care (see Chapter 12).

In ethical decision making, the physician has a responsibility to educate the patient, family, and nursing home staff about the implications of various therapeutic options (Purtilo 1984).

Research in LTC

Research in the LTC setting provides the physician with useful tools for education. Studies conducted within the nursing home can be used to improve the type and quality of care provided, and improve patient outcome. For instance, studies conducted on the patterns of infection within a facility can highlight problem areas and serve as a basis for further in-service training on infection control. Studies on the prevalence of urinary incontinence in an institution can provide a data base for intervention and nursing assessment of this problem. Likewise, surveys on personnel satisfaction can provide useful suggestions on how to improve job satisfaction of the nursing home professional and ancillary staff.

The Physician's Role as Educator

The physician plays a key role in education in long-term care. As an authority and resource on the medical problems of the aged, he or she should disseminate information to patients and their families, members of the nursing home staff, and, where present, to students and residents. Education in specific geriatric physical diagnosis should be a major responsibility of the LTC physician.

Rounds in the teaching nursing home should reflect the multidisciplinary team approach, cover difficult patient management cases and unusual or specific geriatric syndromes, and include the physician, director of nursing, pharmacists, and any trainees. This comprehensive team approach allows the physician to teach physical assessment and the art of history taking from the older patient at the bedside. Nurses should be asked to provide pertinent data on the patient and to offer their insights into particular problems. The pharmacist should be asked for information on the appropriateness of certain drugs and the potential for drug interactions. The physician should encourage this team decision-making process to facilitate an active exchange of ideas and to foster both an educational atmosphere and better patient care.

It is not practical to assume that such a comprehensive team-directed approach can be adopted by every physician who has patients in a long-term care facility. In a non-teaching nursing home, the medical director or house physician, because of his responsibilities, is best suited to initiate and direct such teaching rounds.

Geriatric grand rounds are monthly or bimonthly conferences dealing with particular geriatric topics or special case presentations. These grand rounds should take place in the nursing facility so that all members of the multidisciplinary team, and nursing home personnel, can attend.

Specialty rounds can be scheduled to make it cost-effective for the consultant, by waiting until there are at least two or three people for the consultant to see. The patient should be available for the consultant (i.e., not be engaged in an activity), and the attending physician should provide pertinent points of the medical history in a clear and concise note. After the patient is evaluated, the consultant should communicate his recommendations to the attending physician. Several subspecialty services are of particular importance in the institutional setting. Dermatologists can teach the principles of proper skin care for older people and early recognition of malignant skin changes. The orthopedist can illustrate the proper way to recognize and treat fractures. The neurologist can identify the subtle changes of stroke and can establish principles for the appropriate workup of gait disorders and mental status alterations. The general surgeon can recommend certain aspects of post-operative care. The consultant psychiatrist can offer tips on the early diagnosis and treatment of depression and can establish goals for the treatment of agitation and depression. The dentist can teach principles of oral hygiene and proper denture fit. Finally, the physiatrist can educate the staff on appropriate evaluation of the patient's rehabilitation potential and selection of treatment.

The physician in long-term care can also use his committee responsibilities as an avenue for teaching and as a way to influence institutional policy. The physician on the utilization review committee, which supervises the appropriateness of admissions and services for the individual patient's needs, can teach others about alternatives to institutional care and the availability of resources for the nursing home patient. The physician on the quality assurance committee, which formulates standards and criteria for assuring quality of care, can instruct staff in such issues as decubitus ulcers, incontinence, infection, medication side effects, immobility, dehydration, personal care activities, diet, nutrition, and the quality of environment. Out of such discussions should come periodic in-service training for nurses and aides to improve the management and monitoring of such conditions. Infection control committees review infection policies in the facility and establish standards to prevent and manage the spread of infections. Pharmaceutical committees survey drug prescribing policies and practices in the institution and recommend interventions in prescribing and monitoring to improve medical care and patient outcomes. In every case, the physician's understanding, interest, and willingness to teach others can have a major impact on institutional policy.

Education of Ancillary Personnel

Cooperation and input from nurse's aides, care staff members, dietitians, and activities personnel are essential for successful long-term care. They can and should contribute to the treatment plan for each resident. While aides comprise only 43 percent of the total nursing home staff, they deliver more than 90 percent of direct patient care (Waxman 1984), and are a major source of emotional support for the resident, often shouldering the responsibility of providing for the patient's personal, emotional, and even spiritual needs.

The annual turnover rate for nursing home aides is between 40 and 75 percent (Kasteler 1979). Nursing home wages are lower than those for jobs of similar description and responsibilities in hospitals or government institutions. Poor working conditions, inadequate training, heavy patient care activities, and excessive workloads contribute to the high turnover rate. Frequently, there are not enough professional nurses to provide backup and resources for the aides, increasing their frustration.

Despite the nurse's aide's critical role in providing quality care to nursing home residents, there are currently no federal regulations requiring them to complete a training course prior to working in a long-term care setting, and only 17 states currently require some type of training program. These requirements vary from a low of 20 hours in Nebraska to a high of 150 hours in California (Institute of Medicine 1986). LTC administrators are often reluctant to offer preservice training for aides because of the high turnover and the perceived lack of cost-effectiveness. However, a majority of nurse's aides cite a lack of training as their source of job dissatisfaction and a primary reason for leaving their jobs (Kraus 1974).

The physician or Medical Director can contribute to education of other LTC personnel by reviewing courses and content, and by providing ongoing information and instruction. This can be done in a variety of ways:

Orientation. Ideally, the physician would meet with new personnel during their orientation, but this is not usually possible. However, the physician can convey his philosophy and approach to the staff through a short handout or videotape that outlines important aspects of quality care, and reflects medical interest in providing such care.

In-service programs. The physician working in long-term care should assist the nursing home staff by participating in educational in-service programs on such topics as skin care, infection control, reporting of changes in a patient's condition, and dealing with hearing- and vision-impaired residents. The physician does not always need to be physically present, but may help identify appropriate educational materials such as slides, videotapes, articles, and printed lectures.

Workshops. Periodic workshops can be offered to aides and nurses, focusing on clinical problem areas and other major issues in geriatric care. The physician should suggest certain areas where additional training might prove beneficial, such as: managing behavioral problems in dementias, urinary incontinence, bladder training, and decubitus care.

Question and answer sessions. By being available to answer any questions that the staff may have with respect to patient care, the physician establishes himself as an additional resource and support person for the nursing staff and reinforces the importance of the nursing staff in patient care. Recognizing the contribution of nurse's aides, seeking their input, and answering their questions, can improve morale and reduce job dissatisfaction. Explaining treatment decisions helps nurses and aides participate more intelligently in patient care.

Patient Education

The physician has a responsibility to educate elderly patients. Indeed, for health care plans to work, the affected patients must, as best they can, understand them.

In the nursing home, the health care team has the opportunity to provide preventive, maintenance, and therapeutic care without the usual barriers facing physicians who care for the elderly. The pattern of physician travel to the residence of the institutionalized patient resembles the house calls of doctors of the past. However, many older persons are reluctant or unable to use available medical knowledge to their benefit.

Preventive medicine may seem less important in the face of complex medical problems, and it may be difficult for medical practitioners to focus on prevention when the care of the current problems is overwhelming. In addition, physicians remain skeptical about the benefits of denying the older patient the satisfaction of his bad habits, when the future benefits of changing them are uncertain. However, although studies are limited, some data suggest that old people can improve their function with certain interventions or lifestyle changes, such as diet, exercise, and behavioral modification. A study from Sweden demonstrated that previously untrained 70-year-olds could increase their maximum oxygen consumption markedly, increase their muscle strength, and lower their heart rates after exercise simply from the institution of a simple exercise regime (Anianson 1980). In addition, improvement in memory scores has been noted in elderly subjects after trials of mental stimulation (Langer and Rodin 1976). Preventive medicine can perhaps improve the *quality* of life, which depends on function, even if it does not *prolong* life.

The Patient as Decision-Maker

Research has demonstrated that well-informed residents equipped with the information necessary for problem-solving are better adjusted and more cooperative (Institute of Medicine 1986). It is therefore essential that the residents themselves receive necessary information for self-care. Practicing medicine in the chronic care setting takes on new dimensions as goals are adjusted from curative to supportive, including maintenance efforts.

When decisions need to be made about choices concerning care, the physician's responsibility is to educate the patient or proxy objectively about the nature of a disease or problem, so that the competent patient or proxy can make an informed decision regarding appropriate care.

Community Education

Public Education

The physician's role as educator does not stop with health care professionals, patients, and patients' families. With the surge of public concern for LTC issues, physician input is often solicited on quality assurance issues, ethical decisions, and reasonable expectations for patient care. Public education can be accomplished through lecture series or symposia conducted at hospitals, community centers, or LTC facilities, through print or mass media, or by testimony on pending legislation. In addition, the physician can serve as an advisor or board member of health or social organizations dedicated to the care of the elderly.

Professional Education

As a professional, the physician in long-term care can provide ongoing education for other physicians as well, either informally — through interactions regarding patients or consultations — or formally, by speaking at medical staff meetings, seminar series, or other continuing education programs.

Quality Assurance Assessment in Education

Quality assurance assessment is an important educational tool in long-term care. In every facet of long-term care, quality assurance should promote a critical awareness of patient condition and needs. The concept of quality assurance, covered in detail in Chapter 6, extends to quality assurance assessment for educational purposes and as a means for assuring that the resident in the LTC setting receives quality care.

Quality assurance assessment in long-term care is the process by which professionals obtain data on the health and status of the elderly, record this data in certain retrievable and repeatable ways, and develop strategies to correct any related problems (Institute of Medicine 1986). In addition, physician and trainee involvement in quality assurance assessment is an important means of learning geriatric medicine and physical diagnosis, and teaching it to other health care professionals, by comparing performance with those standards, and demonstrating associations between interventions and outcome. Finally, it provides an easily accessible data base for research purposes.

Among the pertinent areas of physician care are the history and physical, admissions and transfers to and from hospitals, ongoing evaluations, physician visits, and progress notes. For example, hospital transfers should be reviewed periodically. A pattern of recurrent hospital transfers should prompt an investigation into the circumstances leading to decompensation to determine if these transfers were appropriate. Appropriate staff education on early disease detection and observation for subtle changes in residents' status can then be implemented.

The physician's progress notes are vital components in providing quality care to the LTC patient, and should reflect the patient's physical, mental, and functional status, and identify short- and long-term treatment goals. Periodic reassessment of these observations should be documented in the physician and nurse notes as well, and successes and failures identified. With such a systematic approach to the patient's problems, the physician can use these notes to provide information for a patient data base in longitudinal follow-up studies. These notes should be clear enough so that other physicians (attendings, residents, and students) can understand treatment objectives and interpret results. They can also be used to educate nurses about the medical problems of their patients, and to help them understand why certain interventions were made. Physician problem lists and problem-oriented orders can be used similarly.

Excessive use of mood-altering drugs, including tranquilizers and antipsychotics, is considered to represent poor quality care (Institute of Medicine 1986). Monthly drug reviews by the physician or pharmacists should attempt to correlate the physician's problem list with the drug list. Each drug should be matched with the appropriate diagnosis; the use of those drugs without an appropriate diagnosis should be reconsidered. Start dates should be identified and reviewed periodically, and the number of medication errors associated with each drug should be noted. Such an organized plan of review assists in the educational process by facilitating a more thoughtful approach to prescribing for individual medical problems. Reports of adverse drug reactions can also educate physicians and nursing home staff, and influence future drug prescribing patterns.

High incidence of decubitus ulcers is another indicator of poor quality care. Protocols should be developed to document the presence or absence of skin breakdown, the severity of the breakdown, and the intervention used. Proper analysis of these records can determine which methods of therapy are most effective for different degrees of ulceration. Over time this information can help to ascertain whether the care in the facility is deteriorating, staying the same, or improving.

Since loss of function often precipitates institutionalization, assessment of functional impairment is very important to help gauge patient outcomes. The patient's ability to perform activities of daily living, his ability to ambulate and communicate, his need for skilled nursing care, and the presence or absence of urinary incontinence should all be measured. Patient performance and functional classification should be done according to measurable criteria (Kane 1981). Some states also use this information in making their Medicaid payment determinations. The data obtained from these assessment instruments can be used for longitudinal studies of patients, interventions, and outcomes. This information can subsequently be used to formulate guidelines for medical and nursing care, and by administration to help formulate institutional policy. For example, if incontinence is identified as a problem on an initial functional assessment, the treatment plan might include a toileting schedule (assuming all reversible or treatable conditions have been ruled out). On follow-up, resolution of the patient's incontinence with the toileting schedule would suggest that a routine toileting schedule may be an effective means of treating incontinence. If success can be demonstrated in other patients with similar characteristics, the information may be used to formulate institutional policy, such as ensuring an adequate number of staff to implement such a toileting schedule, or to try to convince third-party payors that such staffing levels are ultimately worthwhile.

Summary

Effective medical care of the aged in the LTC setting requires a special data base in geriatric medicine. Age-related changes in physiology predispose the older patient to chronic disease, which leads to functional impairment. Disability can also be accelerated by the presence of medical or psychiatric problems, such as depression or dementia, that often have subtle presentations in the elderly. Long-term care physicians must develop adequate strategies for detection and treatment of these disorders.

Physicians must also be aware of the role of social and economic factors in determining outcomes for LTC patients, and utilize the appropriate social support services.

The LTC physician also has the opportunity to be an educator as well as a care provider. He should disseminate information to patients, families, institutional staff, and professional trainees. Physician participation in such an educational network can help to assure better quality care and ultimately a better quality of life for the LTC resident.

References

Andres, R., E.L. Bierman, and W.R. Hazzard. 1985. *Principles of geriatric medicine.* New York: McGraw-Hill, Inc.

Anianson, A. et al. 1980. Physical training in old men. *Age and Aging* 9:186-187.

Bergman, H.D. 1975. Prescribing drugs in a nursing home. *Drug Intelligence and Clinical Pharmacy* 9:365.

Butler, R.N., and M.I. Lewis. 1977. *Aging and mental health.* St. Louis: C.V. Mosby.

Finch, C.E., and E.L. Schneider. 1985. *The handbook of the biology of aging.* New York: Van Nostrand Reinhold Company, Inc.

Goodnick, P., S. Gershon, and C. Salzman. 1984. Dementia and memory loss in the elderly. In *Clinical geriatric psychopharmacology,* edited by C. Salzman. New York: McGraw-Hill, Inc.

Gordon, K.G., and R. Stryker. 1983. *Creative long-term care administration.* Springfield, IL: Charles C. Thomas, Inc.

Institute of Medicine. 1986. Committee on nursing home regulation. *Improving the quality of care in nursing homes.* Washington, D.C.: National Academy Press.

Kane, R.A., and E.R. Kane. 1981. *Assessing the elderly: a practical guide to measurement.* Lexington: Lexington Books, D.C. Heath and Company.

Kasteler, J.M., et al. 1979. Personnel turnover: A major problem for nursing homes. *Nursing Homes* 28:20-25.

Kottke, F.J., G.K. Stillwell, and J.F. Lehman. 1982. *Krusen's handbook of physical medicine and rehabilitation.* Philadelphia: W.B. Saunders Company.

Kraus, E.A. 1974. Study reveals reasons for personnel turnover rates. *Modern Nursing Home* 11:48-50.

Lamy, P.P. 1980. *Prescribing for the elderly.* Littleton, MA: PSG Publishing.

Langer, E.J, and J. Rodin. 1976. The effects of choice and enhanced personal responsibility: A field experiment in an institutional setting. *Journal of Personality and Social Psychology* 34:191-198.

Leventurier, M.F., and R.B. Talley. 1977. The incidence of drug-drug interactions in a Medi-Cal population. *California Pharmacist* 20:18.

Melton, L.J., and B.L. Riggs. 1983. Epidemiology of age-related fractures. In *The osteoporotic syndrome*, edited by L.B. Avioli, New York: Grune and Stratton.

Ouslander, J.G., R.L. Kane, and I.B. Abrass. 1982. Urinary incontinence in elderly nursing home patients. *Journal of the American Medical Association* 248:1194-1198.

Purtilo, R.B. 1984. Social justice in chronic illness and long-term care. In *Geriatric Medicine*, edited by C.K. Cassel and J.R. Walsh. New York: Springer-Verlag, Inc.

Resnick, N.M., and S.V. Yalla. 1985. Management of urinary incontinence in the elderly. *The New England Journal of Medicine* 313:800-805.

Rice, D.P., and J.J. Feldman. Demographic changes and health needs of the elderly. Presented at the annual meeting of the Institute of Medicine, National Academy of Sciences, Washington, D.C. October 20, 1982.

Rowe, J.W., and R.W. Besdine. 1982. *Health and disease in old age.* Boston: Little, Brown and Company.

Rowe, J.W., and K.L. Minnaker. 1985. Geriatric medicine. In *Handbook of the biology of aging*, edited by C.E. Finch and E.L. Schneider. New York: Van Nostrand Reinhold Company.

Swanson, A.G. 1979. The role of geriatrics in medical education. *Journal of Medical Education* 54:59-61.

Wade, D.T., R.L. Hewer, and C.E. Skilbeck. 1985. *Stroke.* Chicago. Year Book Medical Publishers, Inc.

Waxman, H.M., E.A. Carner, and G. Berkenstock. 1984. Job turnover and job satisfaction among nursing home aides. *The Gerontologist* 24:503-509.

Wilkins, C.E., and M.S. Khurana. 1985. Digitalis withdrawal in elderly nursing home patients. *Journal of the American Geriatrics Society* 33(12):850-851.

Williams, M.E., and F.C. Pannil. 1982. Urinary incontinence in the elderly. *Annals of Internal Medicine* 97:895-907.

Williams, T.F. 1986. *Aging Research and Training News* 9:49-56.

Williams, T.F., et al. 1973. Appropriate placement of the chronically ill and aged: A successful approach by evaluation. *Journal of the American Medical Association* 226:1332.

For Further Reading

Periodicals

The Journal of the American Geriatrics Society. Elsevier Science Publishing Co., Inc. 52 Vanderbilt Ave., New York, NY 10017. This monthly journals deals primarily with clinical issues and has sections for original articles, clinical experience, law and public policy, and monthly book reviews. Emphasis is on clinical research.

The Journal of Gerontology. Gerontological Society of America, 1411 K Street, N.W., Suite 300, Washington, D.C. 20005. This bimonthly journal includes sections on biological, psychological, social sciences, and clinical medicine. A section of book reviews and book briefs is also included.

The Journal of Chronic Diseases. Pergamon Journals, Inc., Maxwell House, Fairview Park, Elmsford, NY 10523. This monthly international journal deals with the problems and management of chronic illnesses in all age groups. The majority of the articles deal with research (methods, content, or both) in chronic disease.

The Gerontologist. Gerontological Society of America, 1411 K Street, N.W., Suite 300, Washington, D.C. 20005. This bimonthly journal reports mainly on social and health services research. *The Gerontologist* also provides book reviews on gerontology and audiovisual reviews.

The Clinical Gerontologist. Haworth Press, Inc., 75 Griswold Street, Binghamton, NY, 13904. This quarterly journal of aging and mental health focuses on psychological and psychiatric topics. An extensive book review section is included in this journal, as well as a brief section devoted to media and software review.

Geriatric Consultant. Medical Publishing Enterprises, 15-22 Fair Lawn Avenue, Fair Lawn, NJ 07410. This bimonthly journal offers concise reviews of important clinical topics in the care of the aged. A geriatric update with highlights on upcoming events and professional meetings is also provided.

Age. Journal of the American Aging Association, 42nd and Dewey Avenue, Omaha, NE 68105-1063. Published quarterly, this journal offers rapid publication for papers pertinent to biomedical aging research, primarily on basic science topics.

Geriatrics. Modern Medicine Publications, Inc., 7500 Old Oak Boulevard, Cleveland, OH 44130. This monthly publication addresses the clinical management of the elderly patient. A monthly geriatric quiz and abstract section is included; it also contains highlights of clinical presentations at major national meetings.

Journal of Geriatric Psychiatry. International Universities Press, Inc., 315 Fifth Avenue, New York, NY 10016. Published semiannually, this journal is the official publication of the Boston Society for Gerontologic Psychiatry. Several major topics are addressed in each issue with case studies and a book review section.

Age and Aging. Baillere Tindall, 1 Vincent Square, London, SWIP2PN. Published bimonthly, this is the official journal of the British Geriatrics Society and addresses gerontology and geriatrics, especially the clinical, epidemiological and psychological aspects of medicine in old age.

Textbooks

Principles of Geriatric Medicine. 1984, Andres R., E.L. Bierman and W.R. Hazzard. new York: McGraw Hill, 992 pages. This book, prepared under the sponsorship of the Gerontological Society of America, is a comprehensive review of information in disciplines relevant to the geriatric practitioner. This first part of the book deals with biological, behavioral, and social aspects of gerontology. Normal and pathological changes with aging are evaluated in detail in the section entitled "Disease of the Organ Systems." The book closes with chapters on terminal care and the prospects for the future of geriatric medicine. This is an excellent reference work.

Geriatric Medicine. 1984, Cassel C.K. and J.R. Walsh. New York: Springer-Verlag, 1168 pages. This is a comprehensive two-volume set with up-to-date information on principles of geriatrics and gerontology. Volume I is entitled *Medical, Psychiatric and Pharmacological Topics* and reviews the fundamentals of geriatric medicine with emphasis on selected geriatric medical disorders. An enlightening section on psychiatric disorders and pharmacologic dilemmas in the geriatric patient is a highlight of this volume. Volume II is entitled *Fundamentals of Geriatric Care* and deals with the demographics and social aspects of aging. Excellent chapters address elder abuse, drug abuse, terminal care, sexuality, and spiritual care. The third part of this volume deals with legal and research issues in geriatric medicine. An "Appendix of Resources for the Health Care of the Elderly Persons" closes this volume.

Annual Review of Gerontology and Geriatrics. This is an annual review of relevant geriatric topics published by Springer Publishing Company, Inc. Each year, reviews are undertaken in a specific field of geriatrics and gerontology. In alternate years, volumes address either biomedical or psychosocial topics. Selected topics are reviewed in depth. For example, in 1984, Volume 4 contains sections on podiatry, oral care, aging, and neoplasia and psychomotor performance with aging.

Geriatric Medicine Annual. Published by Medical Economics Publishers, Oradell, NJ 07649, this is an annual review of clinical geriatrics subjects and controversies in geriatric medicine, especially for the practicing primary care internist and family practitioner with a significant elderly patient population.

Essentials of Clinical Geriatrics. 1984, Kane R.L., J.G. Ouslander, and I.B. Abrass. New York: McGraw-Hill, 369 pages. This book, published under the direction of the American Geriatrics Society, is prepared for the primary care clinician and addresses topics such as history taking in the elderly, principles of the management of dementia, falls and rehabilitation, and sensory impairment.

Care of the Geriatric Patient in the tradition of E.V. Cowdry. 1983 (6th edition), Steinberg, F.U.. St. Louis: C.V. Mosby, 651 pages. This book deals primarily with medical topics in geriatric care, but also includes a section on nursing and home care. An excellent chapter on rehabilitation is also contained in this volume.

Clinical Aspects of Aging. 1983 (2nd edition), Reichel W. Baltimore: Williams and Wilkins, 642 pages. A practical volume that includes over 40 authors discussing the foremost medical, psychiatric, social, and ethical problems of the elderly patient. Perspectives on sexual intimacy in older adults, professional nursing care of the aged, and long-term care options are highlights.

Prescribing for the Elderly. 1980, Lamy P.P., Littleton, Mass.: PSG Publishing Company, 696 pages. This book deals with pharmacologic principles and practices pertinent to the elderly population. Topics such as drug sensitivity, altered pharmacokinetics, and adverse effects of drugs in the aged are explored.

Improving the Quality of Care in Nursing Homes. 1986. The Committee on Nursing Home Regulation, Institute of Medicine. Washington D.C.: National Academy Press, 415 pages. This is a landmark volume which will be influential in future regulation and policy making in this area. Chapters on regulatory criteria, performance monitoring, and quality assessment and assurance are highlights of this book. Practical suggestions on federal, state, local, and institutional policies are offered. Extensive appendices of statistics on nursing homes by state are included.

Conferences in Geriatrics and Gerontology

Continuing education opportunities exist for the long-term care physician in the form of courses in geriatric medicine. Every year, a diverse selection of conferences is offered. A listing of some of these follows:

1. The American Geriatrics Society and American Federation of Aging Research jointly sponsor an annual four-day meeting.

2. The annual meeting of the Gerontological Society of America, for five days each November.

3. Intensive Course in Geriatric Medicine offered annually (usually in January) by the American College of Physicians.

4. Recent Advances in Geriatric Care offered annually in October by the Division on Aging, Harvard Medical School.

5. Clinical Management of the Elderly Patient for the Practicing Physician and other Health Professions – an annual conference (usually in March) cosponsored by the American Geriatrics Society and the Health and Education Council and held in Orlando, Florida.

6. Annual meeting of American Medical Directors Association, each fall.

Associations

American Aging Association (AGE), College of Medicine, University of Nebraska, Omaha, NE 68105. Consists of laymen and scientists in the biomedical field conducting aging studies with the goal of slowing down the aging process. This association also informs the public on aging research and how to live long, healthy lives.

American Federation for Aging Research (AFAR), 335 Madison Avenue, New York, NY 10017. This group consists of physicians or scientists involved in research in aging or associated diseases. Its purpose is to stimulate and fund research on aging and to award research grants.

American Foundation for Aging Research, 117 Tucker Hall, University of Missouri, Columbia, MO 65211. Its purpose is to support research and educational opportunities for the study of age-related disease and the biology of aging. It also awards undergraduate scholarships, graduate fellowships and postgraduate fellowships.

American Geriatrics Society (AGS), 770 Lexington Avenue, Suite 400, New York, NY 10021. This is a society of health professionals, mainly physicians, interested specifically in the clinical and research problems of the aged. Membership benefits include subscriptions to the monthly journal and newsletter.

Gerontological Society of America (GSA), 1411 K Street NW, Suite 300, Washington, DC 20005. This group includes professionals from all disciplines interested in improving the well-being of older people by promoting and publishing scientific study of the aging process. Membership benefits include subscriptions to the *Journal of Gerontology, The Gerontologist* (a newsletter), and reduced rate for the annual conference.

American Medical Directors Association (AMDA), 1200 15th St., N.W., Washington, D.C. 20005. This group consists of physicians and allied health personnel providing care in nursing homes and other LTC facilities. This group sponsors continuing medical education in geriatrics. It also publishes an AMDA newsletter three times yearly.

International Association of Gerontology, Duke University Medical Center, Durham, NC 27710. Promotes gerontologic research in biologic, medical, and social fields, fosters cooperation between international gerontologic societies, and sponsors international congresses and regional meetings.

National Geriatrics Society (NGS), 212 W. Wisconsin Avenue, 3rd Floor, Milwaukee, WI 53203. This group consists of staff from various long-term care institutions—public, voluntary, and proprietary. It promotes maintenance of proper operational standards and qualified administration of facilities caring for the aged.

National Association of Area Agencies on Aging, 600 Maryland Avenue, SW, West Wing, Suite 208, Washington, DC 20024. Members of this association are the area Agencies on Aging established under the Older Americans Act of 1965. This group promotes a national policy on aging and communication among the members of the network on aging.

National Association of State Units on Aging (NASUA), 600 Maryland Avenue S.W., Suite 208, Washington, DC 20024. This is a public interest organization which provides information and technical assistance to State Units on Aging. It also distributes information on social policy to respond to the needs of older adults.

Regional Organizations. These organizations sponsor annual conferences and periodic special conferences. Their appeal is to interdisciplinary groups of health professionals, educators, and service providers:

- *Mid-America Conference on Aging* - 9400 State Avenue, Kansas City, Kansas 66112.

- *American Society on Aging* - (founded in 1954 as Western Gerontological Society) 883 Market Street, Suite 516, San Francisco, California 94103.

- *Northeastern Gerontological Society* - c/o Rhode Island College Gerontology Center, 600 Mt. Pleasant Avenue, Providence, RI 62908.

- *Southern (Southeastern) Gerontological Society* - University of Georgia. Department of Adult Education, 420 Tucker Hall, Athens, Georgia 30602.

- *Southwestern Society of Aging* - Box 36445, Dallas, Texas 75235.

Newsletters

Gerontology News. Gerontological Society of America, 1411 K Street NW, Suite 300, Washington, DC 20005. Information on public policy, program guides to federal funding, annual meeting news, and a job clearinghouse are included.

American Geriatrics Society Newsletter. American Geriatrics Society, 10 Columbus Circle, New York, NY 10019. Policy statements, meeting highlights, committee reports, fellowship reports, and members in the news are featured.

Topics in Geriatrics. Department of Psychiatry, Massachusetts General Hospital, Boston MA. Correspondence: Managing Editor, *Topics in Geriatrics,* PSG Inc., 545 Great Road, Littleton, MA 01460. Briefly reviews clinical topics and research in geriatrics with references to current literature. Offers concise summaries on pertinent topics.

Geriatric Medicine Letter. The Center for Aging and Adult Development, New York Medical College, Valhalla, NY 10595. Quarterly newsletter. Discusses one or several topics in depth per newsletter.

Aging Services News. Business Publishers, Inc., 951 Pershing Drive, Silver Springs, MD 20910. Biweekly newsletter. Provides updates on federal legislation pertinent to funding for aging services and information on privately funded programs.

Aging Research and Training News. Business Publishers, Inc., 951 Pershing Drive, Silver Spring, MD 20910. Monthly newsletter devoted to research and educational issues in geriatrics and gerontology. Grant program announcements and award information are listed.

Other Sources for Geriatric Information

Index Medicus. This is the major index to all medical periodical literature. The new series began in 1960. The index appears monthly and cumulative annually. Published by the National Library of Medicine, it indexes over 2500 journals in medicine and health-related topics. Further information can be obtained from the National Library of Medicine, Building 38A, Rm. 4N421, Bethesda, MD 20894.

Medline. This is a computerized searchable data base that is equivalent to the following indexes: *Index Medicus, Index to Dental Literature* and the *International Nursing Index.* This data base uses the same subject categorization as does the *Index Medicus* and is available at regional medical libraries. Software packages for microcomputers (BRS colleague, Grateful Med, etc.) are available and sufficiently inexpensive to make this technology accessible in the home or office.

Health, Planning and Administration Line. This is equivalent to the *Hospital Literature Index.* This is a joint data base between the National Library of Medicine and the American Hospital Association (840 North Lake Shore Drive, Chicago, IL 60611). Information concerning health care issues, hospitals, and other institutions and topics dealing with administration are available.

Chapter Eleven

Legal, Policy, and Regulatory Issues

Kay E. Jewell, M.D.

Chapter Objectives

This chapter will:

- Summarize the general legal principles relevant to the LTC physician

- Examine liability concerns of the medical director

- Consider legal elements of the medical director's contract

- Provide an overview of the legal foundation of the medical director's responsibilities

- Present legal considerations in the patient decision-making process

- Consider other significant legal issues of LTC practice

- Discuss the regulatory process in the nursing home and pertinent regulations and rules

Both legislation and regulation increasingly affect all aspects of medical care, from mandating services and standards to determining eligibility for payment. Neither medical direction nor the practice of LTC medicine can be considered apart from applicable laws and regulations.

As Kapp and Bigot (1985) note, law may be either constitutional, statutory, administrative, or common. All four forms are relevant to physicians and medical services.

Constitutional law refers to the organization, plan, and principles of government. The individual right to privacy, which forms the basis of legal protection for the individual exercise of the right to refuse medical care, is an example of a right derived from constitutional law.

Laws enacted by legislatures (*statutory law*) are termed statutes on the federal and state levels, and ordinances or codes on the local level. "Statutory law must be written, expressed in general language, and promulgated or published so that affected individuals are put on notice regarding what is expected of them. A statute may be addressed either to the entire society or to a specified group" (Kapp and Bigot 1985, 8). Laws may not violate the constitutions which empower the legislatures that enact them. Judicial decisions which interpret the meaning of specific laws, or parts of those laws, become part of statutory law. Medicare and Medicaid laws are examples of statutory law.

Administrative laws are rules, regulations, or orders enacted by administrative agencies, part of the executive branch of government, as a result of general instructions or powers granted by legislatures. Administrative laws fill in the details of expected actions that statutory laws usually only address in generalities.

For example, a state law may require that NHs should provide quality care. The state department of licensing and certification then must create rules and regulations that explain what this means and what NHs must do to comply with those standards. Failure to conform to regulations is therefore considered a violation of the law.

Finally, *common law* is made by judges or courts and is based on social custom, tradition, history, usage, or legal or judicial precedent.

All four forms of law may also be either federal, state, or local. All levels of government have both *police powers*, to protect general health, safety, welfare, and morals; and *benevolent powers* to protect the welfare of those who cannot or will not protect their own interests. An example of police powers is state support for appropriate commitment of the mentally ill. Benevolent powers are exemplified by statutes related to provision of protective services for those who cannot manage or care for themselves.

Health law may be further classified according to five different but related functions (Kapp and Bigot 1985):

- prohibition of conduct injurious to health, such as sanitation laws, or laws requiring wearing of seat belts

- authorization of programs and services to promote health, such as laws establishing programs of care for the elderly

- provision for public financing of health care, such as Medicare and Medicaid

- regulation of the production of resources of health services, such as health manpower and state certificate-of-need laws

- surveillance over quality of care.

The LTC physician, especially, the medical director, is most concerned with statutory and administrative law, and somewhat with constitutional law. This chapter will focus on important statutory and administrative issues. Other chapters consider various aspects of patient care, as required by law and regulation, including:

- bylaws requirements to ensure physician compliance (Chapter 3)

- policies and procedures for various physician practices (Chapter 4)

- quality assurance and utilization review mechanisms (Chapter 6)

- financial and reimbursement issues (Chapter 8)

- maintenance of adequate information (Chapter 9)

- determining patient competence and deciding on care choices (Chapter 12)

- managing trainees and patient rights in the teaching NH (Chapter 13).

Liability of Medical Directorship

It is important to distinguish between negligence and liability, and problems discovered under quality assurance or peer review. In contrast to the latter, "negligence" and "liability" issues must be resolved within the legal system. Negligence refers to conduct performed without due care under specific circumstances. Legal action regarding alleged negligence is usually initiated by a patient or family and is specific to events in one case. Proving negligence requires proof of four key elements:

- a duty to care existed

- a breach of duty (i.e., the duty is not satisfied or fulfilled)

- causation (i.e., an injury was sustained)

- damages (i.e., the injury suffered was the direct result of the failure to act in accordance with duty owed the injured party).

Usually a jury decides if the challenged behavior has met the standards expected of a reasonable person in similar circumstances.

On the other hand, quality assurance and peer review refer to evaluations of all care delivered within a facility, using individual cases and review and comment made by professional colleagues at a local or state level. The actions and consequences of such reviews, defined by bylaws or policies, may range from an educational program to the denial of privileges or the reporting of the individual practitioner to the state medical examining board for further review.

Peer review also refers to review by physicians. It may occur as part of a survey or inspection of care at a state level, or as a Peer Review Organization (PRO) review as defined in federal rules and regulations.

In this section, we will focus on the legal aspects of liability. To date, there have been no reported cases of a medical director charged with liability or neglect. But with the growth of the long-term care (LTC) industry and the increasing involvement of corporations in nursing home (NH) care, the medical director must be aware of the potential issues.

Facility responsibility

There are four ways in which a facility may be liable for negligence.

Failure to retain a medical director. The facility has a general obligation to provide coordinated and quality care commensurate with individuals' needs, and to protect patients from harm by careless physicians, nurses, and other professional staff. A key issue is whether this duty requires a medical director. While legal precedent and experience supports the position of a facility's duty, the only statutory or licensure requirements for a medical director are for those facilities which voluntarily participate in Medicare.

Selection of a Medical Director. Generally, anyone with a valid medical license to practice in that state may serve as a medical director. A facility should select a competent and "suitable" person. To do otherwise is to place patients at an unreasonable risk of harm, and therefore create a greater liability risk. (See Chapter 4 for a discussion of the qualifications and background of a medical director.)

Review of performance. The facility must assess a medical director's performance, and take action in the event of inadequate performance or inappropriate conduct. Failure to do so increases liability risks.

Vicarious liability. The *"respondeat superior"* doctrine holds an employer responsible for an employee's negligent conduct, if the negligent conduct occurred while the employee was acting in the course of and within the scope of employment.

The liability of facilities for negligence is a relatively new legal concept, and such liability depends on whether the medical director is an employee of the facility. In determining this, the courts consider: (1) the amount and nature of control exercised by the employee and employer; (2) the professional status of the employee or the activity; (3) where the work is done; (4) the ownership of the equipment used; (5) the method of compensation; (6) the opportunity for profit; and (7) pertinent customs in the field.

Medical Director's Responsibility

There are several distinct areas of individual liability for medical directors, including personal negligence, responsibility as "captain of the ship," and intentional torts.

Personal negligence. While medical directors have faced negligence charges as practicing physicians, negligence as an administrator is not yet a legal issue, but may become one as expectations increase.

Liability resulting from application of the <u>respondeat superior</u> <u>doctrine</u>. Though the facility may be held responsible for an employee's negligence, the wrongdoer may be legally obligated to the employer for losses resulting from his negligent conduct. If the medical director is negligent, the facility may recover damages.

Intentional torts. A tort is a wrongful act which results in injury to another person, or another person's property or reputation. An intentional tort results when a person intentionally commits a wrongful act. For example, certain actions by a medical director to restrict the scope of a physician's practice, or to deal with inadequate care, might be challenged on the grounds of intentional interference with the business of the attending doctor-patient relationship—as an invasion of privacy or as a breach of confidentiality. Protection against such charges can be enhanced by adequate and appropriate policies, procedures, and bylaws, evenly and fairly applied to all physicians.

Liability Insurance

In the past, physicians have sometimes assumed erroneously that their current malpractice insurance will also cover them as a medical director, only to find that their insurance carrier may make a clear distinction between actions taken in treating patients, and those taken in an administrative capacity. A second assumption, that they are covered by a facility's insurance, may not be true unless it is specifically agreed to under contract.

One consideration of personal liability insurance is the types of risk to which the medical director's duties expose him (as described above). A second concern is that of representation by the insurance carrier in case a claim is filed. Since insurance companies generally assume control over the defense in case of a lawsuit, the medical director should know if he can choose other representation, if desired. A third consideration is the amount of coverage to be obtained, since the company is only responsible to the limits of the policy. Considering recent trends, it would be wise to carry a $1,000,000 per occurrence/$3,000,000 total occurrences minimum.

A final choice is between insurance and an indemnity contract. Insurance is a contract whereby one party agrees to compensate the other for a specific loss due to specified perils. In health insurance, for example, the company pays for certain defined coverage for hospitalization or procedures. Under an indemnity contract, one party agrees to indemnify the other against loss or damage arising from some act or from the claim or demands of a third party. In health insurance, for example, the company pays the individual a set amount according to an agreement if the individual requires hospitalization or undergoes a procedure.

The Medical Director's Contract

In the past, service as a medical director was often voluntary. Today, it is much more important for physicians who serve in this capacity to have a written contract to help both sides focus on the expectations and mutual responsibilities. It may be as simple or as complicated as necessary (See Tessaro [1974] and Chapter 4).

Duties of the Medical Director

This section focuses on the legal aspects of several major duties of the medical director which have been discussed earlier (see Chapters 3 and 4).

Medical Staff Bylaws

One of the medical director's major tasks is to develop the Medical Staff bylaws. Legally, the process is similar to that used for hospital staff. Bylaws constitute a legally enforceable agreement between the facility and attending physicians. Since changes in bylaws require formal approval according to authorized procedures, it is advisable to keep the medical staff application, duties and responsibilities, and any other physician agreements as separate processes and forms.

Once bylaws are developed and approved by the medical staff, they should be reviewed and approved by the governing board, after which they become the standard by which physicians services will be reviewed.

Credentialling procedure. One of the most neglected areas is the processing of the application, including the verification of the information and a review by a credentialling committee. In the 1980 case of *Johnson v. Misercordia*, the court determined that the facility must use reasonable care to evaluate its applicants and to request information about sanctions or denied privileges elsewhere.

Responsibilities of the attending physicians. Any designation of physician privileges and requirements must conform to certain state and federal requirements, including those governing admission, the history and physical, and the physician plan of care and its review, and scheduled patient visits. Consequences of failing to meet these requirements should be specifically defined.

The Conditions of Participation for physician services, and the interpretive guidelines issued by the Department of Health, Education, and Welfare (HEW) Office of Long Term Care in 1974, which remain in effect at this writing, specifically address attending physician responsibilities in facilities receiving Medicare and Medicaid. Briefly, they require that:

- the patient is admitted by order of a physician and remains under a physician's care

- prior to or at the time of admission, patient information should include current medical findings, diagnoses, and orders from a physician for immediate care of the patient

- at the time of, or within 48 hours of, admission, information about the rehabilitation potential of the patient and a summary of prior treatment shall be made available to the facility

- patients shall be under the supervision of a physician who shall prescribe a planned regimen of total care based on the medical evaluation of the patient's immediate and long term needs, including medications, treatments, rehabilitative and specialized rehabilitation services, diets, precautions for activities, and plans for continuing care and discharge

- the medical evaluation should be based on a physical examination done within 48 hours of admission (if it has not been performed within 5 days prior to admission), which should pay special attention to sight, oral, speech, hearing and foot problems, and emotional and social adjustment

- each physician shall make arrangements for the medical care of his patients in his absence

- in the first 90 days after admission, the patient is seen by the attending physician at least once every 30 days, and that during a visit, the physician should review the total program of care, including the medications and treatments, write and sign a progress note, and sign all orders

- after the first 90 days, an alternate schedule for physician visits may be adopted, where the attending physician determines that the patient's condition does not require every 30-day visits, and justifies this in the medical record. The alternate schedule may not exceed every 60 days

- this visit schedule should apply to all patients in the facility, including private-pay patients, although a private patient may refuse such services without creating a deficiency for the facility.

Additional conditions may be added by individual state regulations.

Interpretive guidelines require a statement of those actions to be taken in the event that these requirements are not met. The medical director should notify a facility administrator of such delinquency and should take steps personally to correct the noncompliance, first informally by communication with the attending physician. If informal action is ineffective in obtaining compliance, the administrator should inform the physician in writing of the facility's policy concerning patient supervision, the facts of the delinquency and action pending continued failure to provide timely visits. Attending staff should also be notified of any reports of reviewing agencies, especially when these include physician services.

For details of the Conditions of Participation, see *Medical Directorship* (1986).

Due Process. A due process procedure should be developed and described in the bylaws for the attending physician, including five basic components:

- Standards by which the individual will be judged must be known.

- The individual must be informed formally and adequately of any wrongful or inappropriate conduct.

- Notice and opportunity must be given to attend a hearing on the matter.

- The individual has the right to be present and participate in the presentation of evidence reviewed at the hearing.

- The individual has the right to appeal an adverse finding.

Patient Care Policies and Procedures

The medical director is legally responsible for two areas of policies and procedures: patient care policies for the facility, and those specific to the medical staff and its function.

For example, the single issue of alternate coverage for an attending physician would require policies for the *patient* (e.g., any patient agreement on admission should include the facility's policy on this topic); *nursing* (their actions in the event the attending and the alternate physicians are not available); the *medical director* (how he will be involved); and finally the *medical staff* (the attending's responsibility to designate an alternate provider and the procedure if that person is not available).

The Conditions of Participation require patient care policies and procedures to include the following:

- admission, transfer, and discharge policies and categories of patients accepted and not accepted

- physician services

- nursing services

- dietetic services

- rehabilitative services

- pharmaceutical services

- diagnostic services

- care of patients in emergencies, including critical illness, communicable diseases, and mental illness
- dental services
- social services
- patient activities
- medical records
- transfer agreement
- utilization review
- personal and property rights.

These must be written and available on request to anyone, including patients, family, and the public. They are to be developed by the medical director or the organized medical staff, in conjunction with registered nurses and representatives of administration and other clinical services. They must be reviewed by the medical director and revised as necessary, at least annually. Minutes of meetings should reflect such activity.

Medical record documentation, confidentiality, and patient access. Some important specific legal requirements for medical records exist. The law views medical record documentation as a reflection of quality of patient care (Kapp and Bigot 1985, 43). The medical record also has great importance as a document in court, and for payment, or denial of payment, by third-party payors; review of care in cases of malpractice actions; claims for disability benefits under public entitlement programs; and personal injury lawsuits. Some record keeping and documentation requirements are mandated by federal Medicare and Medicaid statutes and regulations. The recommendations in Chapter 9 for information and documentation thus serve legal as well as patient care purposes.

In the NH, the attending physician is responsible for medical documentation, and the medical director for ensuring the adequacy and appropriateness of such documentation. Responsibility for medical documentation should not be delegated to nurses or physician assistants unless the physician is prepared to cosign the note, and thereby assume responsibility for its contents.

From a legal standpoint, LTC medical records should be accurate, truthful, timely, complete, legible, and thorough. Corrections should be limited, and initialed and dated by the person making them.

The LTC medical record should contain the following items relevant to legal matters:

- information relating to direct patient, or to proxy, consent, and reasons why proxy consent was needed

- some indication of the foundation for conclusions about patient competence

- appropriate consent forms, signed and witnessed as indicated

- explanations of decisions to withhold or to withdraw medical treatment, including no-code orders, and listing of those who were consulted

- reasons for the nontreatment of abnormal test results

- justification of the recommendations for, or performance of, potentially risky procedures or tests

- explanation of why consent was not obtained or sought (as in an emergency)

- documentation of patient actions against medical advice, such as refusing medications or leaving a facility prematurely.

Many states and the federal government support the rights of patients or families to gain access to the medical record. However, this does not have to mean uncontrolled access. It is appropriate to establish policies whereby the attending physician or medical director reviews the record with the patient or family present. This can help prevent misinterpretation and reflect a willingness of the physicians, or the facility, to communicate fully and adequately.

Health care professionals, including physicians, are obliged to maintain patient confidence, except in specifically prescribed instances such as reportable communicable diseases or disclosure of information necessary to ensure payment for care. Especially in the teaching NH, policies should cover the preservation of such confidentiality, and the protocol for access to such records, in light of the significant number of transient medical and other trainees and faculty reviewing or using the medical record for various clinical and research purposes. Disclosures should be accurate and limited, both to protect the patient's privacy and to protect the practitioner or facility from potential liability.

Telephone communications. As noted in Chapter 4, policies clarifying telephone calls and assessments made over the phone are important. Such calls can create potential legal problems for the physician, even if someone else has made the error (e.g., the nurse mistakenly transcribes the wrong medication strength even though the physician authorized the correct one).

Documentation should include symptoms and signs which have been identified, the nurse's assessment of the situation, and the plan for nursing action and for notification of the physician. Further documentation should cover what was told to the physician, the physician's assessment of the problem, and the recommended action, even if it is merely to observe the patient further.

Besides helping to clarify the reasons for various physician decisions, the documentation of telephone exchanges is important in today's legal climate.

Committees. Besides patient care policy committees, the federal Conditions of Participation also include requirements for infection control, pharmacy and therapeutics, and utilization review.

Utilization review activity in the skilled nursing facility is governed under Medicare (405.1137) and Medicaid regulations (456.250-.338, .346-.348). Under the Medicare regulations and the Conditions of Participation, this committee is assigned the responsibility for assuring that there is appropriate and efficient use of health care services and high-quality patient care. For details of these regulations and guidelines, see *Medical Directorship* (1986).

The Patient Decision-Making Process

The medical director plays an important role in protecting patient rights in the areas of decision making and consent, and must ensure that physician decisions consider the patient's vulnerability, especially when institutionalized.

The substantial number of nursing home patients with some cognitive impairment or other psychiatric diagnoses necessitates an adequate assessment to establish capacity for decision making on matters ranging from finances to health care.

While not intended to be all inclusive, the following offers an overview of the range of issues and activities involved in the medical director's multifaceted role:

- obtaining legally valid decisions about care options (informed consent)

- ensuring the patient's participation in the decision-making process

- evaluating patient competency (decision-making capacity)

- making decisions on behalf of the incompetent individual

- creating supportive care plans for critical and terminal illness, and resuscitation

- complying with documentation requirements.

Informed Consent

Informed consent is a legal reflection of the ethical principle of considering and protecting individual autonomy to the greatest possible degree. A medical decision should involve not only medical facts, but also a person's values and goals. The patient is free to authorize or to refuse the administration of medical treatment (Mariner and McArdle 1985). As an outgrowth of the post- World War II Nuremberg trials, the term originally referred to research issues, but today it alludes to all decisions regarding care. This is especially relevant to long-term care, because of frequent individual difficulties in receiving, processing, and reacting to information.

The ultimate objective is a process which "protects the residents' bodily integrity, privacy and right to make a decision" either for or against a procedure or treatment, free from coercion and with "adequate information so that the decision can be made intelligently" (Meisel, Roth, and Lidz 1977, 287). The elements necessary for a legally valid decision are: (1) voluntariness, (2) provision of adequate information, (3) competency, (4) understanding, and (5) communication of a decision (Meisel, Roth, and Lidz 1977).

Two important exceptions to the disclosure requirement are emergencies and "therapeutic privilege" (that is, the argument that disclosure would so upset the patient as to render rational decision making impossible). This latter contention should be used cautiously, and certainly much less often than in the past, when it was often erroneously assumed that old people in general cannot manage bad news. "While the law may now accept the withholding of information under certain limited circumstances, it will not condone clear-cut misrepresentation" (Kapp and Bigot 1985, 41). No health care professional has yet been sued successfully for disclosing the truth, but some have been sued for withholding or misrepresenting it.

The consent process. *Express consent* refers to direct oral or written statements. *Implied consent* is that which is not stated directly, but suggested by circumstances, such as emergencies. The standards for implied consent are not less than, but only different from, those for express consent, since appropriate conditions for obtaining consent must be met in each case. Express consent should be obtained whenever there is doubt.

For the elderly, with their sight and hearing limitations, any consent form should not only contain comprehensible information, but should also be readable, perhaps through the use of color or larger type. Language should be simple and clear, and terms adequately explained. The request for consent should be discussed in a setting as free as possible from distractions. The elderly individual should, where possible, have the time to consider and discuss the information before a decision is reached. See Kaufer, Steinberg, and Toney (1983) for additional information and samples of consent forms.

The issue of coercion often arises when consent in NH patients is considered. All health care professionals must guard against suggesting that the patient is obliged to consent to requests in exchange for his ongoing care. The Nursing Home Action Group has developed guidelines to evaluate the effect of the NH setting on the freedom and voluntariness of a person's consent (Hoyt and Davies 1984, 104). These include questions about whether:

- the facility's nursing and medical care, and social services, meet state and federal standards

- the environment encourages meaningful supportive interactions between residents and others

- residents have available, and are encouraged to participate in, meaningful, life-enriching activities

- residents' civil and human rights are fully protected and the residents are encouraged to exercise those rights

- residents are free from the effects of any medications which might reduce activity, motivation, or communication, or cause other undesirable side effects.

The physician is responsible for obtaining consent for specific medical interventions, having a duty to disclose "the relevant risks and benefits, which the patient might be expected not to know" (Mariner and McArdle 1985, 68). This requires that "physicians describe to their patient, in nontechnical language: (a) the nature of any therapy and its expected benefits, (b) serious risks or side effects of that therapy, (c) alternatives to the recommended therapy (including no therapy) and their benefits and risks, and (d) any additional information that physicians would disclosure in similar circumstances as a matter of good medical practice, or that the patient requests" (Mariner and McArdle 1985, 69). In the absence of negligence, properly obtained consent generally protects the physician from liability. However, substandard care cannot be defended by claiming that the patient gave his consent.

Regarding consent, then, the attitude and techniques of the individual(s) presenting the information are just as important as the capacity of the individual to consider it. Other than for routine matters, it is imprudent to delegate the responsibility for obtaining consent to other professionals, such as asking nurses to get patient or family consent for a special procedure or operation. It is, however, useful for physicians to work with other professionals caring for the LTC patient to help explain to patients what is to be done, to answer their questions, and to alleviate their fears.

The medical director must establish a process which ensures that such decisions are legally valid. The NH itself could be held liable if an employed physician, such as the medical director, violates the patient's right to consent or refuse treatment. In the future, under its obligation to provide quality care and to monitor that care, it could even be held liable for the failure of an independent contractor, such as a nonsalaried medical director or attending physician.

Competence

Competence is both a legal and an ethical issue. Under the law, all adults are presumed to be competent unless they have been adjudged incompetent. Incompetence may be *de facto* (apparent through examination or observation) or *de jure* (determined by a court after judicial proceedings). While only a few states explicitly authorize substitute consent for those not yet legally determined to be incompetent, most physicians in practice use this method for dealing with *de facto* incompetent elderly. Some now advocate use of the phrase "decision-making capacity" in place of *"de facto* incompetence," to avoid confusion.

In determining competence (see also Chapter 12), the physician collects data from various sources, including the patient, family, caregivers, and the medical records. The evaluation should consider "psychodynamic factors, accuracy of historical information conveyed by the patient, accuracy of information disclosed to the patient by others, the stability of the patient's mental status over time, and environmental factors" (Baker 1986, 1091).

As discussed by Applebaum and Roth (1982), four levels of standards relevant to legal considerations of competence are:

- evidencing a choice
- factual awareness of issues
- rational manipulation of information
- appreciation of the nature of the situation.

Evidencing a choice, the least rigorous standard for competence, refers to the individual's expression of an interest in taking part. The simplest test is whether the individual responds to the questions posed, signs a consent form, or cooperates with a procedure (Applebaum and Roth 1982, 953).

Factual awareness has been the most widely accepted standard for competence. The individual must show awareness of the nature of the procedure or treatment, its risks and benefits, and facts about other alternatives. A broader application of this standard requires that the individual also show awareness of the risks and benefits of other options, the consequences of signing or not signing a form, the fact that there is a choice to be made, and who and where he is.

Rational manipulation of information, including the ability to rationally consider the alternatives and their potential consequences, goes one step beyond the ability to understand the existence of that information, to involve the capacity for reality testing and judgment.

Appreciation of the situation, the strictest standard for determining competence, requires that the individual be able to rationally manipulate information, *and* have an emotional appreciation of the situation.

Choosing a standard. In assessing the competence of the LTC patient, it may be appropriate to use a different level of standards, depending on the situation. Simple issues, such as obtaining a blood test, can be decided by using the lowest standard. More complex issues, such as decisions about resuscitation, require application of a higher standard (full appreciation of the situation).

The medical director should work with attending physicians, administrators, and a facility's legal counsel and (where present) ethics committee to determine which standards should be applied in individual or general cases.

Determining competence. The judicial determination of competence is a time-consuming and often costly process. State statutes, and the criteria they use, vary significantly. *"Causal link"* statutes, such as Ohio's, require demonstration that a person has a diagnosis or condition causing the socially disapproved behavior. Thus, someone able to care for himself, but who failed to do so, would not be declared incompetent.

The *uniform probate code*, of which the Utah statute is typical, emphasizes the lack of cognitive and communicative ability as a necessary criterion for incompetence. 'Incapacitated person' means any person who is impaired by reason of mental illness, mental deficiency, physical illness or disability, advanced age, chronic use of drugs, chronic intoxication, or other cause (except minority) to the extent that he lacks sufficient understanding or capacity to make or communicate responsible decisions regarding his care" (Utah Code

Ann 75. 1978, 1.20.[18]). Because interpretations of this code vary among states, the physician must determine his state's guidelines.

The *functional or therapeutic approach*, such as that adopted by New Hampshire, is a broader one, based on function, rather than on diagnosis:

> Incapacity means a legal, not medical disability and shall be measured by functional limitations. It shall be construed to mean or refer to any person who has suffered, is suffering, or is likely to suffer substantial harm due to an inability to provide for his personal needs for food, clothing, shelter, health care or safety or an inability to manage his or her property or financial affairs...
> "Functional limitations" means behavior or conditions in an individual which impair his or her ability to participate in and perform minimal activities of daily living that secure and maintain proper food, clothing, shelter, health care or safety for himself or herself (N.H. Rev. Stat. Ann. 1983, 464.A:2[VII], [XI]).

To support the determination of incompetence, some evidence of behavior which reflects such incapacity must be proved beyond a reasonable doubt at the hearing.

Nolan (1984) describes the elements of a functional evaluation pertinent to competence and guardianship proceedings.

Options for Decision-Making with the Incompetent Patient

The states use various approaches in making decisions for incompetent individuals.

Alternate decision making. Alternate decision making may take any of three forms:

- transmitted or advance directive
- substituted judgment
- best interest standard

With a *transmitted or advance directive*, a substitute decision is unnecessary, because the individual made a decision previously while still competent (e.g., via a living will).

Substituted judgment is designed to preserve individual rights of self-determination and is usually applied when an advance directive or conversations regarding these issues failed to address the particular situation. This would follow the format of "if the person were competent, he would ..."

The *best interest standard* considers what is in the individual's best interest, including: (1) medical good: which includes the effects of medical intervention and the natural history of the disease; (2) the patient's preference and value system; (3) the quality of the person's life; and (4) the good of last resort; that is, the unconditional value of life itself.

When there is no clear indication of the incompetent person's wishes, it is suggested that the "best interests" approach be used (Gutheil and Applebaum 1985, 64).

Alternate authority of decision-making. Three common legal forms of alternate decision-making authority are guardianship, power of attorney, and durable power of attorney. Each has advantages and disadvantages and will be briefly discussed.

Guardianship. After judicial proceedings, a guardian is sometimes appointed for incompetent persons substantially incapable of managing their own personal or financial affairs.

The process usually begins with the filing of a petition to the court through an attorney of the family or a friend. The court appoints a *guardian-ad-litem* whose sole purpose is to advocate on behalf of the alleged incompetent. The *guardian-ad-litem* evaluates the need for guardianship. A physician or psychologist is usually asked to examine the alleged incompetent to confirm the conclusion. A court hearing is then held to review this information, to determine competence, and to decide on appropriate living arrangements. The guardian is appointed and appropriate protective placement is arranged. The guardian must file a periodic report with the court regarding the individual's financial, medical, and social condition.

Guardianship is involuntary, and the court determines the conditions of the guardianship. Protective placement must be preceded by certification that the proposed placement is the least restrictive appropriate to the circumstances. The guardian has access to medical records and can consent to treatment.

Power of attorney is a voluntary designation of another person, (the attorney-in-fact), to act on someone's behalf in specific areas. It typically involves business-related activities, such as managing accounts, collecting and depositing funds, purchasing items, and transferring real estate. The actual document conferring power of attorney details the specific powers and responsibilities of the attorney-in-fact. Any competent individual can appoint (or be appointed) an attorney-in-fact. In some states, this document is also considered appropriate to cover decisions regarding medical conditions.

The *durable power of attorney* refers to a power of attorney which remains valid even after the person becomes incapacitated or disabled. It can also specify that the individual wants the attorney-in-fact to serve as a guardian, if that should become necessary.

Special Legal Issues for the Nursing Home Patient

Three special areas of concern to NH patients and their physicians are: hospitalization, consent for medical treatment, and the state of being hopelessly or terminally ill.

Hospitalization. In general, there is no problem if both patient and family agree to hospitalization. If the patient is in agreement but is significantly cognitively impaired, it is reasonable to notify the next of kin of the decision.

If the patient is evidently impaired in judgment and comprehension and refuses a clearly necessary hospitalization, some states permit the next of kin to consent to hospitalization. In an emergency, involuntary hospitalization may occur, with or without consent of next-of-kin (Baker 1986, 1091).

Supportive and terminal care issues. Among individual rights is the option not to have cardiopulmonary resuscitation (CPR) or advanced life support (ALS). Each facility should clarify for its patients, families, and medical and nursing staffs its policies and procedures covering resuscitation, critical care and the terminal care plan.

The traditional informal approach is legally inadvisable. The mere omission of treatment may raise questions of whether adequate physician care was rendered, and can create both ethical and legal problems for staff members who are expected to carry out these informal orders. After all, staff members are legally obligated to identify and assess changes in a patient's condition and to notify the physician of changes which may require treatment, unless there is a specific order not to do so.

Given the extent of external review of NH care, the record should reflect that the individual received care appropriate for his condition and goals. It should describe how these decisions were reached.

An LTC facility which chooses to provide *cardiopulmonary resuscitation* (CPR) and/or *advanced life support (ALS)*, should make this clear. Though a NH is a health care facility, it is not yet widely expected or required that CPR and ALS are standard nursing home operating procedure, as they are in the acute care hospital. This is potentially more relevant to someone in for a short stay (e.g., respite care).

Long-term care facilities increasingly take the position that if a witnessed loss of consciousness and cardiorespiratory arrest develop, CPR will be instituted unless there is a documented decision and order to the contrary. When the event is not witnessed, however, the chance of irreversible loss of function from an unknown time delay is thought to outweigh the possible success of resuscitation and CPR is therefore not initiated.

Once the facility has determined its policy, it must then define how to communicate it to the patient upon admission, how the decision of code status will be determined and recorded, how nursing will carry out this order, and how physicians will be involved.

The trend with *critical care plans* is to discuss the patient's wishes regarding further hospitalizations and procedures in advance. Legally, the patient always has the right to reverse a previous decision not to be hospitalized, when an acute event actually occurs.

There is increasing support for creating *terminal care plans* for patients, including a definition of which conditions will be considered in initiating such a plan. The plan can meet requirements for informed consent, depending on how thoroughly it is developed and documented. Regardless of differences among states as to the legal status of living wills and other such plans, health care staff should still have some indication of what the patient desires in certain situations.

After the policy is created, its implementation must be considered. Medical staff should participate in drafting these procedures. A terminal care plan should address each aspect of care to be implemented or altered when the plan takes effect, including diet, activity, pastoral care, routine laboratory/X-ray orders, and the use of analgesics and other medications. There are two approaches to implementation. One is to define specifically each aspect in the policies, as a facility-wide standard. A second option is to designate by policy those items to be addressed in the order sheet, but to leave the details to the individual physician.

The *living will* is a written document prepared by a competent person specifying "the circumstances under which he would want extraordinary treatment to be discontinued if an illness or accident renders him incompetent to express his wishes." (Baker 1986, 1092). As of 1986, 40 states had passed laws authorizing living wills (see also Chapter 12).

In summary, then, facility policies regarding supportive and terminal care should cover:

- who will determine the patient's competence (decision-making capacity)
- who will discuss such conclusions with patient or family
- what information will be provided about the medical condition
- what the risks and benefits are of various treatment options
- how the treatment decisions will be recorded in the chart
- how this decision will be transmitted to other facilities and staff.

Medical input in each of these areas is important. Each LTC physician should be aware of his state's laws regarding these issues. However, because a consensus on appropriate management is still evolving, many laws do not yet address all the various aspects of these issues which confront physicians. Some local medical societies and state hospital associations have developed useful guidelines. The Society for the Right to Die can also provide information and references on current and past practices (see "For Further Reading and Information").

Documentation

As stated earlier, adequate documentation of these discussions and decisions is critical in conforming with legal standards.

Such documentation should include the following:

- the patient's legal and competency status
- how and by whom the competency was assessed, including the existence of any conditions which might affect competency, such as depression or medications
- evidence that the patient made the decision freely and without duress
- who was present for the discussion
- the patient's understanding of these conditions
- the options, and their risks or benefits, especially in light of the patient's underlying conditions
- the patient's understanding of these options
- the patient's decision
- who was, or will be, notified of the decision
- a written order consistent with the decision.

Legislative and Regulatory Surveillance of Care

The federal government has played a major role in legislating standards for the health care industry and in deciding what to delegate to the states.

LTC physicians must understand the differences between laws and regulations and between federal, state, and local authority. Otherwise, attempts to clarify or modify such laws and rules become difficult, if not futile.

Laws, Regulations, and Rules

Laws are enacted by legislative bodies under the authority of the constitution and are usually a broad statement of a principle or goal. A law is relatively permanent, and can only be amended by the same legislative body.

Regulations are rules governing future actions of a specified group of people or organizations, issued by an executive agency of the government under authority granted by the legislative body. Regulations are reviewed regularly and may be rewritten more rapidly than can laws.

Rules are designed to specifically implement, interpret or prescribe laws or policies. Examples of rules in LTC are the Medicare and Medicaid Standards and Conditions of Participation. *Substantive rules* are equivalent to law and can be enforced as such. *Interpretative rules* are an agency's interpretation of statutory requirements or of its own rules and regulations. *Procedural rules* describe the process by which the agency function (e.g., procedures for hearings, applying for grants or contracts, and handling of complaints).

Guidelines provide advice offered to those who are regulated. Since guidelines are not mandatory, they can be observed or ignored. Compliance with guidelines usually, but not necessarily, implies that an agency will be less likely to dispute an action, since to do so would be to act against its own guidelines.

Jurisdiction

Besides federal jurisdiction over facilities receiving Medicare or Medicaid funds, each state also has a code to govern the skilled and intermediate nursing facility, to help fulfill its responsibility to enforce both federal and state rules and regulations. In addition, the state has the authority and responsibility to begin decertification proceedings for Medicare eligibility, if indicated.

The current regulatory and legal climate in LTC is the result of a long struggle among many public officials, elected representatives, and interest groups such as consumers and physicians over many years and through many legislative sessions, responding to events and concerns identified in hearings and committee investigations. These standards, laws, and regulations will certainly continue to evolve and LTC physicians should play a major role in their modification.

Government Monitoring of Care in the Nursing Home

Each state is responsible for monitoring nursing home care under the Medicare and Medicaid regulations. Nursing home performance is monitored in three ways: (1) nursing home surveys; (2) inspections of care (IOCs); and (3) *ad hoc* investigations of specific complains. Generally, surveys are conducted by the state health department, and facilities are reviewed annually for compliance with regulations. The IOC is conducted by a state Medicaid health facility licensing and regulatory agency, or by a Peer Review Organization (PRO). This type of inspection focuses on utilization review and quality of care issues. *Ad hoc* investigations address specific concerns about individuals, such as claims of patient abuse or inadequate care.

When a facility is found to be out of compliance during a survey or IOC, a "Notice of Violation" is issued, describing the unsatisfied standard and the magnitude of the act or omission. Fines may be imposed for each day of each violation, especially if they are repeat offenses. These violations may be appealed to the state, both formally and informally.

Substantial criticism of these current methods of review have centered on the following:

- *Predictability*: The facility could predict the time of the survey or IOC and could take steps to prepare for it in advance.

- *Inefficiency*: Regardless of the past record, each facility is reviewed to the same extent.

- *Paper compliance*: It is possible to meet many conditions on paper, without ensuring that the patient care and outcome have been improved.

- *Insensitivity to patient needs*: Residents have not been directly involved in the survey process.

- *Inconsistency*: Standards are inconsistent and unevenly enforced, both within and between states.

- *Irrelevance*: Though other means of monitoring care are being utilized in some states and settings, the results of these activities are not included in this process.

A major review of the quality of care in nursing homes, carried out by the Institute of Medicine (1986), detailed the problems listed above. The Institute, therefore, recommends that the nursing home survey process be redesigned, as follows:

- The Medicaid and Medicare survey procedures should focus on disruptive events in the life of a facility, such as a change in ownership.

- A two-stage survey approach should be employed, which should include a screening, followed by an in-depth survey and resident assessment.

- There should be case-mix referencing, initially based on patients' physical and mental characteristics. For example, instead of checking each patient for bedsores, only those at risk, according to specific characteristics, would be checked.

- Key indicators of quality should be used. If the facility is found wanting, the surveyor would then look further to determine whether the failure was based on a deficiency in that facility's quality control or on some other condition. Examples of appropriate areas for key indicators are decubiti, dehydration, medications, rehabilitation, mental status, urinary tract infections, management of incontinence, and nutritional status. Medically related indicators include number of medications, medication errors, and physician involvement in the plan of care.

- A system for scoring the results should be developed to ensure a more objective and reproductive review.

- A survey data source should be developed.

- There should be coordination of survey efforts with those programs which address complaints.

- Consumers should be more involved in the process of review.

- Positive incentives should be developed. The current system has negative ones.

- The survey process should be continually reviewed and improved.

Judicial precedents. The 1975 case of *Smith vs. O'Halloran* began the process which culminated in the August, 1986 implementation of a new survey tool. The suit, filed on behalf of a group of nursing home residents in a Denver, Colorado facility, alleged poor care and claimed that the government violated the residents' rights by failing to monitor the nursing home adequately.

In 1982, the case was tried, and Federal District Court decided (1) that deficiencies did exist; (2) that the survey was facility-oriented, not resident-oriented; and (3) that HHS could develop a new system that was resident-oriented, but had no duty to do so under Medicaid regulations.

In 1984, the 10th Circuit Court of Appeals decided that the law *did* obligate the Secretary of HHS to establish a system which would evaluate whether facilities receiving federal money are actually providing quality care, based on outcome.

Patient Care and Services (PaCS). As a consequence of this decision, the Medicare and Medicaid Long-Term Care Survey of Patient Care and Services (PaCS) was developed and implemented in the summer of 1986.

The four components of this approach are:

- Evaluation through direct observation of certain aspects of the physical environment, including cleanliness, space, equipment, infection control, and disaster preparedness

- Detailed review of the care provided to a sample of residents, through observation, interviews, and medical record reviews

- Evaluation of meals, dining, and eating assistance by observing meal service

- Observation of drug administration for a sample of residents.

While acknowledging the advances which the PaCS survey tool represents, the Institute of Medicine report (1986) identifies key issues which this new survey does not address, including: (1) lack of a formal protocol for sampling the residents for detailed reviews of care; (2) continued reliance on an unguided surveyor's judgment to make important decisions about problems with care; and (3) absence of a requirement that facilities maintain standard resident assessment data to facilitate data collection.

So while the process has become more resident- and outcome-oriented, room for improvement still exists.

Summary

All levels of government attempt to influence the practice of medicine through laws and regulations. Both the practice of geriatric medicine and medical administration in LTC must conform with these broad standards and requirements.

The medical director needs to be aware of four basic areas of law and regulation: personal responsibility and liability, patient decision making and protection of rights, reimbursement for care and accompanying standards and requirements, and monitoring and regulation of actual patient care. In each case, this involves the medical director's personal practices and protection, supervision of the practices of attending physicians, and facility compliance with essential governmental policies and requirements.

In addition, LTC physicians will want to attempt collectively to influence the legislative bodies and regulatory agencies. There is a balance to be struck between inadequate care and protection of vulnerable elderly, and the imposition of excessively costly and time-consuming requirements that do not actually improve standards or quality of care. Finding and maintaining that balance requires constant vigilance and physician participation.

Awareness of these laws and regulations may be gained from federal, state, and local agencies, published sources of legislation and regulatory activity, local and national medical societies and organizations, and hospital and NH administrators. Some of these sources are further identified in the references below.

References

Appelbaum, P.S., and L.H. Roth 1982. Competency to consent to research: A psychiatric overview. *Archives of General Psychiatry* 39:951-958.

Baker, F.M. 1986. Legal issues affecting the older patient. *Hospital and Community Psychiatry* 37(11):1091-1093.

Gutheil, T.G., and P.S. Appelbaum. 1985. The substituted judgment approach: Its difficulties and paradoxes in mental health settings. *Law, Medicine and Health Care* April: 61-64.

Hoyt, J.D., and J.M. Davies. 1984. A response to the task force on supportive care. *Law, Medicine, and Health Care* June: 103-105.

Institute of Medicine. 1986. *Improving the Quality of Care in Nursing Homes.* Committee on Nursing Home Regulations. Washington, DC: National Academy Press.

Kapp, M., and A Bigot. 1985. Geriatrics and the law. New York: Springer.

Kaufer, D.S., E.R. Steinberg, and S.D. Toney. 1983. Revising medical consent forms: An empirical model and test. *Law, Medicine and Health Care* September: 155-162.

Mariner, W.K., and P.A. McArdle, 1985. Consent forms, readability, and comprehension: The need for new assessment tool, *Law, Medicine and Health Care* April: 68-74.

Medical Directorship: Regulations and Guidelines. 1986. Owings Mills, MD: National Health Publishing.

Meisel, A.L., Roth, L.C. and Lidz. 1977. Toward a model of the legal doctrine of informed consent. *American Journal of Psychiatry* 134(3):385-289.

N.H. Rev. Stat. Ann. 1983, 464.A:2 (VII), (XI).

Nolan, B. 1984. Functional evaluation of the elderly in guardianship proceedings. *Law, Medicine and Health Care.* October: 210-218.

Tessaro E. 1974. The medical directorship. *Journal of Long-term Care Administration,* Winter 1974-75.

Utah Code Ann. 75. 1978, 1.20.(18).

For Further Reading and Information

Adams, C.E. 1981. Considerations in Regard to Physicians in Nursing Homes, *Proceeding of a Conference held May 23-24, 1981.* Washington, DC: National Foundation for Long Term Health Care.

American Medical Association. 1977. Guidelines for a medical director in a long-term facility, in *The Medical Director in the Long-term Facility.* Chicago, IL: American Medical Association.

Estes, C., and Newcomer. 1983. *Fiscal Austerity and Aging.* Vol 152. Beverly Hills, CA: Sage Library of Social Research.

———. 1986. *Federal Regulatory Directory,* 5th Edition, Congressional Quarterly Inc.

Fox, T. 1977. The medical director - questions and answers, in AMA *The Medical Director in the Long-Term Facility.* Chicago, IL: American Medical Association.

Furrow, B.R. 1984. Informed consent: A thorn in medicine's side? An arrow in law's quiver? *Law, Medicine, and Health Care.* December: 268-273.

HEW Office of Long Term Care Standards Enforcement. Status of medical director with respect to membership on a facility's utilization review committee. Policy Memorandum No. 14B, August 11, 1976. *Medical Directorship Regulations and Guidelines*. Owings Mills, MD: National Health Publishing. I. Appendix D/1.

HEW Office of Nursing Home Affairs. Implementation of conditions of participation 405.1122—Medical direction. Policy Memorandum No. 14, February 2, 1976. *Medical Directorship, Regulations and Guidelines*. Owings Mills, MD: National Health Publishing. I. Appendix C/1-5.

——. Legal requirements of selecting and supervising the medical staff. *Medical Directorship, Regulations and Guidelines*. Owings Mills, MD: National Health Publishing. I. Appendix E/1-E/7.

——. Medicare Standards. Conditions of participation: Medical staff— 482.22. (a) Standard: Compositions of the medical staff, (b) Standard: Medical staff organization and accountability, (c) Standard: Medical staff bylaws, (d) Standard: Autopsies. *Medical Directorship, Regulations and Guidelines*. Owings Mills, MD: National Health Publishing. Sept. 1986. 27: 1-9.

——. Medicare Standards. Skilled nursing facilities. Patient care policies— 405.1121(1). Medical director standards—405.1122. Physicians services— 442.346. *Medical Directorship, Regulations and Guidelines*. Owings Mills, MD: National Health Publishing. Sept. 1986. 27: 9-15.

——. Medicare and Medicaid Quality Standards. Skilled nursing facilities. 405.1100's. *Medical Directorship, Regulations and Guidelines*. owings Mills, MD: National Health Publishing.

——. Medicare Regulations. Utilization review. Skilled nursing facilities. 405.1137. *Medical Directorship, Regulations and Guidelines*. Owings Mills, MD: National Health Publishing.

Moss, B. 1977. Medical direction in long-term care facilities, *The Medical Director in the Long-Term Facility*. Chicago, IL: American Medical Association.

Page, C. 1977. Facts and suggestions regarding the medical director. *The Medical Director in the Long-Term Facility*. Chicago, IL: American Medical Association.

Page, C. 1981. Is medical direction needed in nursing homes? *Proceeding of a Conference held May 23-24, 1981*. Washington, DC: National Foundation for Long Term Health Care.

Pattee, J. 1983. Update on the medical director concept. *The American Family Physician* 28(6):129-133.

Pattee, J. 1980. Utilization review committee as a peer review mechanism. *Journal of the American Geriatrics Society* 28(4):144-145.

President's Commission for the Study of Ethical Problems in Medicine and Biomedical and Behavioral Research. 1983. *Deciding to forego life-sustaining treatment.* A report on the ethical, Medical and Legal Issues in Treatment Decisions. March.

Regan, J.J. 1985. Process and context: hidden factors in health care decisions for the elderly. *Law, Medicine and Health Care* September: 151-152.

———. *Regulations and health: Understanding and influencing the process.* National Health Council, Inc. Governmental Relations Handbook Series, No. 7. November 1979.

Rogers, W.W. 1980. *General administration in the nursing home.* New York: Von Nostrand Reinhold Company.

Shaughnessy, M. 1977. The role of the medical director in the nursing home. *The Medical Director in the Long-Term Facility.* Chicago, IL: American Medical Association.

Southwick, A. 1978. *The law of hospital and health care administration.* The University of Michigan: Health Administration Press.

Task Force on Supportive Care. 1984. The supportive care plan — Its meaning and application: Recommendations and guidelines. *Law, Medicine and Health Care* June: 97-102.

Tessaro, E. 1977. The medical directorship. *The Medical Director in the Long-Term Care Facility.* Chicago, IL: American Medical Association.

Turner, A. 1981. Medical directors in multi-facility organizations. *Proceeding of a Conference held May 23-24, 1981.* Washington, DC: National Foundation for Long Term Health Care.

Williams, T. et al. 1977. The medical directors' group. *The Medical Director in the Long-Term Care Facility.* Chicago, IL: The American Medical Association, Division of Professional Relations.

The Federal Register and the Code of Federal Regulations, both available at major libraries, provide actual regulations and interpretations of same. State medical societies often have staff who can assist physicians in obtaining relevant material.

The *Federal Register* is a daily publication (except for weekends and federal holidays). It includes four parts: documents issued by the President, final rules, proposed rules, and published notices of hearing; investigations; and delegations of authorities.

Code of Federal Regulations (CFR) is an indexed and codified compilation of all current substantive rules. These rules are divided into 50 "titles" which cover a major functional or administrative areas of government. For example Title 21 - Food and Drugs; Title 40 - Protection of the Environment; Title 42 - Public Health; and Title 45 - Public Welfare. The Code of Federal Regulations helps in locating those rules of specific interest. The *Federal Register* publishes changes in the regulations since the last publication date of the CFR and includes background information, comments and responses. They cross-reference each other. Each title in the CFR is divided into levels covering progressively a narrower range of programs or administrative areas. The Index of the CFR refers to these levels: Titles; Subtitles; Chapter; Subchapter (roman numerals); Part; Subpart; and Subsection. For example, 42 Part 405 refers to Title 42, part 405. Material cited in legal form shows the Title first, the reference CFR and then the part, subpart and subsection numbers. 42 CFR 405.1101 refers to Title 42, Code of Federal Regulations, Part 405, Subsection 1101.

Federal departments and agencies playing a major role in programs and services for the aged include the following:

- Department of Health and Human Services (HHS), 200 Independence Avenue S.W., Washington, DC 20201 (programs, services, funding, long-term care standards, physician and facility reimbursement, monitoring of care). Much of the HHS responsibility for programs and services for the elderly is carried out within an HHS agency, the Health Care Financing Administration (HCFA).

- Department of Agriculture, The Mall, 12th and 14th Sts., Washington, DC 20250 (food stamps)

- Department of Housing and Urban Development, 451 7th St. S.W., Washington, DC 20410 (Housing for the elderly and handicapped, housing subsidies)

- Department of Labor, 200 Constitution Ave. N.W., Washington, DC 20210 (jobs and employment)

- Department of Transportation, 400 7th St. S.W., Washington, DC 20590 (mass transport, handicapped services)

- Veteran's Administration, 810 Vermont Avenue N.W., Washington, DC 20420 (medical care, compensation and pensions, education and research)

- Commission on Civil Rights, 1121 Vermont Ave. N.W., Washington, DC 20425

For further information on terminal care issues contact the Society for the Right to Die, 250 W. 57th St., New York, New York 10107.

Chapter Twelve

Managing Ethical Issues in Long-Term Care

Steven A. Levenson, M.D.

Chapter Objectives

This chapter will:

- Review some major ethical concerns for the LTC physician, and suggest how to handle them

- Discuss policy and procedure issues for competency determinations, patient expression of wishes, consent, living wills, terminal and hospice care, and no-code orders

- Consider the purpose of an ethics advisory committee, and the medical role on such a committee

Introduction

Nowhere has the recent increase in physician attention to ethical issues in medicine been more substantial, relevant, or critical than in geriatrics. Despite the proliferation of medical literature on ethical issues, many physicians are still uneasy about the subject, viewing it as unscientific, subjective, and fraught with unanswerable questions and legal hazards. Much of the extensive literature and debate on the subject still comes not from practicing physicians, but from medical academicians, lawyers and politicians. Ultimately, this is inadequate, since physicians must participate actively and intelligently in both medical and ethical decision making for the older individual.

Clinical and ethical issues are as intimately interrelated in the elderly as in any group. In fact, the similarities between clinical and ethical decision making are much closer than they at first glance appear to be. Both require certain underlying general principles, which must be applied to individual cases. Both require the best possible job of data gathering prior to attempting to reach conclusions. And both often require that we proceed in the face of uncertainty, trying options and reconsidering our conclusions in the light of the results of those trials. Thus, the uncertainties of ethical decision making should be no more formidable than those in the clinical decision-making process. Still, the physician must have: 1) an understanding of the issues; 2) some guidance in tactics and tools for dealing with actual cases; and 3) lots of practice. This chapter will touch on the first and focus on the second, and necessarily leave the third to the reader.

Goals of Ethical Decision Making

Ultimately, intelligent ethical decision making should *not* be based on complying with rules or avoiding lawsuits, but rather on enhancing the quality of life and fulfilling the rights of the individual. A central guiding principle in our society is the exercise of autonomy, implying that each person should be allowed to be free to make his own moral choices, unless there is some condition that clearly interferes with his decision-making capacities, or some greater social good that clearly overrides them.

If each qualified person has the right to autonomy, then others have the ethical duty to respect that right, and to try to promote its exercise. When a person reaches a decision seemingly not in his best interests, we must wonder whether that person has a different set of values from us, or that person is incapable of making such decisions, and should therefore have others make the decisions for him. We must be careful not to jump to the second conclusion without entertaining the first.

Watching Our Criteria

Above all else, in trying to make ethical decisions, physicians must be wary of their criteria. In other words, they must recognize their underlying assumptions and rules for deciding what is right and wrong, true and false, and reliable or unreliable, and how such criteria relate to their conclusions, and those of others.

This advice is especially pertinent in several issues relevant to the elderly LTC patient: quality of life and competency.

One study of physician decision making examined differences between physicians deciding to treat, or not to treat, a terminally ill patient. Private practitioners were much more inclined to intubate such patients than were residents or attending physicians. In all groups, those more likely to decide to withhold therapy were also those who placed more value on social information about the patient. Religion, degree of faith, and ethical attitudes were not correlated with these decisions, but physician characteristics, attitudes, and information management were important independent variables. Decisions often depended on which factors the physician took most into account; for instance, the nature of the acute problem, the patient's quality of life, or the natural history of the illness. There were noteworthy differences in interpretation of the meaning of the phrase "quality of life," and in how different practitioners arrived at such conclusions as estimated survival time (Pearlman and Jonsen 1985).

The authors of this study suggest that the responsible use of the phrase "occurs when clinicians attune their interactions with patients to the values and goals of the patient."

Quality of life considerations are sometimes seen as a choice between life itself (quantity) and personhood (quality). But in practice, the distinction is hard to make because quantity is often a part of quality (Pearlman and Speer 1983). "Quality of life" advocates see this as including such things as the ability to communicate with others, self-determination, and relative freedom from pain and excessive suffering. Quality depends greatly on individual values. Attempts to develop a "calculus" or standardized criteria for quality of life persist.

Quality of life considerations should not be confused with a person's social worth because they are not equivalent. Many older persons have lost some or all of the utilitarian criteria for social value. Findings suggest that physicians may tend to link quality of life, curability, and valuation of life. For instance, immobility and pain in a nursing home resident make nontreatment of fever more likely (Brown and Thompson 1979). This is not always appropriate.

Medical decisions about older patients which consider "quality-of-life" issues should therefore be based, whenever possible, on the patient's own assessments. When the patient is unable to express his feelings, however, it is recommended that quality of life be a decisive factor only when the patient's quality of life falls below a "minimum standard," such as the complete loss of sensory and intellectual activity, and extreme physical debilitation (Pearlman et al., 1985).

The Ethical Decision-Making Process

With so many opinions and attitudes, and no hard and fast rules to guide conclusions, how is the LTC physician to decide what to do, or to guide a patient's or family's thinking?

In an attempt to make ethical decision making a more systematic and rational activity, the following steps are recommended:

- Use the team approach, rather than trying to make ethical decisions alone.

- Gather as much information as possible before trying to draw conclusions.

- Present the options carefully and systematically to maximize understanding and to minimize conflict.

- Be flexible about evaluating and reevaluating situations, and changing approaches based on changing circumstances.

- Keep in mind the goals of LTC and of the patient, as well as the medical objectives.

Let us examine some of these in more detail.

The Team Approach

Most older patients now die in hospitals or LTC facilities, rather than at home. Though many professionals contribute to their care, the physician has traditionally been the main decision maker. Nonphysician professionals increasingly expect to be included in such decision making. The team approach is highly useful to encourage different viewpoints, to obtain consensus, and to make staff more comfortable with the care they must deliver or withhold as a result of that decision. This is also consistent with the multidisciplinary approach essential to the care of the geriatric patient (see Chapter 7).

The team approach also means including patient and family in the discussions and decisions. The old paternalistic "doctor knows best" approach, whereby the older person was presumed to not have an interest, or an ability, to participate in such discussions, was never appropriate. Including the patient does, of course, depend on his capacity for handling such situations, a problem to be discussed later in this chapter.

Eventually, however, decisions must be made, and one course of action must be taken at any given time. After the aforementioned discussions with the patient and family, the LTC physician must still be responsible for authorizing the specific elements of the plan.

Gathering the Information

Both clinically and ethically, the decision about what to do or not to do is the *endpoint*, not the beginning. It must be preceded by the gathering and analysis of relevant information. This includes medical, ethical, social, psychological, functional, and legal information.

Medical information is the cornerstone of this process, and the physician's unique expertise as gatherer and interpreter of such information makes his role central. The fundamental questions in any situation are: "What is the condition and the prognosis?" and, "What are the probabilities that a given treatment or nontreatment will yield a given result?"

Ethical information refers to the values and wishes of, and the goals for, the individual patient. A patient's "value history" is just as important a piece of information as their medical history (Mc-Cullogh, 1984). Upon a person's admission to an institution or program, referral sources should be asked about knowledge of any statements or other evidence of the wishes of patient or family concerning care in the event the patient is or becomes unable to express such wishes subsequently. Such a history should be recorded in advance, while a person is still able to express it. Even if the physician does not personally obtain this information, he should nonetheless make himself aware of it and include it in any subsequent decision making. When decisions about whether to treat could reasonably go either way, information about past preferences and values should be a major factor in the decision, all things being equal. In this way, general ethical rules and clinical prescriptions can be better individualized to the case at hand.

When the patient himself is unable to represent his wishes or values, these may be obtained through statements of others who knew of previous expressions, or by actual statements previously recorded by the patient himself. The most tentative source of such information is conjecture by those who know or knew the individual about what that person *would* have said or *might* have wanted if he were now able to express such wishes. Though fraught with uncertainties, such conjecture is sometimes the *only* information we have to go by.

Social information refers to the setting in which the patient lives and functions, his interrelationships with other people, the effects of the medical problem or condition on such function, and the prospects for improvement or change of such a condition as a result of choosing one particular option or another.

Psychological information includes assessments of an individual's capacity to absorb, process, and communicate information. Ultimately, such information is used to decide on a person's *decision-making capacity* or *competence*. It is helpful to include in any preadmission assessment an evaluation of whether the patient has shown previous evidence of being capable of participating in discussions and decisions related to his medical care. These concepts will be further explored shortly.

Functional information includes an individual's *current* and *potential* capacity to perform the tasks which he is expected or required to perform for himself or others within his particular setting. These may range from shopping, to keeping financial records, to caring for a spouse, to simply showing up for activities or leaving a NH on a given day by himself.

Legal information refers to the laws of a state or local government, or the regulations of federal, state, or local agencies, concerning proper procedure to follow in all such cases. For example, there are laws covering the proper way to offer a "living will," regulations to protect individuals who are asked to consent to participate in a research project, and policies or regulations regarding the withholding of treatment in the terminally ill. Compliance with these must be a part of the considerations.

Presenting the Options

Once the information is gathered and reviewed by professionals, options for care or treatment must be presented to patient or family, or other representative. Several issues concerning presentation of options to patient and family include: whom to approach, when to approach them, what to say, and how to say it.

Whom to approach. Sometimes, either the patient has definite opinions on care issues, while the family does not, or vice versa. Sometimes, patient and family do not agree on these issues.

The competent individual is assumed by law to have the right to speak on his own behalf, regardless of what others, including close relatives, want for him. Once a person is deemed legally incompetent, he has no such support.

It is simply impractical to go to court for every decision about the competence of LTC patients. Therefore, some system is needed to determine and follow the *decision-making capacity* of these patients, as a basis for subsequent clinical decisions.

If the individual possesses decision-making capacity, the procedure is quite clear: Approach that individual. The family can certainly be included in the discussion, or can be approached separately, but the patient's wishes should take precedence, unless he requests otherwise. If the individual clearly does *not* have decision-making capacity, then it is helpful to approach family or other significant person from the beginning (on first visit to an assessment center, or on admission to a NH) for any specific instructions or information to use as a guide for subsequent decision making about care issues.

Sometimes, neither patient nor family is interested in discussing the subject, in which case it may be prudent not to pursue it until a later time, after they have become adjusted to their setting, or they indicate their interest.

In situations where there is disagreement between patient and family, or among individual family members, it is extremely helpful to request that they decide among themselves who will represent the family, or with whom the physician should communicate. Doing this helps to reduce chaos. When this is not possible, the physician may need to consult personal or institutional legal counsel to help him determine exactly who should be involved in the decision.

In the vast majority of cases, appropriate physician management of family, patient, and staff discussion of these issues can lead to appropriate decision making with minimal conflict, and make judicial intervention unnecessary.

What to present. Instead of presenting the patient or family with a difficult issue for them to resolve, it may be helpful to first engage them in a general discussion of their feelings or wishes on the subject. This can be a part of the aforementioned *information gathering.* One approach is to present them with the option to issue a "Statement of Wishes" (See Figure 12-1), a general set of options encompassing more than just a living will. One has a choice to complete some, all, or none of it.

If there is some interest in a "living will" or similar more formal statement concerning specific wishes about *terminal care*, patient or family can be provided, as appropriate, with a copy of a prototype "living will" document consistent with state requirements, and assisted in considering and completing such a document.

Such signed statements or requests should be considered a part of the permanent medical record, and stored in the chart. At the patient's request, or as a matter of policy, such directives should be sent with other chart materials at the time of transfer to another program or facility. Similar information received from others should be included in a patient's current record. If such materials are not transferred, the receiving facility should at least be notified that these statements exist.

What to say and how to say it. There are some common-sense rules for physicians discussing ethical issues with patients and families, unfortunately often commonly violated, which can help facilitate lay consideration of the issues, and minimize confusion and conflict:

- Avoid the "everything or nothing" approach.
- Always present the facts of the case as clearly as possible.
- Lay out the options and present the likely outcomes of each.

STATEMENT OF WISHES ABOUT CARE IN THE EVENT OF CHANGES IN MY CONDITION

At this time, I am capable of rationally discussing with my doctors decisions regarding my care. However, I recognize that there may come a time in the future when, because of illness or some other problem, I am no longer able to express my wishes or thoughtfully discuss my care.

If this should occur, I would like the following to guide those who will be making such decisions for my care: (Circle or write in those which are desired; cross out those which are not.)

1.   If I am terminally ill (as certified by my own doctor(s)), I wish to be allowed to die with dignity and comfort and not be kept alive by artificial means or heroic measures.

2.   If I should be on a respirator or other mechanical support equipment, and my condition continues to deteriorate despite such treatment, and there is not a strong probability that continuing such treatment would help me to recover, I would wish such treatment be discontinued and that I be allowed to die with dignity and comfort.

3.   I hereby request _____ to speak on my behalf to assist my physicians and other caretakers in deciding on my care, and to consent to appropriate treatment.

4.   If I am transferred to another facility, I request that this information be sent with my records to the receiving facility.

5. Other Statements:

Date:_____   Signature _____

                              Witness _____

Reprinted courtesy of Levindale Hebrew Geriatric Center and Hospital; Baltimore, Maryland

Figure 12-1 Statement of wishes form.

- Allow ample time for questions and explanations.

- Respect the rights of people to think things over or defer discussions to a later date.

- Point out that what is started can also be stopped.

- Don't be afraid to use the "If it were me. . ." approach.

"Everything" or "nothing." Today, it is always possible to do *something* for almost every patient, even if it is just to alleviate pain or promote a comfortable death. These options should never be mistakenly presented as "doing nothing." When they are, family members may be reluctant to agree to reasonable restraint of treatment, out of fear that they are hurting or even killing a loved one by refusing to allow *anything* to be done. The search should be for a middle ground. For instance, an older person with advanced heart disease may not be a candidate for an ICU or for intubation or respirators, but may nonetheless deserve some medical therapies on a regular hospital unit, or in a NH.

The facts of the case. Don't confuse lay people by telling them, for example, that someone has had "an inferior myocardial infarction with lateral extension, and has poor cardiac output with evidence of progressive myocardial failure, and what would you like us to do?" Explain the situation in the simplest possible terms without grossly oversimplifying. Where appropriate, use diagrams and drawings. Explain why certain results are likely or not likely to occur, despite or without treatment. Speak in terms of probabilities and likelihoods, not absolutes. Don't offer explicit prognoses (e.g., "only three days to live unless you agree to surgery") without substantial confidence in the reliability of such specifics. And don't confuse the facts of the case with your own interpretations of likely outcome (The fact that someone has pneumonia should not necessarily be presented as "She's going to die soon because she has pneumonia.")

The options. Options should be selected *by* the patient (or proxy) *for* the doctor, not vice versa. Few doctors can make guarantees, but most people are not looking for them. Therefore, as with discussion of prognosis, presentation of options should be done in terms of likelihoods and probabilities, not absolutes. People should have the opportunity to compare options, and the likelihood of outcomes.

What is started can be stopped. Choices of options should *not* be presented as irreversible ("Once we put him on the respirator, we won't be able to take him off until he's brain-dead"). Patients and families should be given the opportunity to let doctors try one course, and then review the results, to consider whether another course might then be more appropriate. Such flexibility may require physician advocacy to change existing laws and policies.

"If it were me. . . ." There is nothing wrong with assisting people in reaching conclusions about ethical issues, as long as we take care to provide them with alternatives, and avoid suggesting that we insist on one decision over another. Many times, people both request and appreciate the assistance of an attending physician who says, "If this were my mother, I would decide. . .for these reasons. . ." and then explains why. The conclusion is not necessarily as important as the reasoning process used to get there. Do acknowledge, however, that ambivalence is a normal response at such times.

When a conclusion is finally determined, it should be documented in the medical record, and communicated among all shifts and patient caretakers, to facilitate a consistent approach to the patient.

Competency Issues

Competence is becoming the central ethical issue in geriatrics, for it is the basis of most other areas of ethical concern. In short, the judgment of competence is a document of individual freedom. It is a widely accepted article of faith that a person's best interests are served through informed choice. The declaration of *incompetence* has substantial social and personal ramifications—perhaps most importantly, a loss of certain individual freedom. Once an older person is labeled "incompetent," much of his personal freedom is gone for good.

While the terms "competence" and "incompetence" have been used freely, few have given careful thought to their meaning and implications. Since the physician has a major role in competence determinations, he must be aware of the pitfalls in making such determinations.

The LTC physician can take a number of steps to improve the competence determination process and enhance the individual autonomy of the older individual. These are as follows:

- Know the definitions of competence and incompetence.
- Consider what we are asking or expecting of the individual.
- Appreciate that competence can fluctuate with time.
- Consider physical causes of mental status change which may affect competence.
- Use, but don't abuse, the tools.
- Be aware of the criteria we are using.
- Appreciate that competence is *not* a fact, but a conclusion.
- Try to maximize the rational foundation for the determination.

Definitions of "Competence"

There are legal, ethical, and psychological definitions of "competence," each of which employs different criteria. The *legal* definition primarily looks at how a person fits in with a defined status; for example, age, citizenship, or soundness of mind. For instance, a person is generally considered legally incompetent to consent to treatment if he is unconscious or suffering from the effects of drugs or alcohol, dementia, or mental illness, or if he is below a certain stipulated age.

A central issue to all legal determinations of competence is whether one can reasonably understand the condition, nature, and effect of the proposed treatments, and the risks of choosing or not choosing those treatments. Thus, the law makes a presumption that if you are 24 years old and not legally incompetent, you are capable of carrying out certain legally delineated tasks—writing a will, for example. Conversely, a person who does not meet the legal definition for competence is considered incapable of legally performing the act. Thus, if you are 13, you are not considered competent to write a will, even though you may have more understanding of the process than someone three times the age.

In contrast, the *psychological* concept of competence relates more to the specific mental and behavioral capacities needed to perform a certain task. Thus, though a 12-year-old might be considered legally incompetent to manage his own financial affairs, he might nonetheless be perfectly capable of the most intricate mathematic computations. Or, an elderly individual might be legally competent, yet unable to properly make decisions on his own behalf because of certain thought disturbances.

From the ethical viewpoint, competence depends on actions being voluntary (uncoerced), intentional (goal-directed), and authentic (consistent with values). As the President's Commission for the Study of Ethical Problems in Medicine and Biomedical and Behavioral Research states: "Decision making capacity requires, to greater or lesser degree: (1) possession of a set of values and goals; (2) the ability to communicate and understand information; and (3) the ability to reason and to deliberate about one's choices." (President's Commission 1982, 57)

For convenience, "competence" is sometimes classified as follows: (1) the capacity to conduct business and financial affairs, (2) the capacity to make decisions on medical care, and (3) the capacity to function in activities of daily living.

Practical Affairs and Competence

Competence is *not* on all-or-none thing; that is, you are not *either* competent or incompetent. Rather, it largely depends on what we expect a person to do, and on the setting in which we expect him to function. An elderly individual, especially an institutionalized one, might be involved in certain situations or need to perform any number of tasks for which some determination of competence would be highly relevant:

- writing or revising a will or estate

- managing personal financial affairs, or those of others

- consenting to or refusing food or treatment

- consenting to become an experimental subject

- disruptive behavior and the need for institutional staff to control it

- assessment of changes in mental status

- guardianship and proxy consent

- wishes regarding treatment in time of terminal illness

- being admitted to, or desiring discharge from, a hospital or LTC institution.

Even seemingly simple issues can present competence questions. For instance, a fairly common problem at LTC facilities concerns the right of patients to refuse to adhere to their diets, to knowingly eat foods which the physician says are bad for them, or to refuse to eat or take medicine at certain times.

The urgency and seriousness of the need for competency determination depends on the seriousness of the task at hand. A patient's choice of clothing or of lunch options is not likely to adversely affect health, life, or safety. A decision to have surgery or to participate in a research project most certainly will. Many determinations of competency have traditionally been blanket declarations: a person is declared either competent or incompetent—period. Current thinking on the issue has begun to reflect a different orientation; specifically, that competency determinations ought to be based on practical situations. Figure 12-2 shows a sample competence evaluation form to help in making such determinations.

Fluctuating competence. No one is equally capable of the same level of task performance at all times. For example, try performing a skilled act right after having been aroused at 4 A.M. from a deep sleep. So, too, even the incompetent older person is not necessarily equally incompetent at all times. Such fluctuations should, however, be taken into account, both in judging competence and in choosing the time to approach an individual to explain options or to try to obtain consent.

Physical factors. Before anyone can process, ponder, and decide upon information, he must have a comparatively intact *physiological* system. It is important not to condemn a person to the label of incompetence until we rule out certain physical causes of dementia

Figure 12-2 Determination of individual decision-making capacity.

This form is for recording information about the people, tests, or conclusions relevant to a person's decision-making capacity (DMC).

I. The Tests and the Examiners

The conclusions below are based on the following information, tests, or examinations, found in the following locations (e.g., patient chart, medical records, doctor's office, administrative offices, etc.):

INFORMATION/RESULTS   *LOCATION*   *DATE*

____ Attending physician
____ Psychiatric evaluation
____ Mental status examination
____ Depression rating scale
____ Psychologist's assessment
____ Social work assessment
____ Other psychological testing
____ Other tests, observations, or
      examinations, as follows:

II. Extent of Decision-Making Capacity

This individual's decision-making capacity (DMC) is considered to be as follows:

____ The individual has the capacity to decide on simple inconsequential issues with only short-term significance
____ The individual has the capacity to decide on simple low-risk issues with longer-range consequences
____ The individual has the capacity to decide on major decisions, with long-term effects, and some possible life and death impact
____ The individual has the capacity to decide on high risk life-and-death issues
____ The individual has DMC for all the above conditions and circumstances
____ The individual has DMC, but resists or refuses making decisions on his/her behalf
____ The individual has DMC but clearly prefers that others make the decisions for him/her (specifically:)
____ The individual lacks DMC for all circumstances, under all conditions

These conclusions about this individual's DMC were reached by the following individual(s), on the dates indicated:

NAME   *DATE*

Dissenting opinions (if any, name and reason):

III. Duration of Any Incapacity

If the individual is deemed to have less than full DMC, the likely duration of the deficiency is:

____ Unclear or undetermined
____ Less than 1 month
____ Less than 3 months
____ Less than 6 months
____ Indefinite
____ Permanent

Figure 12-2, continued.

IV. Prior Relevant Judicial Actions or Decisions

The following are previous judicial determinations regarding this patient:

ACTION	DATE	DECISION	REASONS
Competence:			
Protective services:			
Guardianship:			
Other:			

V. Proposed Protection, Restrictions, or Substitute Decision-Making

Based on the above conclusions, this individual needs:

____ Selection or designation of a proxy consenter
____ A court-appointed guardian
____ A power-of-attorney or durable power-of-attorney
____ Application for protective services
____ Other:

VI. Existing Documentation of Patient Wishes

The following documents or statements of patient wishes exist:

DOCUMENT	DATE	LOCATION
Living will		
Power of attorney		
Statement of intent		
Others:		

VII. Proxy Consenters

For those for whom proxy consent is necessary, the following individual(s) is/are the appropriate contact person for decisions requiring proxy consent for this individual:

Name	Address/	Phone No.	How Designated

VIII. Review Dates

These determinations have been reviewed on the following dates:

DATE	ITEM REVIEWED	PEOPLE INVOLVED

and delirium, including infections, fluid and electrolyte imbalances, drug toxicity, thyroid dysfunction, severe anemia, heart disease, or stroke.

Use, but don't abuse, the tools. To evaluate competence, we often use tools designed to evaluate various aspects of mental function, such as the mental status examination and various scales of anxiety or depression. After asking the patient certain questions, or having him perform certain tasks, the information collected is used for various assessments. But these tools do *not* measure competence, and the findings of such instruments should not be confused with measurements of competence. In fact, they test aspects of mental function, emotions, or behavior, more or less relevant to the issue of competence. The results should be among the facts used to assess competence, but are not sufficient in themselves to reach such conclusions.

Therefore, written assessments such as, "Mental status: patient incompetent" are neither accurate nor appropriate. Competence relates to functional capacity to perform various tasks. Mental status is not a single measurement, but rather a collection of assessments of specific aspects of behavior and thought. Mental status is comprised of signs and symptoms, not diagnoses. Mental status is a description; competence is a label, based substantially on the findings of the mental status examination.

Competence is not a fact, but a conclusion. In the end, the conclusion about a person's competence is *not* a fact, but an opinion, based on a variety of information, ranging from a comparison of current actions with past inclinations, to the results of a mental status examination. Therefore, such statements are *always* necessarily relative to underlying personal and social standards and criteria. That does not make them worthless, but only tells us that we should do everything possible to make this a rational, rather than an arbitrary, process.

It is possible, and not uncommon, for a belligerent, uncooperative older person to be labeled incompetent because he will not accede to the suggestions of the physician or family. Not infrequently, the competence of an older person is not called into question until that individual disagrees with some recommendation. Therefore, it is a good idea for competence to be assessed *before* recommendations are made or decision-making situations arise. In addition, lack of information has been shown to lead to refusal to accede even to routine tests; thus, professionals may be responsible for provocations which they inappropriately turn around to interpret as deficiencies of the patient.

Consent — Original and Substitute

Requirements for medical consent are based on the legal principle of assault and battery, which states that each person has the right to be protected from being touched except in ways he authorizes. "Assault" is considered a threat to touch which causes another person to fear battery, and "battery" is the actual act of unauthorized intentional touching. Performing a procedure other than the one to which the patient originally consents may or may not constitute battery, depending on the situation. A doctor's judgment as to the medical necessity for the deviation may or may not be sufficient defense, even when that judgment is medically sound.

Similarly, a competent individual has the right to refuse to authorize a procedure, regardless of how arbitrary or incorrect his assumptions, fears, or concerns. The individual or institution rendering the service has the obligation to prove that valid consent was obtained.

Again, competence is a necessary prerequisite for consent. "The essential determination to be made is whether the patient has sufficient mental ability to understand the situation and make a rational decision as to treatment. In terms of mental capacity to consent, the test may be stated as: Does the patient has sufficient mind to reasonably understand the condition, the nature and effect of the proposed treatment, attendant risks in pursuing the treatment, and not pursuing the treatment." (Rosoff 1981, 233)

In contrast to the legal rationale, the ethical basis for consent is the enhancement of individual autonomy, decision-making capacity, and personal well-being.

The President's Commission for the Study of Ethical Problems in Medicine and Biomedical and Behavioral Research defined consent as an ongoing process of information exchange and shared decision making, rather than the signing of a document required to protect practitioners from legal liability (President's Commission 1982).

Although in the strictest sense, there may not be such a thing as "fully informed" consent among laymen, this does not necessarily make such consent impossible. It only means that we must try harder to obtain the most informed consent possible from a given individual. The physician, however, is never strictly an impartial supplier of information and is likely to show some personal preference or inclination.

The judicious process for obtaining informed consent in LTC therefore involves a number of steps:

- Determine competence before requesting consent.

- Formulate the presentation of the information to accommodate limitations of the patient, such as hearing deficits or lessened attention span.

- Consider using a family member or patient advocate to help interpret the information.

- Record the consent in the medical record.

- Make allowances for a change of heart.

- Don't confuse refusal to consent with incompetence.

The individual always has the privilege to waive his right to informed consent, and either give the decision-making power to the physician (or someone else), or request only certain limited information that he feels comfortable receiving.

Proxy Consent

Many elderly patients are unable to give consent for a variety of reasons, and physicians must therefore obtain proxy consent.

There are several different types of proxy consent.

1. specific authorization, whereby the patient directly instructs to do or not do something

2. general authorization with instructions, wherein the person tells a proxy agent, "Here are my general values; offer consent consistent with those guidelines"

3. general authorization without instructions, wherein the agent is merely authorized to act

4. substitute judgment, whereby the agent says, "Here is the judgment the patient would make if he could"

5. deputy judgment, whereby the agent simply makes a decision for the patient without regard to any particular claims, instructions, or values.

At one time or another, every LTC physician will encounter each one of these circumstances. Wherever possible, doctors should encourage and facilitate explicit directives, documented appropriately and in a timely manner, to simplify and expedite subsequent decision making, especially at times when the individual is no longer able to participate in the deliberations.

The Judicial Role

The courts are *not* the best place for substitute judgments to be made routinely, because this route is cumbersome, costly, and not timely. Therefore, the physician should do everything possible to resolve the question among physician and patient representatives without resorting to the courts.

Increasingly, the law is approving of proxy consent without preliminary court-appointed guardianship, when the proxy consenter is a close relative or associate acting in the patient's best interest. The guarantor (the one responsible for paying the bill) is not necessarily the patient's appropriate consenter.

The physician and other professionals should first check to see if a patient has indicated a specific person or order of preference; if so, those requests ought to be honored, unless they are legally inappropriate. Otherwise, the generally accepted sequence for obtaining consent is:

- spouse, or if not reasonably available,
- an adult child, or if not reasonably available,

- a parent, or if not reasonably available,
- an adult sibling, or if not reasonably available,
- a grandparent, or if not reasonably available,
- an adult grandchild.

As always, the laws of specific states may dictate otherwise.

Before proxy consent is sought, the treating physician should in-dicate on the appropriate forms or sections of the medical record that the involved patient is not capable of offering his or her con-sent, and the reasons why not.

When proxy consent is obtained for various purposes, the physician and other professionals should complete appropriate forms or progress notes, verifying the nature of the discussion with the proxy consenter, the date and time, any special comments or considerations, the witnessing of a signature of the proxy consenter, and the medical verification that such consent was necessitated by the patient's lack of decision-making capacity.

Living Wills

The living will is one way in which a person can express his wishes and issue directions for his care prior to the time he reaches a state where this is no longer possible.

The living will provides a legal insistence that a person's wishes about terminal care *must* be honored by the attending physician. However, patients do not require a living will in order to have those wishes honored.

Each state that has passed a "living will" law has issued some specific guidelines regarding a proper procedure and format for such a document. The physician should consult his own state's law, the local medical society, the state hospital association, or the American Hospital Association for further information and guidance on his state's specific requirements. (A typical living will declaration is illustrated in Figure 12-3.) Descriptions of the in-dividual state statutes are also available in a handbook from the Society for the Right to Die (1985).

If at any time I should have an incurable injury, disease, or illness certified to be a terminal condition by two (2) physicians who have personally examined me, one (1) of whom shall be my attending physician, and the physicians have determined that my death is imminent and will occur whether or not life-sustaining procedures are utilized and that where the application of such procedures would serve only to artificially prolong the dying process, I direct that such procedures be withheld or withdrawn, and that I be permitted to die naturally with only the performance of any medical procedure necessary to provide comfort and care, or alleviate pain. If I am unable to give directions regarding the use of such life-sustaining procedures, it is my intention that this declaration shall be honored by my family and physician(s) as the final expression of my right to control my medical care and treatment.

I, _____, being of sound mind, willfully and voluntarily direct that my dying shall not be artificially prolonged under the circumstances set forth in this declaration.

Other Instructions

_____

_____

I am legally competent to make this declaration, and I understand its full importance.
Declaration made this _____ day of _____ (month, year).

Signed _____
Address _____

* *

Statement of Witnesses

Under penalty of perjury, we state that this declaration was signed by: _____ in the presence of the undersigned who, at his/her request, in his/her presence, and in the presence of each other, have hereunto signed our names and witnessed it this _____ day of _____, 19___, and declare: The declarant is personally known to me and I believe the declarant to be of sound mind. I did not sign the declarant's signature to this declaration. Based upon information and belief, I am not related to the declarant by blood or marriage, a creditor of the declarant, entitled to any portion of the estate of the declarant under any existing testamentary instrument of the declarant, financially or otherwise responsible for the declarant's medical care, or an employee of any such person or institution.

Signature_____ Address: _____

Signature_____ Address: _____

Reprinted courtesy of Levindale Hebrew Geriatric Center and Hospital; Baltimore, Maryland

Figure 12-3 Sample living will declaration.

In general, the following steps are appropriate for the LTC physician in dealing with a patient who wishes to draft a living will:

- Determine and document the patient's capacity for executing such a document (see previous discussion on competence).

- Make sure that proper procedure is followed, according to state laws.

- Verify with the patient that a copy is to be a part of the record.

- Confirm whether the individual wishes information about his preferences, or the actual document, to be sent with him if he is admitted to a hospital, or otherwise transferred within the LTC system.

- Make known to an acute hospital, and to other professional staff, the existence of such a document when the individual is admitted to a facility, especially where required by law.

- Cover the appropriate circumstances of limiting or withdrawing treatment with pertinent orders.

Limiting or Withdrawing Treatment

There is always a need for decisions in LTC regarding the limiting or withdrawing of treatments, regardless of whether an individual has drawn explicit guidelines for professionals to follow.

Such decisions should be just as much a part of the plan of care as the treatment, test, and medication orders. Seen in this way, they do not have the same ominous sense of "doing nothing."

Making the Decision

The decision to withhold or withdraw care should be made by the physician in consultation with patient (where possible), patient representative, and other professional staff. The reasons for the decision should be documented appropriately. The possibility for reevaluating a situation and changing the approach should be left open, where indicated.

Implementing the Decision

Appropriate orders should be left for other staff to follow (see discussion under *No-Code, Do Not Resuscitate (DNR) Situations*, following). These do not necessarily cover only the case of resuscitation, but may include other specific guidelines about nonresuscitation events. Therefore, one DNR order may *not* be sufficient to cover all such possibilities. Some sort of classification system may be helpful, specifying the components of a given level of care (for example, transfer to an acute hospital, or nothing, except measures for comfort and pain relief). Such a classification is not an order, but a plan of care. It serves as general guidelines, and may vary depending on the individual case. For example, the fact that antibiotics *may* be indicated does not necessarily mean that they should or will be ordered or administered in a given instance (see the Appendix).

The "no-resuscitation" classification should be covered by a signed physician's order, clarified by an appropriate policy (see discussion below).

No-Code, Do Not Resuscitate (DNR) Situations

No-code orders have only recently been widely accepted. They specifically refer to whether and to what extent attempts at resuscitation should be made in the event a person suffers cardiopulmonary arrest.

Several studies have found that individuals who are made "no-code" patients are often given less treatment for other nonterminal illnesses. As noted above, it may very well be appropriate to distinguish the two circumstances, either by policy or through specific orders in individual cases, so that no-code patients will receive some appropriate treatment and supportive care.

For example, a bedridden, immobile uncommunicative NH resident would almost certainly be a "no-code" patient, but might well still deserve treatment for a bout of pulmonary edema or a urinary tract infection. Or, an alert functional older person might be a "no-code" patient as a result of having written a living will, but would still desire and deserve substantial medical therapy for acute illness, short of resuscitation.

Every medical staff should cover itself with an appropriate DNR policy. Cardiopulmonary resuscitation (CPR) should be defined to include all physical, mechanical, electronic, or chemical intervention used to try to help a patient recover following spontaneous cessation of cardiac or pulmonary function. When a no-code, no-CPR, or DNR order is written, none of these methods should be used in the event of sudden spontaneous cessation of cardiac or pulmonary function. The following are some suggested guidelines:

- The attending physician should decide when to write the DNR order after consultation and agreement with patient or family.

- The attending physician should write the DNR order directly, except under extraordinary circumstances. A verbal DNR order should be witnesses and documented by two nurses, and should be countersigned within 24 hours.

- Documentation should include: a summary of the person's condition; the names of persons involved in the decision leading to the DNR status; and, a brief description of the wishes of the patient or authorized proxy.

- The attending physician should review the DNR order periodically after reassessing the patient's condition, to ensure that the order remains appropriate.

Terminal Care and Hospice Consent

Any facility or program providing terminal care should have certain policies covering the various aspects of that care. Above all else, a physician should certify that the individual has a terminal condition, for which only the relief of pain and the maintenance of personal comfort are appropriate. Although such patients can receive appropriate terminal care in any LTC setting, many will opt to participate in a hospice program. Hospice care provides a comprehensive approach to terminal care using formal guidelines and standards (see Chapters 2 and 5). Individuals who desire admission into a hospice program can be requested to agree to certain conditions and guidelines, which may be presented in a hospice consent form (see Figure 12-4).

When used, this form should be presented to the patient or family on the day of admission or at the earliest opportunity. If the patient is determined to be capable of making decisions, the physician should review diagnosis, prognosis, care and treatment plan, and assure understanding and acceptance.

If the patient is not capable of offering consent, the attending physician should so indicate, and should help present the information and form to the proxy consenter.

Using Ethics Advisory Committees in LTC

Ethics committees are becoming increasingly common in acute hospitals, and occasionally in LTC settings. They are also known by such other names as human values committees, medical-morals committees, bioethics committees, and ethics advisory committees.

Among others, the President's Commission for the Study of Ethical Problems in Medicine and Biomedical and Behavioral Research, which produced its report in 1982, suggested that health care institutions experiment with such committees. In the process, though, it is important to clearly define the roles and responsibilities of such committees.

Functions

These committees may serve one or more of these functions:

- allowing forums for discussion among various professionals on bioethical issues

- making recommendations to professionals on their options in various cases, and reviewing decisions already implemented to see how things might be done differently in similar future circumstances

- educating staff and community on various bioethical issues

- assisting in the development of administrative, board, medical, and patient care policies

(Complete only revelant sections. Cross out others.)

Name of Patient: _____

Date of Admission: _____

1. Patient's Statement

I,_____, request admission to Levindale Hebrew Geriatric Center and Hospital's Hospice Program. I understand that I have a terminal illness for which cure is no longer a possibility. I request that I be allowed to die with dignity and comfort and not be kept alive by artificial means or heroic measures. I understand that the Hospice Program will provide physical, psychological, social and spiritual support to myself and my family. This form has been fully explained to me and I am aware of its content and significance.

Date: _____   Signed: _____
                                                                                     (Patient's Signature)

Witness:_____

2. Physician Confirmation of Patient Statement

I, _____ am the attending physician to the above named patient. I hereby certify that the above directive represents the sentiment of the patient and that this individual is competent at this time to make such a statement on his/her own behalf.

Date:_____   Signed: _____
                                                                                     (Physician's Signature)

Witness:_____

3. Proxy Statement (Where appropriate)

I (we),_____, am (are) related to the above-named individual as follows: _____

At this time, this person is, according to his/her caretakers, unable to competently express his/her wishes regarding care and treatment. I (we) understand from the attending physician (s) that he/she has a terminal illness for which a cure is impossible. I (we) believe that this person wishes to die with dignity and comfort and to not be kept alive by artificial means or heroic measures. I (we) furthermore believe that this individual does not wish to be resuscitated if he/she should be found without pulse or respirations. I (we) also believe that this is what this person would request if he/she could express himself/herself at this time.

Date:_____   Signature _____

Witness:_____

4. Physician Confirmation of Proxy Statement

I agree that this patient has an incurable terminal illness, and that the above statement represents the wishes of the proxy consentor (s).

Date:_____   Signature: _____

Witness:_____

Reprinted courtesy of Levindale Hebrew Geriatric Center and Hospital; Baltimore, Maryland

#1028

Figure 12-4 Sample hospice consent form.

- assessing institutional experiences on various specific bioethical problems

- reviewing the current literature, state and federal laws and regulations, and the experiences of others, and adapting these to the specific setting.

The committee should feel free to involve consultants and to meet with the patient, professionals, families, or any other interested or concerned individuals. As necessary, it should search the literature, or avail itself of any pertinent information from other institutions in similar situations.

After due consideration, recommendations of the committee should be made as appropriate to the professionals caring for the patient, and offered to the patient and the family or other proxy decision maker. Those involved in a particular case should generally excuse themselves when that case is discussed.

Regardless of the arrangements, these committees should not be used to force decisions or particular viewpoints on anyone. They are not professional review boards, substitutes for legal or judicial review, or decision-making or policy-making bodies. Instead, they should assist by clarifying issues, explaining options, and facilitating the exploration and convergence of different opinions.

Whether such special committees exist is perhaps not as important as the fact that the relevant activities take place. A number of models are available (Levine 1984). They can be linked to other institutional committees, such as patient care and quality assurance. Minutes of any such committee meetings should be kept to document the process of decision making and the consideration of options.

Representation

Membership should be multidisciplinary and may include doctors, nurses, social workers, clergy, ethicists, administrators, attorneys, and patient advocates. Some of these may be better used as consultants rather than as standing committee members. A typical LTC ethics advisory committee consists of two physicians, including the medical director, two representatives of nursing, one social worker, and the chaplain of the facility.

Physician Role

The physician role on the committee is similar to that in individual cases. The physician should:

- clarify medical issues in specific cases, such as prognosis and likely outcome of treatment options

- explain and interpret technical medical terms and procedures, such as those involved in life support or resuscitation

- represent the questions and concerns of attending physicians

- help educate those physicians about concepts in ethics and the recommendations of the committee

- help the medical staff draw enlightened patient care policies, such as those regarding hospice care or DNR orders, based on such recommendations.

When the committee is unable to reach a consensus to advise on resolving a difficult case, it should still issue its report and various opinions to the administration to assist in further deliberation about appropriate management.

Appendix 12-A Example of Long-Term Care Treatment
Classification System

Classifications

Terminal and Critical Illness

Class A — Maximum therapeutic effort.
Transfer to chronic hospital or nearest hospital without hesitation, if necessary.
Patient is candidate for intensive care unit (ICU), respirator, if necessary.

Class B — Maximum therapeutic effort within limits of his institution.
Transfer to chronic hospital, if necessary (where reevaluation may occur).
Not an ICU candidate.
Some invasive procedures, special tests may be appropriate.
Try to avoid transfer to hospital.

Class C — Limited therapeutic measures.
X-rays, blood tests may be in order.
IVs may be appropriate.
Antibiotics should be used sparingly.
Invasive procedures and transfer to hospital for special tests should be avoided.
Change to Class B or D depends on patient's response to initial treatment.

Class D — No therapeutic effort.
Only that which enhances comfort and minimizes pain.
No X-rays, blood tests, and antibiotics.
IVs ought not be instituted unless they are to enhance comfort or minimize pain.

ON ADMISSION, PATIENTS SHOULD BE TREATED AS CLASS A OR B UNTIL FURTHER DESIGNATION IS MADE.

This patient should be considered Class ____ if critically ill. "Critical illness" means an illness which could lead to imminent death, but might respond to treatment, i.e., pneumonia, pulmonary embolus, M.I., etc.

(Reprinted by courtesy of Levindale Hebrew Geriatric Center and Hospital; Baltimore, MD.)

This patient should be considered Class ____ if terminally ill. "Terminal illness" means an illness which will result in imminent death regardless of treatment, i.e., metastatic cancer, certain neurologic diseases, etc.

Resuscitation

Class 1 — Maximum resuscitative effort, within limits of this institution.
　　　　Transfer to nearest hospital if needed. Full-fledged code.

Class 2 — Limited effort
　　　　A period of appropriate drugs may be tried.
　　　　Full-fledged code until physician says otherwise.
　　　　If patient survives, transfer to nearest hospital, if needed.

Class 3 — No resuscitative effort.
　　　　Do not call a code.
　　　　Do not send to hospital.

If this patient should suffer witnessed cardiopulmonary arrest because of an accident, choking, or other emergency, do attempt to stop bleeding, clear obstructed airway, etc. If a continued resuscitative effort appears needed, treat this patient as Class ____.

If this patient is found to be apparently dead, (that is, without pulse or respirations) and the event is unwitnessed, he or she should be considered a Class ____ patient.

In all cases, unless the patient is Class 3, the Nursing Staff should initiate resuscitation and thereafter contact the attending or on-call physician for further instructions.

References

Brown, N.K., and D.J. Thompson. 1979. Non-treatment of fever in extended care facilities. *New England Journal of Medicine* 300:1246-1250.

Levine, C. 1984. Questions and (some very tentative) answers about hospital ethics committees. *Hastings Center Report* 14(3):9-12.

McCullogh, L.B. 1984. Medical care for elderly patients with diminished competence: an ethical analysis. *Journal of the American Geriatrics Society* 32:150-153.

Pearlman, R., et al. 1982. Variability in physician bioethical decision-making: A case study of euthanasia. *Annals of Internal Medicine* 97:420-425.

Pearlman, R., and J.B. Speer. 1983. Quality of life considerations in geriatric care. *Journal of the American Geriatrics Society* 31:113-120.

Pearlman, R.A., and A. Jonsen. 1985. The use of quality-of-life considerations in medical decision making. *Journal of the American Geriatrics Society* 33:344-352.

President's commission for the study of ethical problems in medicine and biomedical and behavioral research. 1982. *Making health care decisions, Volume 1.* Washington, DC: Government Printing Office.

Rosoff, A.J. 1981. *Informed consent.* Rockville, MD: Aspen Systems.

Society for the Right to Die. 1985. *The physician and the hopelessly ill patient.* New York: Society for the Right to Die.

For Further Reading

Periodicals

Hastings Center Report. A bimonthly publication of the Hastings Institute (see below). Offers a wide variety of reports and commentaries on the spectrum of biomedical issues and concerns. Available with membership.

Hospital Medical Ethics. A recent publication of the American Hospital Association, designed to provide much of the same information as the above.

Medical Ethics Advisor. A newsletter providing a broad range of information on ethical issues of current interest, diverse opinions, recent court cases, and advisories. Available by subscription from American Health Consultants, Atlanta, Ga. for $148 a year.

Also, many issues of the *Journal of the American Geriatrics Society* and *The Gerontologist*, and some issues of the *Annals of Internal Medicine* and *The New England Journal of Medicine* have articles of interest on ethical issues in geriatrics.

Books

The following books provide a nucleus of interesting and helpful information on bioethical issues pertinent to the practice of the LTC physician:

American Hospital Association. 1985. *Values in Conflict: Resolving Ethical issues in Hospital Care.* A report of the Special Committee on Biomedical Ethics, with a number of ideas and opinions that can be just as useful in LTC as in the hospital setting.

Beauchamp, T.L, and J.F. Childress. 1983. *Principles of Biomedical Ethics.* New York: Oxford Univ. Press. A clear, concise overview of the principles underlying biomedical ethics.

Brody, H. 1981. *Ethical Decisions in Medicine.* Boston: Little, Brown. One of the pioneering books in the field, this is an interactive case-oriented workbook which helps demonstrate the ethical decision-making process, and clarify the issues and principles.

Doudera, A.E., and J.D. Peters. 1982. *Legal and Ethical Aspects of Treating Critically and Terminally Ill Patients.* Ann Arbor, Mich.: AUPHA Press. A very comprehensive discussion of legal and ethical principles and precedents for the management of the critically and terminally ill.

Kapp, M.D., Pies, H.E., and A.E. Doudera. 1985. *Legal and Ethical Aspects of Health Care for the Elderly.* Ann Arbor, MI: Health Administration Press. Published in cooperation with the American Society of Law and Medicine, this covers the spectrum of issues from both legal *and* ethical standpoints, showing how the two often mesh, and sometimes diverge.

Pellegrino, E.D., and D.C. Thomasma. 1981. *A Philosophical Basis of Medical Practice.* New York: Oxford University Press. A readable discussion of the ideas and principles underlying the issues and decisions of medical ethics.

Siegler, M., Jonsen, A., and W.J. Winslade. 1982. *Clinical Ethics.* New York: Macmillan. A well-indexed, case-oriented handbook that strives to offer both practical and theoretical guidance and support for the spectrum of ethical problems that the practicing physician might encounter in everyday practice.

Additional Resources

Hastings Institute (Institute of Society, Ethics, and the Life Sciences). A center for the study of all ethical issues, especially in society, politics, and the biomedical sciences. Also, a vast information resource for organizations, governments, students and fellows, and interested individuals.

Kennedy Institute of Ethics. A center for bioethics information, and the study of the issues, founded in 1971, and based at Georgetown University. Among its programs is the National Reference Center for Bioethics Literature, located on the main campus. The library houses the world's largest collection of material related to ethical issues in medicine and biomedical research. *Bioethicsline*, produced by the Bioethics Information Retrieval Project of the Kennedy Institute, is a comprehensive online bibliographic data base supplied by the Institute to the National Library of Medicine.

Medline. The National Library of Medicine's online citation service can include a search through the medical literature for any topic of interest, including bioethics.

Chapter Thirteen

The Teaching Nursing Home

Jane F. Potter, M.D. and Susan G. Scholer, M.D.

Chapter Objectives

This chapter will:

- discuss the teaching nursing home concept and the academic geriatric medical center
- provide an overview of the educational opportunities in long-term care
- describe the program components and various roles for physicians
- discuss the program's organizational structure
- consider the advantages and disadvantages to the community and elderly patients
- review the possible arrangements for patient care in a teaching setting
- evaluate the experience with teaching nursing homes in the U.S. to date
- consider various modifications of the teaching nursing home concept

History

Organizations to support study and research in aging were started in the early 1940s, among them, the American Geriatrics Society (1942) and the Gerontological Society of America (1945). It is significant that the early research and patient care programs that followed (1950-1970) were centered at not-for-profit nursing homes and that the first training program in geriatrics at a U.S. medical school was based in a skilled nursing facility (1972). In 1975, the first organized fellowship program in geriatrics in the U.S. was started at the Jewish Institute for Geriatric Care in Stony Brook, Long Island, New York. During the last decade, the number of training programs has increased to fifty-four. Ten of these programs were established by the Veterans Administration as Geriatric Research, Education and Clinical Centers (GRECCs); the remainder are based in teaching programs of internal medicine and family practice. In 1986, many geriatric fellowship programs joined the nationwide matching program.

Today, several practical reasons favor basing geriatric education and research programs in long-term care facilities (LTCFs). The residents of LTCFs display a vast array of pathology. LTC wards allow teaching in a traditional hospital style. Since LTC is generally underserved by physicians, the training programs help ensure access to physicians' services. Thus, teaching nursing homes are evolving as the home base for academic geriatrics, the vehicle for teaching, service, and research.

Why Are Teaching Nursing Homes Needed?

Teaching nursing homes (TNHs) are highly appropriate sites for teaching and research in geriatrics. They are the clinical laboratories for research into chronic disease, health policy, markers of disease and disability, the pathophysiology of aging, and the delivery of health care to the older population. During the first half of his century, medical investigation focused on acute reversible illnesses affecting people of all ages. Improved longevity has resulted in a very large older population with the attendant chronic diseases of old age. Whether or not people are reaching old age more disabled, or in a generally healthy condition, is a subject of current debate (Brody 1985). In either case, the burden of chronic illness is substantial. Many such illnesses result in institutionalization of the elderly and contribute heavily to the limitations of individuals still in the community. Advances in the treatment of chronic illness now lag far behind those of acute disease.

Though medical training has been based in acute care hospitals since the time of William Osler, the 1980s have witnessed a shift away from the hospital setting for two reasons. First, acute illness is no longer the major cause of morbidity and mortality. Secondly, third-party payors now set limits on the use of expensive acute care services. Adequate patient subjects for training will require some use of chronic care beds, projected to increase in number to 2 million by the end of this century, while the number of acute care beds will decrease at the same time from 1.1 million to 0.9 million. The Institute of Medicine (1978, 54) recommends using LTCF sites because the medical problems of old age cannot be taught adequately on the acute hospital wards. In addition, attitudes towards old people and the objectives of their care can be much better communicated to the trainee in the more relaxed and residential environment of the LTCF.

Properly developed TNHs will help bridge the major philosophical and financial gaps between acute and long-term care (Aronson 1984). Perhaps as many as 40% of all old people will spend some time in a nursing home (Kane 1981). The enormous public expense created by the physician's misunderstanding of LTC has been addressed elsewhere (Williams 1985). Unless students and house officers learn that nursing home care can be, and often is, transitional, they will tend to view nursing homes as warehouses rather than as places for recuperation and rehabilitation, leading ultimately to improved function or to discharge.

Implementing medical interventions to improve function, rather than high-technology acute intervention to treat illness, will bring LTC into focus for physicians without violating the supportive, residential nature of long-term care, and should improve the care and management of chronic illness.

The reimbursement gap between acute and long-term care is obvious to anyone who works in both settings. More physician involvement will, however, require better reimbursement for service. Studies in long-term care should attempt to demonstrate which services can be delivered more cost-effectively in long-term care, as opposed to in the hospital, and to identify those services hospitals could offer to ultimately reduce the cost associated with long-term institutionalization. Especially important are services that improve function and allow patients to be cared for at lower and less costly levels.

Robert Butler (1981) has suggested that just as teaching hospitals have created models for community hospitals, so too TNHs could create the model for physicians (and other health professionals) functioning in LTCFs. The ultimate goals of the TNH are to positively influence public policy, medical practice, and physician training; to improve the care of older patients in nursing homes and physicians' practices; and to design services and strategies for postponing or preventing institutionalization and for rehabilitating patients and returning them to their homes.

The Academic Geriatric Medical Center

The struggle to describe new ideas always produces new terminology. The words "academic geriatric medical center" are used in place of teaching nursing home (TNH) to imply a wide range of services and commitment to innovative programming and research. While the old concept of the nursing home suggested permanent admission for terminal or lifelong care, the new concept includes admission for various acute, subacute, or exacerbated chronic problems, with the desired outcome of functional recovery and discharge to the patient's home or to a lower level of care. To be effective in teaching these concepts, the academic geriatric medical center must expose trainees to the continuum of care, and must therefore have either reliable access to that continuum, or provide many of them itself. This continuum must include a full range of home services, including those necessary for care of totally dependent patients.

The academic geriatric medical center itself can contribute special inpatient and outpatient services to meet specific needs of older patients, yet which are less likely to be found in a traditional LTC setting. This includes, for example, emergency admission to help patients and families deal with a crisis. While generally available in most medical communities, geriatric rehabilitation programs are better centered in the academic geriatric center because of the available support of experts in geriatric medicine and geropsychiatry. Less well-established programs, such as postacute care following hospitalization, are also suited to the academic center. Health services research should try to demonstrate cost-effectiveness of new or partially established services and to work towards appropriate reimbursement for those services. Although postacute care of older patients incorporates the same approach as a rehabilitation program, it addresses the needs of a much broader group of patients.

The academic geriatric center should develop a sufficient referral base for specialty clinics designed to diagnose and treat certain common problems. Appropriate types of clinics would include: geriatric assessment, memory disorders, incontinence, maintenance rehabilitation, osteoporosis, low vision, and foot care. Which clinics are needed will depend on existing strengths in the medical community.

From the outset, the academic geriatric medical center must be prepared for the costs of teaching and training. The ultimate objective of such care is lower cost and better age-specific treatment for selected patients and problems (Libow 1984).

Opportunities for Research

The physician's role at the TNH, as in any academic program, is to lead research efforts to formulate and answer questions that increase knowledge in geriatrics. An academic program is distinguished by the cluster of inquiring faculty who identify important clinical problems for which no routine treatment or approach exists. Out of such an environment emerges a cadre of well-trained students.

As a research environment, the TNH has certain unique features (Maddox 1985). The research population is changing more slowly (as compared with an acute care population), is under constant observation (as opposed to an outpatient population), and is in a relatively controlled environment. The research population is moderate in size, but relatively complex (i.e., increased biological variability with age, and a plethora of pathology). The LTCF is almost unique in providing access to a frail older population which is notoriously difficult to identify in an outpatient setting. The setting, plus the high rates of illness and disability, facilitates multiple separate measures of the desired variables and allows those variables and individuals to be followed for a relatively long period of time, while providing a rich concentration of research opportunities and participants. Although the research programs in the TNH concentrate on illness in inpatients at the end stage of life, much of the new knowledge gained may be applicable to equally affected home-based patients and in understanding those diseases before they reach a relatively late stage.

The LTC research agenda is quite varied and extends beyond the realm of traditional medical research. There must be equal emphasis on better understanding of the diseases of old age and on disability. Markers and predictors of disability must be identified, and efficacious and cost-effective approaches to treatment of disabilities—whether physical, prosthetic, supportive, or behavioral—must be identified. Closely related to this are the issues of how to care for the disabled, and how to promote independence and foster a therapeutic environment. Both the environment and caregivers, be they family or nursing home staff, are also important foci for research. Those providing maintenance or rehabilitative care must be taught to cope through appropriate training.

While the cost of nursing home care in the U.S. is expected to exceed 76 billion dollars by the end of this century (Butler 1981), there are very few data on how we might best meet the needs of those requiring chronic care at the least cost and with the least possible intensity of services. Such data would aid decisions about revising health care policy to limit the total costs of care.

Opportunities for Training and Teaching

As more acute care hospitals become places for treating critical illness and for high technology and invasive procedures, their relative importance in the basic training of health professionals will decline. The acute hospital teaches important aspects of critical care, but is unsuited for training in the basic aspects of patient interview, examination, diagnosis, and education. Shorter hospital stays preclude following patients from onset and presentation of illness through recovery.

There are two logical responses to this critical issue in health professions training (Schroeder 1986). The first option is to integrate students into outpatient clinics and services. The second is to place students in inpatient units of a TNH setting. The latter option has several advantages. First, it emulates the situations which existed previously in acute care hospitals. Training in a TNH also provides a ready supply of patients with multiple problems, extensive histories, and physical findings. The slower pace in long-term care allows for contact between patient and student over a prolonged period, without interfering with scheduled diagnostic studies. We have taught physical diagnosis for medical students in long-term care facilities for several years and have found a broad variety of pathology covering every system. Residents have been pleased to educate the young doctors, to help the attending physician, and to fill a few hours with contact from enthusiastic students. Besides being ideal for beginning students, the long-term care situation also presents challenges for more advanced trainees (e.g., residents of medicine and family practice) who have learned the basic skills and who have not had the opportunity to see chronic disease and its complications. The weekly follow-up of patients with chronic conditions possible in this setting is hard to duplicate elsewhere.

Unlike treating most acute illness, LTC demands a *multidisciplinary* approach, which in turn requires a broader base of information than is presently taught to health professions trainees. In a long-term care facility, trainees interact not only with residents (patients) but also with an interdisciplinary team of health care workers. Such a team approach helps trainees learn the contributions and respective roles of other disciplines—essential information to acquire before facing complex older patients in a more independent practice setting.

The acute care setting usually shows older people at their worst, so that even optimistic trainees may come to view old age as a time of inevitable decline, and the lack of rapid response to medical intervention as reflecting the futility of such intervention. This prejudice against older people, or "ageism" in medicine, is consistent with the broader social view of old age. The TNH, on the other hand, creates an environment where older people are given time and assistance with recovery, commodities that the acute care hospital can no longer afford to provide. Seeing older patients recover their health and function and return to satisfying lives is an inspiration for geriatric practice.

History taking from older patients requires more time and must be supplemented by family, caregivers, and old records. The subacute or chronic setting is better suited to learning these techniques than is the acute setting (Margolis 1981). Similarly, physical diagnosis of the manifestations of normal aging versus illness is clearer in non-acutely ill patients.

Long-term care is also an excellent training ground for managing ethical issues in medical care, because of its slower pace, lack of technology for invasive life-supporting devices, and requirements for an initial evaluation of the patient and interview of the family, which includes expectations for life and death. When not faced with an emergency, patients and families can contemplate and assist in planning their medical care, much as they are already planning estate and funeral arrangements. Where else can young trainees, whose education focuses entirely on saving lives, learn to appreciate that many people do not desire prolonged life in the face of extreme disability? Rather, LTC patients will more likely wish for optimal function.

Another advantage of training in the TNH setting lies in the opportunity to learn to evaluate and treat *functional* problems. For example, a physician in acute care who evaluates an older patient complaining of dizziness and finds no cardiac and neurological causes, would probably reassure the patient and send him home. Unfortunately, this symptom, which reflects a *functional* problem, may lead to reduced mobility, falls, social isolation, and other complications. Because this functional approach is such an important adjunct to traditional medical evaluation, it has been adopted as a technique in geriatric medicine. Trainees mush learn the importance of physical as well as drug modalities of treatment, including rehabilitation medicine.

The disciplines involved in the training programs of the TNH are medicine, nursing, pharmacy, social work and the rehabilitation therapies—physical, occupational, and speech therapy. It is essential that students be involved only under faculty supervision, if there is to be any benefit to the patients and the facilities, as well as to the trainees.

There is a place for many different trainees. Students can be assigned responsibilities appropriate for their level of training. Geriatric fellows and house officers in medicine and family practice can benefit from making rounds with students of medicine and pharmacy prior to the formal rounds by the attending physicians and other faculty. Nursing students should be involved in direct patient care prior to care planning sessions with faculty nursing supervisors and participation in team rounds and conferences. Depending upon the size and nature of the patient population, either a formal geropsychiatry service or a psychiatric liaison service may also be a valuable part of the teaching program. Trainees might include geropsychiatry fellows, psychiatry residents, and medical and nursing students on psychiatry rotations. Participation by educational programs in speech, occupational, and physical therapies can also greatly enhance the overall academic environment. Social work students working closely with faculty supervisors can learn the skills of patient selection for admission, support during stay, family support and counselling, and discharge planning. These students can benefit from multidisciplinary rounds, care planning, and educational conferences.

The list of possible trainees may also include gerontology program students from local colleges and universities, whose special interests will depend on their major degree areas and specific research or course commitments; undergraduate social work students; recreational therapy students; physical education students; and trainees in health administration, counselling, and law.

Program Components

The size and extent of any teaching program are limited by the available resources within the TNH and the existence of other geriatric programs within the affiliated system. For example, the American Geriatrics Society has established recommendations for components of a fellowship training program, copies of which are available on request (see *Additional Resources*). In brief, these guidelines advocate experience in continuity of care, consultation, and primary care. Recommended training sites include acute care, ambulatory care, and one or more levels of chronic institutional care, as well as such chronic noninstitutional settings as day care or home care.

The seven program components described below list certain common educational objectives, other more specific objectives, and ideas about achieving these in the TNH setting. Common to all programs is instruction in the team approach to geriatric care, ethical decision making, functional assessment, and the data base of geriatric medicine.

Inpatient Rehabilitation

An organized inpatient rehabilitation program offers trainees the opportunity to see patients in the posthospital phase of illnesses such as stroke, hip fracture, and amputation. Because of the short-term nature of these problems, trainees admit a number of patients, observe progress, and discharge patients home substantially recovered. This component offers an introduction to physical medicine, including the role of occupational, physical, and speech therapies. Medical students and residents are taught medical monitoring of geriatric patients during rehabilitation, especially respiratory, cardiovascular and endocrine changes during rehabilitation, and certain common complications (e.g., shoulder-hand syndrome, prosthetic hip dislocation, or stump edema).

While Medicare allows inpatient rehabilitation services for very few diagnoses, a large group of deconditioned and functionally dependent individuals could avoid nursing home placement if given adequate posthospital rehabilitation services (Liem 1986). The educational advantages and objectives are the same as in the acute rehabilitation program. In addition, trainees are taught to recognize the danger of deconditioning and to begin early mobilization and physical therapy for acute hospital patients.

Acute Hospital Services

There are several advantages to providing acute hospital services within the TNH. Patients in all of the inpatient programs will occasionally suffer acute illness. If the patient is transferred out of the TNH, the therapeutic program will be interrupted and precious time and therapeutic gains may be lost. For example, a poststroke patient with hemiparesis and depression who then develops a pneumonia needs to continue physical therapy and treatment of the depression as well as to receive antibiotics and oxygen for the pneumonia. Of course, the potential for transfer to a full-service acute care hospital for advanced diagnostics and subspecialty consultation should exist, if needed. Where possible, the hospital to which patients are transferred should be a teaching hospital, to preserve the continuity of care.

Chronic Care

Chronic care at the skilled or intermediate level provides a stable population with a wide range of diseases and disabilities. The specific educational objectives are early recognition of the causes of functional decompensation, and the importance of maintenance rehabilitation during chronic illness. The chronic care program provides a continuing care experience which is otherwise difficult to attain within a training program.

Mental Health Services

Mental health services are another integral part of each program. In certain cases, a primary mental health service or geropsychiatric unit will be a designated inpatient program. A geropsychiatric service will always be an important consultation source for other TNH programs. As a separate component, the geropsychiatric unit treats the cognitive, affective, and behavioral problems of old age. It doesn't matter if these are primary problems or complications of medical illness. The specific educational objectives are: identifying true depression, distinguishing depression from dementia, understanding the role of medical illness and losses in the depression of old age, and learning both psychotherapeutic and somatic treatment modalities for depression. Other less common but equally important psychiatric disorders, such as paranoia, paraphrenia, and anxiety states, represent important diagnostic and therapeutic challenges.

Day Hospital Services

A day hospital provides several important services within the TNH. One is an alternative to inpatient acute care for problems such as recurrent congestive heart failure and the acute phase of stroke. It can provide most of the services of the acute hospital without the hotel function of overnight stays. As such, it leaves crucial support systems intact while assisting family and caregivers with needed medical services. It can also provide ongoing rehabilitation after an inpatient stay, an alternative to inpatient rehabilitation. The day hospital can assist in the transition to home, facilitate earlier discharge, and allow for adjustment to supportive and therapeutic services. Trainees can learn how the very disabled and medically ill can be maintained at home.

Ambulatory Clinics

Ambulatory clinics in the TNH are of two types. One type offers follow-up services to inpatient programs (e.g., geropsychiatry, geriatric internal medicine, and maintenance rehabilitation); the other, specialty services, such as incontinence, geriatric assessment, and low vision. The major educational advantages are the ability to reproduce the outpatient setting representative of most geriatric practice and to teach about specific geriatric problems. The major disadvantage is that few trainees are accommodated, since usually only one or two students per discipline can participate in each clinic.

Home Care

Finally, home visits or home care services are essential for adequate care of the very disabled. This program represents continuity of care for a disabled but noninstitutionalized population. The educational objectives are to learn home assessment and delivery of medical services in the home, and how individuals adapt to disability. The disadvantages are travel time, the few cases that can be seen per unit time, and the difficulty of physician staffing.

Physician Roles

Since most TNH programs are small, a physician is likely to have more than one role. Also, time commitments may change with the phase of program development. Once programs are established, certain administrative functions may be more appropriately delegated to nonphysicians. Five physician roles in a TNH are described below. They include

- program developer

- program manager

- supervisor of trainees

- researcher and

- primary care provider.

Program Developer

The program developer designs programs suited to the training and research needs of the institution. Initially, the job requires identifying programs to be developed. Selected programs must complement, but not duplicate, existing teaching services. The program developer must provide the basic frameworks for the programs and recruit or convene the necessary multidisciplinary team to fully design them. This individual then oversees the team's effort to outline goals, objectives, organization, and physical space requirements. If remodeling of physical space is required, the program developer must work with the architect to ensure that the design fits the requirements outlined by the multidisciplinary team. Another element of the job description is financial, requiring assistance in any plans to raise funds for program start-up, and working with financial analysts to ensure long-term solvency of the program.

The program developer must have administrative expertise and experience in working with geriatric educational programs. Accountability is divided between the academic and service aspects of the job responsibilities. For academic purposes, this individual reports to the director of the academic unit, potentially a section chief in geriatrics or general internal medicine, or the department chairperson of medicine or family practice. For the service program, he reports to the administrator of the long-term care facility serving as the TNH. The time commitment will vary with the intensity of the effort and the time needed to bring the program into operation. For relatively rapid program development, an individual should be allowed 0.5 FTE time commitment during the start-up phase of the program.

Performance monitoring of the program developer also follows the dual lines of job responsibilities. Reviewing the program developer's performance is mainly the responsibility of the administrative head of the long-term care facility. Academic programs use such information as student evaluations and peer judgments in their annual review of faculty performance. Other relevant factors to be noted in performance monitoring include: knowledge of the job, quality of the work, judgment and initiative, the quantity of work, dependability and reliability, courtesy and cooperation, and supervisory abilities.

Program Manager

The second major role for physicians in academic programs within the TNH is as program manager. The manager ensures the smooth day-to-day operation of the program. It is critical from the outset to establish control and clear lines of responsibility and authority. Once the program is running smoothly, many aspects of this position can be handled by a nonphysician, such as an administrative assistant or nurse manager. The job description for the program manger includes monitoring the performance of various professionals in the program and reporting on their performance to the respective major departments. It is especially important to identify changing or new needs within the program and to make the appropriate adjustments in personnel and services. The financial status of the program must be monitored, and it is occasionally necessary to correspond or meet with intermediaries to ensure that the services are appropriately reimbursed. Along with this financial consideration come monitoring of appropriateness of patient triage and discharge planning. Discharge planning is closely tied to the responsibility of arranging and monitoring the program's support services. Another task of the manager is timely and convenient scheduling of personnel and trainees and team meetings.

The skills, knowledge, and abilities of the program manger must include personnel management, administration, finance, community support services, and relevant aspects of geriatrics. For example, in a rehabilitation program, this individual should have had previous administrative experience in similar settings. The physician manger should be accountable to the academic program and to the administration of the TNH.

The time commitment is proportional to the size of the program. An inpatient service with seven-day-a-week operation requires approximately 0.3 full-time employees for program management, with additional time devoted to a professional service role. Later, if an administrative assistant or nurse manager is employed, the physician time for administration can be reduced to 0.1 FTE, although a service commitment would continue at 0.3 FTE or greater.

Performance monitoring again falls to both the academic unit and the long-term care administrators, emphasizing peer judgments and student evaluations, and publications stemming from work within the program. These elements are considered part of the annual faculty performance review. The long-term care administrator's performance criteria center on financial viability of the program, job satisfaction of employees within the program, and continued flow of patients to and from the program services.

Supervisor of Trainees

The third major role for physicians in the TNH is as supervisor of trainees. There must be at least one supervisor per discipline, since a physician cannot adequately supervise students of other professions. Academic appointments are necessary for all supervisors (e.g., at a level of a clinical instructor or assistant professor). The basic job description includes working with the appropriate academic department to schedule trainees, establishing performance standards and expectations for trainees, and clarifying these standards during the orientation of all new trainees. The supervisor provides direct oversight of trainees' clinical data collection and analysis, and plans of treatment and care; integrates didactic teaching with clinical experiences; monitors trainees during conduct of their clinical responsibilities; assesses quality of trainee performance, reporting this to the appropriate academic department; and evaluates curriculum content and effectiveness. The use of pre- and post-testing, and a review of trainee performance on standardized examinations, are two trainee evaluation tools.

The skills, knowledge, and abilities of the supervisor must qualify him for an academic appointment within the respective department, and should include training or extensive experience in geriatrics and knowledge and experience in academic training programs. This individual is accountable to the academic department as described above and to the medical staff of the TNH for the quality of patient care delivered by trainees. The time commitment is 1.0 FTE per 2-3 graduate trainees (residents or fellow) and 2-4 medical students.

Performance of the supervisor of trainees is monitored through the academic unit, and also includes student evaluations and peer judgments, emphasizing evaluation by the program manager in which the supervisor is working. Performance is also monitored by the medical staff of the TNH in accordance with their established bylaws and policies.

Researcher

Another essential role for physicians in the TNH is as a researcher who designs and conducts experimental protocols aimed at reduction of morbidity and mortality in that target population. This individual should hold an academic appointment at the affiliated medical center. The researcher seeks approval for protocols through the Institutional Review Board (IRB) of the long-term care facility or, if the LTCF does not wish to conduct this review, by agreement with the IRB of the academic institution on behalf of the LTCF. He seeks informed consent or assent for participation in protocols from residents, and in most cases, also from guardians or relatives. He should routinely share research findings with the administration and medical staff of the long-term care facility. He should seek funding for research from sources outside the LTCF, which will have a positive spill-over effect on care within the TNH. He must also ensure that the protocols conducted at any given time do not compete or interfere with each other.

Most importantly, the skills, knowledge, and abilities of the researcher in a TNH should include knowledge of the problems of disabled individuals and the important conditions producing morbidity and mortality in this population. The researcher must also know the LTC setting, and the ethics of conducting research with incompetent or partially competent individuals. The relevant research skills are to be identified by the academic institution prior to the individual's appointment with that institution and the TNH. Accountability is to the academic institution for purposes of promotion and tenure. For the conduct of research, the researcher is responsible to the medical director of the TNH and the IRB. The time commitment spent on research is determined by the academic institution where that faculty member's time is routinely allocated between research, clinical, and teaching responsibilities. Performance is monitored by the chairperson of the department in which the academic appointment is held, who must seek review of the researcher's performance by the medical staff and the IRB of the TNH.

Primary Care Provider

The final physician role is as primary care provider. In this role, the physician is an essential member of the medical staff to cover nonteaching units in a large facility or in a facility with a small teaching service. This individual might supervise trainees, when present, and provide primary care in their absence. The job description has four major requirements. The primary care provider must: 1) make timely visits to residents for health monitoring, reevaluation and treatment, and to satisfy the requirements of regulatory agencies; 2) be on-call to see patients with new or emergent problems noted by the charge nurse; 3) evaluate changing levels of care needs, such as increasing or decreasing degrees of dependence, and reevaluate appropriateness of the level of care; and 4) educate patients, families, and nursing staff on the residents' diagnoses, prognoses, and treatment programs. Essential skills, knowledge, and abilities should include training in internal medicine, and training in or knowledge of psychiatry, physiatry, neurology, and the causes of functional decline in old age. This individual is accountable to the medical director and the medical staff. The time commitment is proportional to the number of patients served. Performance monitoring is by the medical staff organization under their bylaws.

Affiliations with Other Institutions

The impetus for establishing a TNH may begin within either the long-term care facility or the academic institution. However, without a strong desire for a TNH program on both sides, the effort is doomed to failure. An academic initiative may provide for the purchase or building of a facility to house programs or for an affiliation agreement with an interested LTCF. The advantage of affiliation is that the cost of management and maintenance of the environment is the responsibility of the LTCF. The major disadvantage is that the academic institution or representatives may not have a formal place in the organizational chart, and will therefore be less able to influence program selection and direction.

If the desire for becoming a TNH arises within the LTCF, it must first have the support of the medical staff. With that support, the next step is to approach academic institutions to ascertain interest in such a program. Unless the academic side is willing to commit substantial resources, the LTCF must be willing to supplement and financially support development of the academic faculty. Even then, the long-term viability of such an academic program will depend on recognition of the importance of clinical service and clinical research in geriatrics by the academic administration.

The ideal situation is a strong commitment by both the LTCF and the academic institution, which must include personnel, space, and a willingness to work through the difference in perspective that these very different institutions bring. The academic institution is highly ordered in levels of responsibility, and it is rare for any decision to be made by a single individual. The LTCF is accustomed to operating under substantial financial constraints and to make decisions based on established operating procedures. Accepting a meaningful academic affiliation complicates and alters established operating procedures. There must be a willingness on both sides to develop a new operating model. This is discussed further in the section entitled *Organizational Arrangements*.

The essential elements of the TNH are, theoretically, simple. There must be a stable environment. Standards of care and mechanisms for quality assurance must be in place, since the aims of the TNH will be defeated if trainees see suboptimal care in the LTC setting. There must be a tolerance for trainees with varying levels of expertise, and the usual academic arrangement of prerounding by trainees followed by the attending physician's rounds. The nursing staff must become accustomed to changing plans of care after attending rounds. Nurses must also be willing to advise trainees based on the nurses' greater knowledge in certain aspects of resident care. There must be an ongoing commitment to the educational and research programs, and a willingness to work through the inevitable problems which will arise. Finally, there must be a close interdependence between the academic and LTC agencies. This interdependence must occur at all levels from the board (which should include individuals from both agencies) down to the level of staff, where cross-appointments must be sought and encouraged.

Other elements are desirable, but less critical. Geographic proximity to the academic center helps to foster recognition of the TNH as an important part of the academic programs, reduces travel time, facilitates educational exchange, and helps to reduce duplication by permitting sharing of resources and services. The further apart the two institutions, the more likely they are to see their missions as separate and distinct. It is also desirable to have the academic offices within the TNH, as this encourages commitment to academic responsibilities in addition to clinical service, and makes the office more available to trainees assigned to the TNH.

Perspectives of Practice in the TNH

Medical practice within a TNH is distinctly different from that in the traditional LTCF and more closely approximates the pattern of practice of a teaching hospital. The perspectives vary for physician trainee, staff physician, medical director, and community practitioner.

For the TNH to be a meaningful experience for residents and fellows, they must have first-call responsibilities to see new patients and to evaluate patient-related problems. The TNH, however, is not an acute care hospital, and trainees must appreciate the different orientation and objectives of care in this setting. They must learn to be less invasive, to focus on function, and to work as members of the team. While physicians continue to be team leaders, they must learn the importance of nonmedical considerations and when to place other priorities ahead of purely medical ones.

For the staff physician in LTC, the TNH programs add teaching responsibilities, which some may not wish to accept. Staff physicians must be avid learners and should view interaction with trainees as a prime source of continuing medical education. They must also be willing to take one step back from primary care responsibilities and allow trainees some latitude in patient management.

The medical director should in most cases have an academic appointment and in every case must have a firm commitment to the training program. The TNH adds another level of complexity to all the usual responsibilities of medical direction. The medical director of the TNH is not only responsible for monitoring permanent medical staff, but must also develop and monitor performance of a constantly changing pool of trainees.

Physicians with busy community practices who occasionally admit patients to the LTCF with a TNH program will find they have reliable on-site coverage for medical problems. It would be to their advantage to have standing orders for trainee evaluation of residents as problems develop. Housestaff will then consult them after the initial evaluation. A drawback of this arrangement is a possible reduction in professional fees because of fewer visits by the community physician. On the other hand, a visit to evaluate a single patient's acute problem is rarely cost-effective for someone in active practice. The practitioner's periodic visits can be devoted to review of trainee evaluations and to treatment and health maintenance for the resident.

Arrangements for Patient Care within the TNH

The inpatient programs within the TNH are of two basic types: either LTC units or short-stay units. Long-term-care units can be staffed by trainees in one of two ways. Trainees can be assigned to either a one-or two-month rotation, or they can be assigned a certain number of patients for longitudinal care responsibilities.

The latter arrangement is the most difficult to achieve, despite its appeal and potential for greater continuity. Just as physicians in practice find it difficult to provide on-site services to LTC patients, so will trainees have difficulty taking time from their acute and ambulatory care experiences to see LTC residents. Even more difficult is providing an attending staff to see patients with the trainees. Assigning a few LTC unit patients for longitudinal follow-up as the sole geriatric experience is not sufficiently intense to teach the necessary information. There is a danger that such an arrangement will foster negative attitudes about LTC if it is viewed as one more burden in an already busy training program. On the other hand, assigning fellows in geriatric medicine a number of LTC patients for whom they provide continuing care during their training, is an essential part of that experience. Such an arrangement, involving a relatively small number of fellows, facilitates formal attending rounds.

Short (1-2 months) rotations on the LTC unit may be more appropriate exposure to LTC for house officers of internal medicine or family practice. Unfortunately, many typical problems encountered in this population (e.g., decubitus ulcers or immobility) take several weeks or months to respond to treatment and are difficult to appreciate with anything less than a two-month rotation.

Short-term stay units, such as the rehabilitation program described above, lend themselves quite nicely to a two-month block rotation. Many patients will be admitted and discharged in that interval, and the intensity of the program demands frequent rounds by trainees and attending staff. This arrangement holds advantages for patients, in that their physicians devote time to their needs while working with experts in discharge planning, who help reintegrate individuals into the community.

Patient Response to the TNH

The basic, underlying tenet of the TNH programs is that there are ways to provide better nursing home care. If this is true, such benefits should be measurable in structure, process, or outcome, and should improve care without disrupting the more difficult to measure, but equally desireable, qualities of patient comfort and support during chronic illness.

At least two controlled studies (Jahnigen 1985; Wieland 1986) demonstrate certain benefits to patients in TNHs and to the community. Of patients who were discharged from the hospital for permanent LTC, those sent to a TNH were more likely to be discharged home, fewer were rehospitalized, and they were more likely to remain at home. Individuals sent to the TNH were more likely to have their medications reduced as compared with control subjects sent to other nursing homes, who were more likely to have the number of medications increased (Jahnigen 1985). In addition to demonstrating similar outcomes, a second study (Wieland 1986) showed improvements in functional status, patient satisfaction, and morale in the TNH. These studies suggest that costs can be reduced and outcomes improved by TNH care without diminishing patient satisfaction with themselves and their lives.

In the future, it will be extremely important to see if key features of the TNH model can be applied to improve care in the nonteaching setting.

Caution must be exercised, however, lest enthusiasm for the concept of the TNH be allowed to "overmedicalize" the nursing "*home*," already so regimented and restricted. Though dissatisfied with invasive, impersonal hospital care, patients tolerate it because it is short-term and viewed as necessary for a better outcome. Residents of LTCFs, however, must sacrifice some of their autonomy on a long-term basis; the TNH must strive to avoid making those conditions worse. TNH personnel must recognize that for many individuals, aggressive, invasive approaches have minimal benefit, and support and comfort must be the first priority.

Legal and Ethical Issues

The legal issues pertinent to the TNH are more straightforward than the ethical concerns, and will be addressed first. The supervisory or attending physician is responsible for the presence and activities of trainees in any setting. Though the attending is legally responsible for the patient, trainees can be, and have been, sued for malpractice, and their home training programs must provide malpractice insurance coverage. The cost of that insurance is part of the overall cost of the trainee and may or may not be reflected in the salary paid by the LTCF for the services of a resident physician.

Ethical concerns within a TNH are complex and can only be introduced here (see also Chapter 12). For an excellent review of this topic, the reader is also referred to a chapter by Cassel (1985). As in every clinical setting, older residents serving as subjects for the teaching of students and house officers become "cases" for study, which to some extent objectifies human individuality. Caution must therefore be exercised to maintain respect and dignity especially among the extremely infirm and disabled, who are often incapable of insisting on such respect. Research in any institutional setting, or with any vulnerable population, presents a number of ethical dilemmas which must be addressed at the outset. The investigator should justify the need to involve the nursing home population. Institutionalized individuals should be asked to participate in research that is *not* relevant to their own condition only if they can provide informed consent (consent by proxy does not suffice) and the research presents no more than minimal risk. As the risk increases, the investigator must provide evidence as to why the research should be conducted on institutionalized subjects, and show that the research is relevant to their clinical condition and is likely to be of direct individual benefit.

While careful consideration must be given to the nature, type, and appropriateness of research conducted in LTCFs, research is not in itself a negative thing. Some residents can find a sense of purpose, new autonomy, meaning, and companionship by being offered the opportunity to participate. Identifying residents to participate is not simply a matter of their legal competence, since many residents have limited ability to provide consent even though their competence has never been denied in court. Others who are declared incompetent may still desire to participate and potentially to benefit. The concept of "assent" to participate, developed by the President's Commission for Ethical Problems in Medicine (1982), allows participation of individuals who cannot fully consent to participate in potentially therapeutic research. A patient who "assents" may not fully understand, but the research and those primarily involved with the individual's care must be satisfied that the individual does not object. In addition, the subject must give tacit, if not verbal "assent" to participate. The President's Commission provides a second very useful concept in dealing with both clinical situations and with enrollment of research subjects: that of "capacity." Because the definition of competence varies by state and serves only narrow legal purposes, the concept of capacity was developed to allow individuals to participate in decisions about their health care on a case-by-case basis. The elements of capacity are (a) possession of a set of values and goals; (b) the ability to communicate and understand information; and (c) the ability to reason and deliberate about one's choices (President's Commission 1982, 57). For purposes of research, assessing an individual's capacity is not the sole domain of the researcher. Rather, it should involve other caregivers with benevolent feelings for the individual being assessed. "Capacity" provides even the legally incompetent patient with a role in decisions about health care and participation in research.

Steps in Putting a Program Together

The essential components for a TNH program must exist both within a university and the LTCF. Within the university there must be a commitment to geriatric programming. At the very least, the colleges of medicine and nursing should be involved, and other disciplines should also be included. The involved colleges should have individuals trained in geriatrics and gerontology. Within the LTCF, there must be a commitment to training health professionals, at both board level and within administration and each of the major departments. There should be an organized medical staff (Garrell

1983), which should make a commitment to support the teaching programs. The LTCF should have a reputation within the community and with regulatory agencies for providing quality care. A teaching program cannot produce quality results where basic quality does not already exist.

Certain key individuals from both the University and the LTCF must be involved. Select individuals from the university include the deans of the colleges, who have the status to negotiate and the ability to commit resources, and major department heads, such as the chairperson of the Department of Internal Medicine or Family Practice. In addition to the Board of the LTCF, the chief executive officer or administrator, and the directors of nursing and social services should be committed to the teaching program and should be involved in the process of program planning.

Both sides should strive to achieve consensus on the objectives and necessary commitments. The academic institution should convene a committee with representatives from all of the involved colleges and teaching programs, preferably chaired by a respected ranking administrator, such as a dean of one of the colleges. Its mandate is to develop a consensus on the goals of the academic TNH. In the process, it must ascertain the level of interest and commitment of the various divisions, and obtain written commitment of resources from the deans and division heads. A written statement of goals and objectives should be produced for exchange and negotiation with the LTCF. The committee should also outline further steps to be taken by the academic institution.

The LTCF must also convene a group of individuals, including those who could be involved in the day-to-day operation of the TNH project, to discuss and reach a consensus on objectives for the TNH, and to describe the steps to be taken by the LTCF to achieve those goals.

After the two sides have decided on their respective goals, they must meet to negotiate, beginning the most critical part of the process. The generally desired outcome—some new, better or improved version of geriatric care—will be easy to agree upon. Much harder to decide are questions on structure and process, especially concerning control of, and responsibility for, the programs. LTCF representatives may have trouble understanding why academics feel they must have some control over the setting, and the academics may find it hard to understand the concern of the LTC side over cost and finances. Regardless of the situation with its unique special problems and considerations, differences in perspective must be acknowledged at the outset, and negotiations must be anticipated.

At least a year should be allowed for the academic and LTC institutions to reach consensus, make contractual relationships, and begin to implement the program. Implementation should begin from the top down; that is, the academic physicians should be brought on board first, followed by graduate level trainees, and finally by students. This allows the academics and the LTC staff to work out problems and develop working relationships. The role of the academic physician in the nursing home should be established and appreciated before it becomes confused with the personalities and approaches of individual trainees.

Depending on the size of the program and services provided, financial arrangements may become exceedingly complex. On the simplest level, the academic program must provide some FTEs for teaching inside the nursing home. Some or all of the cost of those faculty members' time may be covered through fee-for-service arrangements, facility reimbursement for on-site physician services (which may be a reimburseable cost), or as medical director's fees. Because geriatric services are time-consuming, especially in a teaching setting, reimbursement for the time invested will be marginal. The LTCF must also understand the ancillary costs of the training program. Nursing time will be taken for orientation of new trainees every few months, for pre-rounds with trainees, and for attending rounds, easily using 4-8 hours of professional nursing time per teaching service per week. While the biggest impact is on nursing services, other departments will also be affected by the presence of other professional trainees and students.

Organizational Arrangements

A major outcome of the negotiations described above is agreement on how the TNH will be organized and how responsibilities will be shared. To learn how organizational arrangements have developed elsewhere, administrators from four major teaching nursing homes were interviewed by telephone, as were academic physicians from three of these programs (see Figure 13-1). As expected, final arrangements were unique to each situation, but cer-

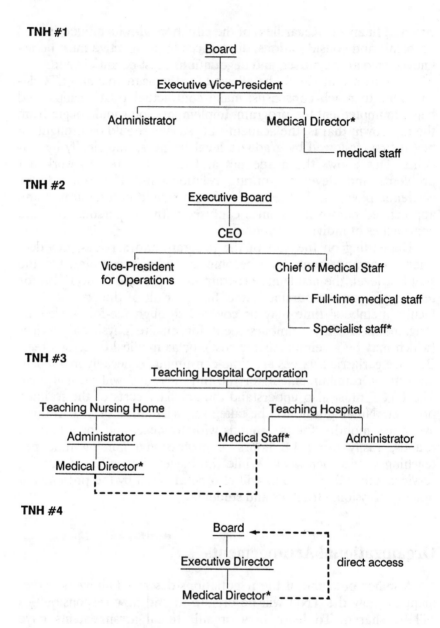

TNH #1

Board

Executive Vice-President

Administrator — Medical Director*

medical staff

TNH #2

Executive Board

CEO

Vice-President for Operations — Chief of Medical Staff

Full-time medical staff

Specialist staff*

TNH #3

Teaching Hospital Corporation

Teaching Nursing Home — Teaching Hospital

Administrator — Medical Staff* — Administrator

Medical Director*

TNH #4

Board ◄ - - - - - -

Executive Director

Medical Director* - - - - - - direct access

*=Academic appointment

Figure 13-1 Basic organization for four TNH programs.

tain recurrent themes appeared. First, the academic physicians all emphasized the importance of direct communication between the academic physician and the board of directors or chief executive officer of the LTCF. This notion is further supported by Gruber (1977) who suggests that a medical director would want some direct access to the board, even while reporting to the administrator for day-to-day operations. A second theme was the need for a closed rather than an open-ended medical staff, as a basic ingredient for quality medical care.

Additional Budget Concerns

The physician in charge of the TNH training program is responsible for securing stipends to cover the cost of residents and fellows training within the TNH. At present, some medical training costs are supported by Medicare's educational adjustment to hospital costs and Medicare extended care services. The future of this support is uncertain, however, and may eventually be eliminated or targeted to support training with a specific geriatric orientation. Reimbursement mechanisms will certainly change over time, and persons responsible for educational programs must keep abreast of these developments (see Chapter 8).

Another, somewhat more hidden, cost of training is space. Space is at a premium in TNHs as in other teaching facilities. The nursing home administration must be willing to maintain teaching space. Space for informal lectures, presentations, and formal teaching conferences must be negotiated and justified. Planning many of these activities as interdisciplinary teaching conferences and as ongoing sources of staff education, may help in negotiation. It may sometimes be necessary to seek a grant or gift to construct or remodel essential teaching space.

Funding Sources for Educational Programs

The National Institute on Aging (NIA), a branch of the National Institutes of Health (NIH), supports six teaching nursing homes. This program is actually a type of program project grant in support of research, with each NIA TNH having a research focus with cooperation among several individual investigators. Because of the NIH focus on research, training is not supported, although research faculty in a TNH can provide training as part of their faculty responsibilities. It is unlikely that additional programs will be funded under this project. NIA TNHs are located at: The Albert Einstein College of Medicine and Montefiore Medical Center and associated chronic care facilities; Philadelphia Gerontology Research Consortium; Case Western Reserve; the Hebrew Rehabilitation Center, Harvard School of Medicine and Boston University School of Nursing ; Johns Hopkins Medical School and Mason Lord Chronic Care Facility; and the University of California-San Diego Schools of Medicine and Nursing. Each center (beginning in 1982, 1983 or 1984) received a possible five years of support. Under this program, each may renew for a maximum ten years' support.

In addition to the TNH program, the NIA is an important source of support for faculty development and research funds in LTC. In general, faculty are eligible for support at most levels, as faculty leaders in geriatrics, as junior faculty under a designated faculty advisor (The Academic Award program), as developers of geriatric curriculum (The Geriatric Medicine Academic Award), and as fellows or junior faculty seeking support for research training (The National Research Service Award). For a concise packet of materials explaining eligibility criteria, level of funding, duration of support, and other information for all of the above programs, request "NIA Training Opportunities in Geriatrics and Gerontology" by writing the NIA, NIH, Bethesda, MD 20205; phone 301-496-1752.

The Veterans Administration supports TNH activities under the Geriatric Research Education Clinical Center (GRECC) program. Research support, facilities, and support for clinical training are part of this program. There are presently 10 such centers located at VA facilities in Durham, North Carolina; Gainesville, Florida; Bedford, Massachusetts; Little Rock, Arkansas; Minneapolis, Minnesota; Palo Alto, California; West Los Angeles, California; St. Louis, Missouri; Sepulveda, California; and Seattle, Washington. Additional sites may be established, depending on availability of funds. For information, write: Office Geriatrics and Extended Care, VA Central Office, 810 Vermont Avenue, N.W., Washington, D.C. 20420.

The Robert Wood Johnson Foundation has sponsored the start-up of twelve TNHs nationwide. These three-year projects were awarded jointly to university-based colleges of nursing and LTCFs. Funds were intended to help establish a working relationship between these two types of institutions, to be continued beyond the funding period. As funding for these projects ends in 1987, it will be interesting to see how and if these relationships will be maintained. An evaluation of quality and cost of care in the TNHs versus nonteaching homes is also forthcoming.

A promising area for funding new training positions in LTCFs appeared as the Graduate Education Act of 1986. This proposal in the Congress targeted four million dollars to expand present programs and create new programs to train physicians who plan to teach geriatric medicine. The bill would have funded one-year training spots for mid-career academic physicians and one- and two-year positions for fellows who had completed training in internal medicine or family practice and who had expressed an interest in teaching. While this bill failed to pass in 1986, it is expected to be reintroduced. This type of program may be extended to the other health professions who serve older patients, such as nursing, pharmacy, physical therapy, and others.

Experience in the U.S. to Date

By the most liberal definition of a teaching nursing home – any LTCF where health professionals obtain training – accurate numbers and descriptions are difficult to ascertain. The American Geriatrics Society's "Directory of Geriatrics Programs" (January 1984) contains descriptions of 55 training programs for residents and fellows in medicine, family practice, and psychiatry. Forty-four of these programs list at least one affiliated TNH. This list includes the Veteran Administration's affiliated GRECCs and the NIA TNHs, but does not include most of the Robert Wood Johnson Teaching Nursing Homes, which are primarily the domain of schools of nursing. Assuming multiple affiliations in some programs, there may be as many as 100 academically affiliated nursing homes in the U.S.

One such program is at the Jewish Institute for Geriatric Care (JIGC), located on the campus of the Long Island Jewish Medical Center, a major clinical campus for the Health Sciences Center at the State University of New York at Stony Brook. JIGC, a 527-bed skilled nursing facility with programs in chronic care and short-term rehabilitation, houses the oldest continuous residency and fellowship training program in geriatrics. Several available options for the graduate training of physicians include 1 to 12 months' residency experience, and 3-month to 2-year fellowships. Newly constructed outpatient facilities house a day hospital/day care center, a long-term home health care program, and clinics for the diagnosis and treatment of dementia, incontinence, and falls. Teaching relationships include multiple affiliations with programs for nursing, social work, physical therapy, occupational therapy, dentistry, physician assistants, medical students, pharmacy, and dental hygiene.

Summary

The extension of health professions education into specialized geriatric centers logically follows the demographic shift in the U.S. population and the need of geriatric patients for subacute and rehabilitational services. The substantial teaching opportunities within academic nursing homes prepare physician trainees for geriatric practice in a variety of settings. An affiliation between an academic center and a LTCF is ideally suited to address important research questions, to provide a service to the LTCF and the community, and to further the academic careers of the faculty in geriatrics. The initial organizational efforts, crucial to the long-term success of the project, must be approached methodically. Leaders from both the academic center and the LTCF must reach consensus on the goals, objectives, and operations of the project. There are at least 100 LTCFs in the U.S. with some type of academic affiliation, a fact which attests to the popularity of such arrangements. In addition, many other NHs serve, or can potentially serve, as sites where some education or training activities occur, by interacting with academic centers, even in the absence of formal affiliations. The substantial variety of these affiliates should help clarify further the essential components of a successful program.

References

Aronson, M.K. 1984. Implementing a teaching nursing home: lessons for research and practice. *The Gerontologist* 24:451-454.

Brody, J.A. 1985. Prospects for an aging population. *Nature* 315:463-466.

Butler, R.N. 1981. The teaching nursing home. *Journal of the American Medical Association* 245:1435-1437.

Cassel, C.K. 1985. The teaching nursing home: ethical concerns. In *The teaching nursing home*, edited by E.L. Scheider, C.M. Wendland, A.W. Zimmer; et al. New York: Raven Press.

Garrell, M. 1983. The organization of a teaching nursing home: an eight year experience. *Journal of Medical Education* 58:482-483.

Gruber, H.W. 1977. The medical director in the nursing home — a catalyst for quality care. *Journal of the American Geriatrics Society* 25:497-499.

Institute of Medicine. 1978. *Aging and medical education*. Washington, D.C.: National Academy of Sciences.

Jahnigen, D.W. et al. 1985. Academic affiliation with a nursing home: impact on patient outcome. *Journal of the American Geriatrics Society* 33:472-478.

Kane, R.L., and R.A. Kane. 1981. A guide through the maze of long-term care. *Western Journal of Medicine* 135:503-506.

Libow, L.S. 1984. The teaching nursing home: past, present, future. *Journal of the American Geriatrics Society* 32:598-603.

Liem, P.H., R. Chernoff, and W.J. Carter. 1986. Geriatric rehabilitation unit: a 3-year outcome evaluation. *Journal of Gerontology* 41:44-50.

Maddox, G.L. 1985. The teaching nursing home and beyond: research objectives for the 1980's. In *The teaching nursing home*, edited by E.L. Schneider, C.J. Wendland, A.W., Wendland, et al. New York: Raven Press.

Margolis, E.J., and S.K. Bishnu. 1981. Nursing home: place for teaching geriatrics. *New York State Journal of Medicine* 1683-1686.

President's commission for the study of ethical problems in medicine and biomedical and behavioral research. 1982. *Making health care decisions, Vol. I*. Washington, D.C.: Government Printing Office.

Schroeder, S.A., and J.A. Showstack. 1986. Residency training in internal medicine: time for a change? *Annals of Internal Medicine* 104:554-561.

Wieland, D., et al. 1986. organizing an academic nursing home: impacts on institutionalized elderly. *Journal of the American Medical Association* 255: 2622-2627.

Williams, C. 1985. Teaching nursing homes: their impact on public policy, patient care and medical education. *Journal of the American Geriatrics Society* 33:189-195.

Additional Resources

For further information on training programs in geriatrics: American Geriatrics Society, 770 Lexington Avenue, Suite 400, New York, NY 10021

For further information on research training opportunities: National Institutes on Aging, NIH, Bethesda, MD 20205; phone 301-496-1752.

For further information on TNH funding opportunities: Office of Geriatrics and Extended Care, VA Central Office, 810 Vermont Avenue, N.W., Washington, D.C. 20420.

For an excellent review of research within the TNH, the reader is referred to Part V: "Research in the Teaching Nursing Home," *The Teaching Nursing Home*, Raven Press, 1985. These chapters describe several examples of research agendas and the NIA-funded TNH research projects, and discuss the strengths and limitations of the TNH as a research environment. General guidelines for establishing research programs are described, as are the implications for public policy.

Chapter Fourteen

The Future of Long-Term Care

Steven A. Levenson, M.D.

Chapter Objectives

This chapter will discuss:

- Future trends in population and demographics of the elderly
- The evolving approaches to LTC, and its future place in medical practice
- The likely goals and accomplishments of the LTC system
- The nursing home of the future
- The future of reimbursement for LTC and physician services in LTC
- The future of hospital involvement in LTC
- The physician's changing role
- Expectations for quality care and monitoring of that care.

Anticipated Demographic Changes

The future of the elderly population in the United States — indeed, in much of the developed world — certainly promises vastly increased numbers, with more people living to advanced old age. Increasingly, more will enjoy high quality of life, with relatively few serious problems. But a substantial minority will also suffer from debilitating physical and mental impairments, requiring multidisciplinary community-based or institutional services.

Statistics on the elderly remain fairly sparse, but efforts to collect such data will expand as government agencies become increasingly aware of the need for additional information to assist future planning. For example, upcoming U.S. censuses will almost certainly include questions specifically directed towards the elderly, their living conditions, functional abilities, and service needs.

As of July 1, 1983, for the first time in history, the number of people in the United States over age 65 was greater than the number under age 25. The mean age of Americans in 1985 was 32, and will be 40 by the turn of the 21st century. In 1986, 1 of 8 Americans was 65 or over; by 2030, this will increase to almost 1 in five. By the year 2000, over 30,000,000 Americans will be over 65, out of a total population of 262.5 million (Department of Health and Human Services 1975), and 49 percent of elderly people will be 75 or older, according to the U.S. Bureau of the Census. By 2020, 31% of the U.S. population is expected to be at least age 55. There are now about 2.7 million over the age of 85, and there will be about 5 million such persons by 2000, and perhaps 16 million—over 5% of the population—by the year 2050 (Senate Special Committee 1986). Of those over age 85, 1 in 4 will be institutionalized at any one time.

Age-adjusted death rates for the elderly fell about 38% between 1940 and 1978. While an individual at the turn of the 20th century had a life expectancy of 57 years, and could expect to spend 3% of this total lifetime in retirement, the average male today has a life expectancy close to 80 years, and can expect to spend as much as 20% of his life in retirement.

Florida will likely continue to have the highest percentage of elderly of any state in the U.S. In 1986, 17.6% of Florida's population was over 65, and in Dade County, Florida, almost 300,000 (almost one-fifth of the population) residents were eligible for Medicare—the same percentage projected for the U.S. as a whole by the year 2020 (Miami's elderly . . . 1986).

New Approaches to LTC

Because of these numbers, LTC will continue to evolve and to occupy an even more important place in medicine. Almost all physicians will be touched in some way by this geriatric explosion.

The LTC system of the future will be distinguished by its *multilevel, multidisciplinary* approach, offering a wide range of services managed or coordinated from a central point, be that a hospital, state agency, NH, private agency, prepaid system, or life-care community. For example, states will look to "channel" older people into the elder care system through single entry points, directed by case managers; while institutional programs will be linked with community- and home-based ones. Hospitals will integrate services vertically, and laws now restricting the use of "swing beds" will likely be modified to allow more flexible use of available resources.

The traditional centers of care, such as NHs and hospitals, will coexist with those offering additional services, such as adult day care, case management, community outreach and education, congregate housing, extended care, foster care, shared housing, and social centers.

These nonhospital organizations will also offer packages of services and programs. Traditional HMOs will extend to Medicare beneficiaries' prepaid medical care, and some additional services such as LTC on a fee-for-service basis. Newer types of HMOs will allow elderly individuals to enroll in prepaid plans that will offer a wide range of LTC services for a guaranteed price, including ambulatory, rehabilitative, and preventive services, and NH care.

Each major component of the LTC system will develop in different ways.

Psychiatry. The proportion of surviving elderly with some degree of mental impairment is increasing markedly, and many of these people are winding up in NHs or mental institutions. The LTC system of the future will be forced to improve and expand its psychiatric services to the elderly, through community-based outpatient psychiatric programs and geropsychiatric day care programs and day hospitals. The NH will go beyond mere custodial care for the mentally impaired, and will offer more comprehensive programs, including mental health and psychiatric specialists, improved diagnosis, ongoing therapies, and more careful management of psychotropic medications. Depressed patients will be offered proper treatment, rather than being grouped with the demented.

Skilled Nursing Facilities (SNFs) and Intermediate Care Facilities (ICFs). These facilities will continue to take sicker and more dysfunctional patients, as acute hospitals must discharge a growing number of those not fully recovered, and still others who can no longer function in the community. This will require them to implement many new and more sophisticated programs, and to rely more on medical direction and services for the care of those patients. Medical and other clinical services will have to be integrated and coordinated far better than at present. Distinctions between SNFs and ICFs are likely to continue to blur, as patients with a variety of needs are offered services at a single site, rather than being moved among sites.

Geriatric evaluation services. Such services, both inpatient and out-patient, have become increasingly available to improve diagnosis, management, and placement of the elderly, especially those with multiple complex problems or illnesses, dementia, incontinence, or other major dysfunction, and those who have not responded to previous attempts at management. While such programs have demonstrated some benefits (see Chapter 5), it remains to be seen just how much they will proliferate, or whether they will justify their cost in the long run. The programs will be staffed mainly by trained geriatricians, along with those in related professions with specific training and interest.

Medical day care. These programs will proliferate as a relatively inexpensive way to care for those who might otherwise have to be institutionalized. Patients will move between such programs and inpatient or acute settings, as their needs dictate.

Day hospitals. These facilities will provide a major means for offering fairly intensive clinical services without the hotel costs of an overnight stay in an acute hospital. Major varieties of day hospital services will continue to include *medical, psychiatric,* and *rehabilitation*. Along with geriatric specialty hospitals, they will provide many of the short-term diagnostic, assessment, and treatment services formerly rendered in the acute hospital.

Rehabilitation services. These will expand because they are a cornerstone of geriatric care, and will include short-term, intensive, goal-oriented therapies in acute or specialty hospitals or day hospitals; maintenance therapies to preserve function and prevent deterioration among the institutionalized elderly; and home-based and ambulatory services that help a person cope with activities of daily living to prevent or delay future institutionalization.

Life care. Unlike some of the other trends in geriatrics, life care faces a somewhat uncertain future, if only because the means of payment are not as secure as they once appeared. Such programs are very expensive to finance, and require a great amount of equity. A more feasible alternative in some settings may be congregate housing, offering housing on a rent/lease basis, without committing providers to offer health care for life.

The Nursing Home of the Future

While still remaining the cornerstone of LTC, the NH will have a dramatically expanded role in the future. Many NHs will provide services formerly centered in acute hospitals, including cardiac monitoring, pulmonary units, incontinence units, geropsychiatric units, and hospice units. Many NHs may in fact become wholly or partly geriatric specialty ("chronic") hospitals. One observer envisions the nursing home's future this way:

> I see the nursing home and geriatric medicine in the 1980s, the 1990s, and the 21st century as analogous to the general hospital and the field of general medicine in earlier years. The hospital was initially seen as a 'pest house,' a place to die. It then evolved as a place where the sick were helped (a place of care) and, at times, healed (a place of cure). The hospital also became a research and teaching focus for the training of all health care professionals. . . . It is also a focus of society's appraisal of moral and ethical values and economic distress.
>
> So, too, the nursing home will move away from its major image as a place to die and to die poorly. It has already become a focus of society's ethical issues and economic distress. It will evolve as a place respected for treating people, not parts. (Libow 1981, 134).

As a result of changes in hospital care, reimbursement, and lengths of stay, plus the aging of the population and the great increase in the "old-old," NH patients will be substantially sicker, with more chronic illnesses, more complex medical and psychosocial problems, and will have more frequent episodes of acute illness. NH patients who have been hospitalized will return sicker and require more intensive follow-up medical and nursing care in the convalescent period. The number of NH beds will continue to expand, even as the number of acute care beds declines.

Reimbursement for LTC Services

The problems of reimbursement for LTC services must be resolved at the individual, professional, institutional, and reimburser levels. Expansion of LTC service capacity will require more adequate reimbursement for LTC service providers, changes in allowable methods of capital financing, and recognition of other alternate services, such as respite care, under Medicare and Medicaid.

Financial trends may include development of private LTC insurance, prospective payment systems for Medicare SNFs, encouragement of personal savings for future LTC needs, and the development of home equity conversions and reverse mortgage programs.

On an individual level, the 15% of current income which the elderly now spend on health care is expected to increase to about 19% by 1990. Currently, as many as two-thirds of NH patients who begin as private-pay patients exhaust their financial resources during their stay, and become Medicaid-eligible. One in 20 elderly Americans faces financial disaster because of inability to pay the costs of LTC.

In 1986, some insurance companies were just beginning to offer LTC insurance. The product is still experimental and likely to change. Typically, the policies cover NH and home health care for at least a one-year period, but not short-term nursing or home health benefits. Many of the policies require prior hospitalization before they will cover skilled nursing services in state-licensed SNFs or ICFs. Many also deny coverage to those with specific chronic conditions and health problems.

Although LTC insurance will probably become more desirable and accepted in the future, the success of employer-provided LTC insurance is still in doubt, since many employers are not eager to add more employee benefits. Employees, however, may be offered the opportunity to begin buying coverage for premiums as low as $5 to $10 a month while still in their early thirties. Emphasis on NH benefits has also had a negative impact on LTC insurance, since people do not want to think about being in a NH. This LTC insurance, like LTC itself, may very well cover many of the noninstitutional services of the LTC spectrum.

Some form of catastrophic health insurance coverage has become a high priority for many Americans, to protect those who exhaust their Medicare hospital benefits. A bill on this type of coverage introduced in Congress early in 1987 stimulated considerable debate, suggesting that this has become a politically important subject, as well. Some form of coverage is likely to be enacted before the 1988 elections.

Reimbursement for Professional Services

Any efforts to control physician fees will have to analyze both cost and utilization, since effective programs will need to control both price *and* volume. Somehow, even as physician fees in the hospital are more tightly controlled, reimbursement for *cognitive* (nonprocedural) nonhospital physician services must improve to the point of providing some reasonable incentives for physicians to spend the time necessary to adequately care for the complex geriatric patient. For example, funding limits for mental health and psychiatric services will have to be liberalized to meet the vast psychiatric needs of the frail and institutionalized elderly at a reasonable level.

Much greater use of physician assistants and nurse practitioners is likely, in an effort to provide much of the essential preliminary assessment and routine follow-up at less cost, especially in the NH.

Almost certainly, physicians will be required to document and justify their management and care plans for their elderly patients, through the efforts of quality assurance and the rules and regulations of third-party payors. Reimbursement may well be linked more closely with measurable outcomes.

Reimbursement for Institutional Care

Important economic issues for financing of institutional LTC services include more uniform standards on eligibility for SNF care, as well as adequate coverage and payment for: hospital-based SNFs; those with catastrophic care needs, who cannot themselves pay the whole bill; and a broader spectrum of LTC services and affiliated noninstitutional services, such as day care and home health care.

Will SNFs and home care come under the prospective pricing system (PPS), and be paid on a case-by-case fixed price basis? They may not immediately, but could at some future time. The problem with prospective pricing is that LTC patients have multiple diagnoses, and primary diagnoses tend to change. In addition, there are currently no widely accepted criteria, standards, or tools available to conduct such reviews. It is nevertheless likely that there will be attempts to use such tools in the future, as costs rise and demand for services grows.

Medicare coverage will need to somehow include better reimbursement to facilities providing home-based and rehabilitative services. We can anticipate some formidable political battles on how this will be accomplished, either by expansion or by cutbacks in other areas.

Reimbursers for Care

Socioeconomic realities are altering delivery of health care radically, especially to the elderly. Government will continue to intervene to assure access to health care and some protection from costs, both for the elderly and for those who have to foot the bills.

Changes are likely to be made to the Medicare and Medicaid programs to ensure their continued solvency and potential to assist the elderly in the future. For example, a number of reforms were proposed by the Harvard Medicare Project (Blumenthal et al 1986) including: reducing deductibles; eliminating the physician's deductible and coinsurance portion; eliminating the requirement for the patient to pay 25% of hospitalization costs after 60 days; charging an additional annual premium to offset lost revenues; expanding coverage to include extended NH care and increasing coverage for outpatient LTC, including home health care and mental health services; and combining Medicare Parts A and B.

Other suggestions by this group include: encouraging enrollment in prepaid health care organizations; paying physicians according to different scales; establishing an annual total expenditure target for physician services; requiring physicians to accept Medicare fees as payment in full; modifying the diagnosis related groups payment scheme; requiring states to make up annual total Medicare costs which exceed certain targets. Which of these actually become adopted will depend on the outcome of ongoing political and social debates over the next several decades.

One almost certain focus will be on the relatively small portion of elderly individuals who use a disproportionate amount of medical care and resources—especially those in the last year of life or who are terminally ill. Those elderly with multiple complex medical and psychosocial problems—the core of the geriatrician's constituency—will also continue to require the most professional time and resources.

Adequate criteria must be developed for decisions on the allocation of resources. Age alone is not a sufficient criterion for including or excluding someone from services or care. Instead, each person's condition and prognosis must be considered on a case-by-case basis. To the greatest extent possible, public policy should continue to permit such decision-making flexibility. Debate will undoubtedly center around such ethical issues as limiting or withholding treatment, and quality of life, in relation to cost and benefit.

As always, before we can decide which treatments and expenditures are appropriate, we will have to define our goals. It will be necessary to fund studies on the application of the new technologies, to see which are genuinely cost-effective in achieving those goals.

Merely tightening the requirements for qualifying services, or arbitrarily establishing levels of payment denial, will not solve the problems in reimbursement for care. As an example, Medicare denials for home health claims increased drastically between 1984 to 1986, apparently in response to pressures to control Medicare costs, even while public discussion continued to focus on the need for institutional alternatives, including home care.

Cost reduction efforts will move beyond publicly funded Medicare and Medicaid to consider privately funded health care reimbursement plans, as well. Excessive services to those in *any* age group should be examined closely, so that funds may be shifted to areas of legitimately greater need. Increases in Medicare coinsurance and deductibles are not likely to be politically feasible beyond a certain point.

The integration of Medicare and Medicaid programs may eventually be necessary to improve efficiency and eliminate cost shifting between the two programs.

Hospital Involvement in LTC

Hospitals of the future will be dominated by capitated systems and comprehensive health service corporations. With the management and capital strength to take on new programs, hospitals will therefore look to diversify, and, where feasible, to vertically integrate their services across the continuum from home-based to institutional.

Hospitals are expected to continue to expand their participation in the LTC industry during the next decade. HMOs and other prepaid programs will ask many hospitals to provide all levels of care. In the future, more hospitals will offer from one site, a continuum of services, from home-based care to postacute care in SNFs.

So far, increased emphasis on discharge planning and new program development have been the major hospital responses to the new imperatives for care of the elderly. In this context, top priorities for hospitals include expanding and refining special services, forming liaisons with NHs and the community, geriatric education, and continuing care case management. Specialized services, such as home health, and coordination, such as case management and discharge planning, are expected to form the foundation of comprehensive hospital-based programs for the elderly.

Because home health and skilled nursing care are currently the fastest moving services within the health care industry, within the next five years, at least half of the hospitals in the U.S. will probably develop or contract for home health care services.

Information and referral services, including emergency response systems, will increase because they help hospitals enhance continuity of care and raise community visibility at relatively low cost. Community-based care focusing on palliative and restorative services for both acute and LTC patients will become increasingly important. Besides home health care, these will include congregate and home-delivered meals, homemaker services, transportation, home visitors, and patient and family education.

The elderly may be cared for in separate medical/surgical acute care units or separate inpatient rehabilitation units. Although many hospitals currently do not have specially organized outpatient departments for the elderly, such outpatient services are expected to grow. In contrast, assessment services are offered most frequently by hospitals. Many hospitals already have certain programs to benefit the elderly, such as hospice or home care, but which are not identified specifically as being for the elderly.

A 1986 American Hospital Association survey of 3,529 hospitals showed that:

- 66 percent plan to develop or expand services for the elderly;

- The most frequently offered LTC service is patient-family educational programs (54 percent);

- The next five most common LTC services are emergency response systems (35.8 percent), home health (33.3 percent), information and referral (33.2 percent), hospital-based SNF's (19 percent), and durable medical equipment (17.3 percent). (*Hospitals* December 20, 1986)

Hospitals are also developing extensive marketing programs to review the needs of their local populations, and to target specific services to their particular needs.

Long-term care of more than 90 days has represented an unfamiliar financial risk to hospitals, primarily because it is mainly reimbursed by Medicaid. More hospitals currently own hospital-based SNF beds and swing beds than any other inpatient LTC services. Today's skilled NHs are often reluctant to take those discharged hospital patients with ongoing medical needs, who are either not ready or unable to return home. Such patients cost more to care for, but bring little or no more reimbursement than lighter care patients. Competition from hospital-owned LTC providers may offer a very stiff challenge to existing nursing homes, many of which have been slow to improve care and services because of continuous occupancy levels in the 90-95% range.

The NH business will also become more attractive with the advent of LTC insurance, which may also reduce state expenditures for LTC, allowing funds for other health care ventures.

Hospitals are both building and buying NHs, in an attempt to capture more of the local health market, and spread financial risks over more areas. Similarly, more centrally managed hospital chains are owning or operating NHs, and the trend is expected to increase. New NHs cost $20,000 to $22,000 per bed to build, and existing ones, as much as $55,000 per bed to buy. But because of certificate-of-need requirements and local market conditions, many hospitals will choose not to build. Those hospitals that do not own or operate NHs or other services will contract with NHs to provide those services, often as part of HMOs, PPOs or managed care networks.

Hospitals have found the continuing care retirement community (life care) market to be more difficult than expected. Hospitals may be best suited for medical model communities, while nonmedical models will be built by such for-profit corporations as insurance companies and hospitality chains. Eventually, however, hospitals may find their niche by providing, under contract, a continuum of services, emphasizing case management.

Political Activities and Public Policy

Future political and regulatory activities concerning LTC will focus on service arrangements, reimbursement, and quality of care issues.

Many state and local governments see *channeling*—that is, establishing a single point of entry for clients in need of health and social services—as the vehicle for improved service delivery. This includes screening, assessment, case management, and a mix of cost-saving services to meet needs, with the goal of providing more efficient, effective, and less costly delivery of needed services.

The Politics of Reimbursement

Most likely, the major American political issue over the next few years will concern the control of huge budget deficits. In geriatrics, political activities will focus on assuring adequate funding for programs and training to provide quality care. At the same time, more laws and regulations ensuring a baseline of quality care and services will be advocated. While regulators and legislators will try to base reimbursement on certain quality standards, the latter remain difficult to define and to apply.

A major political priority for the immediate future should be the review and revamping of the administration of Medicare and Medicaid reimbursement systems. The often arbitrary and highly frustrating process, duly noted by many physicians (Berrien 1987), provides many disincentives, and few incentives, to physicians who take the time to make a thorough assessment and treatment of NH patients and other complex elderly patients outside the hospital. Increased demands for improved care and service are not likely to bring much more willing participation or cooperation without commensurate improvements in the operation of the reimbursement system.

Reimbursement will have to be reevaluated to avoid penalizing those hospitals that offer programs for the care of the elderly with multiple complex problems who exceed the lengths of stay of the relatively healthy. Otherwise, hospitals may be forced to exclude the frail elderly, whenever possible.

Patient Care Politics

More regulations and laws are likely to mandate improvements in care, and physician management of LTC patients. These will prescribe closer patient monitoring, more physician acceptance of responsibility for patient care, and greater accountability of physicians to a medical director or chief of staff. The problem will be to simultaneously provide adequate reimbursement for those quality services.

Better criteria will thus be required to help determine the basis for reimbursement. Traditional criteria have included time spent, amount or intensity of services rendered, and number or type of procedures done. One approach might be to pay for services based on the extent to which they achieve certain realistic objectives for a given patient. Thus, the time spent to accomplish the limited goal of keeping a person pain-free and comfortable would justify the same payment as an equal amount of time spent on achieving the goal of rehabilitation and return to the community, or for example, the time spent by an eye surgeon performing a cataract operation.

Future Regulations

Regulations have always been targeted to the "lowest common denominator;" that is, to force everyone to provide at least a baseline level of care. While government will continue to set minimal acceptable standards for LTC (especially for NHs), these regulatory efforts will need to be more and more voluntary, achieved at reasonable cost and professional time expenditure.

Standards for adequate and appropriate care will become national, rather than local. More of these standards will come from voluntary sources like the Joint Commission on Accreditation of Hospitals (JCAH), rather than from mandatory rules. Regulations will be based more on actual patient results and outcomes of care than on paper compliance, structure, and process.

Regulatory agencies will be forced to coordinate their efforts and regulations to produce an efficient process that will least disrupt ongoing care. Governments at all levels will need to understand that, with few exceptions, a common set of standards and rules will be preferable to local selective regulatory processes.

The Physician's Changing Role

The physician's role in LTC will continue to evolve and expand because of the greater number of old-old with significant medical problems and the much higher expectations for medical intervention to at least improve, if not cure, older patients' problems.

Physicians will be more attentive to proper evaluation, prevention, and multidisciplinary patient management. More complete and accurate preadmission assessments on LTC patients will be needed to help with appropriate placement. Once placed, these patients will need closer ongoing medical monitoring and follow-up care, which must also continue after discharge or transfer.

More physicians in different specialties will be needed to care for the elderly. These will include: primary care providers in internal medicine and family practice; and trained specialists in geriatrics with specific skills and knowledge, who could either train others in academic settings, practice primary care as specially trained individuals, act as physician administrators in specific situations (such as NH medical directors), or provide consultation and evaluation to other physicians concerning their older patients.

The 1980 Rand Corporation study (Beck and Vivell 1984) of manpower projections for the year 2010 calls for approximately a 60 to 70 percent increase in number over the 1977 needs for full-time equivalents (FTEs) to care for and consult on those age 65 or older, and even more for those 75 or older.

The academic community projects a need of at least 900-1600 physicians to serve trainees for medical schools, medical and family practice residents, and other health professionals, in addition to about 450 academic geropsychiatrists, and 1700-2500 researchers (Beck and Vivell 1984, 67).

Unfortunately, this means that for some time, many of those specifically trained in the field will be busy fulfilling their teaching and research requirements, leaving relatively few to provide the clinical care outside of academic centers. It may be necessary to correct this imbalance sooner rather than later, so that more care providers can be trained even before all academic needs are met.

The role of the physician administrator in LTC will continue to expand, as it will in acute care. Formal training for such individuals will increase, as the issues become more complex and their resolutions increasingly time-consuming. More physicians will serve as full-time medical directors in the larger NHs.

Training of geriatric specialists will continue and expand. With the continuing acute hospital trend towards emphasis on complex tertiary care, the ambulatory, outpatient, and NH settings will become increasingly important as training sites. The NH will offer many of the services, and hence many of the learning opportunities, once given in the acute hospital.

Geriatrics will be incorporated into all levels of medical student education. Currently, almost all American medical schools offer some elective or required classroom programs in geriatrics, but not many have clinical requirements, despite the fact that the clinical experience strongly affects attitudes and career choices. Undoubtedly, physicians in training will need to spend more meaningful clinical time with the elderly to fully appreciate their special needs.

Without accompanying adjustments in reimbursement and professional status, it is unclear if the projected substantial physician surplus by the year 2000 will help provide more individuals seriously interested in the field. It could be that more people will simply be forced to do the work out of necessity.

Alternative government funding for developing geriatric medicine programs is unlikely to happen any time soon. Research funding for generalists and reimbursement for the cognitive, nontechnical contributions of geriatrics trainees, will remain limited. Improvement in the situation will require recognizing that clinical services to the elderly are as important as research activities. Likewise, private foundations and agencies will need to continue to support the start-up of trial service programs. Furthermore, funding of graduate medical education will have to originate from sources beyond the hospital.

Clearly, with limits on the number of *people* who can be trained, other ways of improving the efficiency of the *system* will be needed. Better information management, including extensive computerization, will be critical.

Expectations for Quality Care and Its Monitoring

As discussed in earlier chapters, efforts to improve the quality of services and care in LTC have been slow and have been hampered by the inherent difficulty of the task. Nevertheless, as the bills for such services and care become greater, the monitoring will become even tighter. Efforts to improve such care at reasonable cost will require continued development of novel methods and tools.

Some of the sources for improved quality of LTC services will come from increased funding of research efforts and demonstration projects, increased training of LTC personnel and professionals, further revisions of regulations regarding surveys and licensure and certification processes, and more active and appropriate community involvement in LTC facilities.

Previously, regulations in LTC–especially in the NH–have been viewed punitively; that is, violation of the rules is a bad idea, because it brings a citation or punishment from the regulatory agencies. But in the future, a novel concept of quality care in NHs should view such monitoring positively, as an educational tool, with the goal of improving care and reducing costs. This will require a reorientation to long-term care on the part of both professionals *and* regulators.

In conclusion, the future of LTC is exciting and almost limitless in its possibilities. Like other professionals, those physicians with the interest, enthusiasm, energy, and skills will have ample opportunity to make major contributions to the crucial field of geriatric medicine.

References

Beck, J. C., and S. Vivell. 1984. Development of geriatrics in the United States. In *Geriatric medicine (2 volumes)*, edited by C. K. Cassel and J. R. Walsh. New York: Springer-Verlag.

Berrien, R. What future for primary care private practice? *New England Journal of Medicine* 316:334-337.

Blumenthal, D., et al. The future of medicare. *New England Journal of Medicine* 314:722-728.

Department of Health and Human Services.

1975. Publication No. 75-20013. Washington, D.C.: Government Printing Office.

Libow, L. 1981. Geriatric medicine and the nursing home: a mechanism for mutual excellence. *Gerontologist* 22:134-141.

Miami's elderly: the future of health care? 1986. *Hospitals*, 60(6):58-63.

Senate Special Committee on Aging. *Aging America: Trends and Projections (1985-86 edition)*. Washington, D.C. Government Printing Office.

For Further Reading

Hospitals. Journal of the American Hospital Association, with many articles about LTC trends and issues, as well as legal, social, and political matters of importance to hospitals and LTC, and reports on various programs and activities around the country. Available with membership to the AHA, or by subscription from: AHA, 211 E. Chicago, IL 60611.

Modern Healthcare. Privately produced biweekly publication covering many of the same issues as the above. Available by subscription from Crain Communications, 740 Rush St., Chicago, IL 60611.

Senate Special Committee on Aging. *Aging America: Trends and Projections (1985-86 edition)*. Washington, D.C.: Government Printing Office.

Glossary

activities of daily living (ADL) Basic self-care activities (e.g., feeding, bathing, grooming, dressing, toileting, ambulation), frequently measured during the assessment of elderly persons.

acute care medicine Physician services rendered for acute illness, usually in the acute hospital, or in geriatric speciality (chronic) hospitals.

adult day care (ADC) Programs that provide elderly adults with various health and social services in a supervised ambulatory group setting.

alternatives to institutionalization Services in the long-term care spectrum, such as day care or home health care, which offer the elderly needed assistance without the expenses and disruptions of living in an institution, such as a nursing home.

assignment Agreement by which a physician accepts the Medicare-approved charge as the total charge for a service provided to a Medicare-eligible patient.

attending physician The doctor primarily responsible for the care of any patient, whether in the acute hospital, the community, or the nursing home.

board of directors (board, governing body) A high-level body of distinguished individuals from the community, or from business, elected or appointed, responsible for broad policy-making and (in a health-care institution) the overall quality of care and services.

bylaws A formal, legally enforceable set of policies, instructions, and guidelines which define an organization and its relationships with those within and outside that organization.

carriers Organizations which handle claims for services provided by hospitals, skilled nursing facilities, and home health agencies covered under the hospital insurance part of Medicare.

419

case management Services which are a mixture of assessment, referral, and treatment planning, intended to help coordinate the care, placement, and payment for an elderly individual.

case manager The individual responsible for **case management** of a given elderly individual.

certificate of need A certificate issued by a governmental body to an individual or organization proposing to construct or modify a health facility; the intention being to control expansion of facilities.

channeling A concept, used as a starting point for many government-sponsored geriatric services, which establishes a single point of entry for clients in need of health and social services, and which may include screening, assessment, case management, and a mix of cost-saving services.

chief of staff The physician elected or appointed as the president or chief officer of an organized medical staff, equivalent in the medical organization to the chief executive or president of the health-care facility.

chief executive officer (CEO) The president or main administrative officer of a corporation or health-care facility, responsible for major day-to-day policy decision-making, and the hiring and firing of all professional administrative personnel, such as department heads.

chronic hospital A geriatric specialty hospital, licensed in many states, offering acute and intensive chronic medical services to the elderly, but at a less intense level than in the acute hospital.

chronic disease The most common form of ailment in the elderly, characterized by incurability and the possibility for palliation, and frequently causing moderate to marked disability or dysfunction.

clinical information system (CIS) An organized approach at any level (from programmatic to national) to gathering, storing, analyzing, coordinating, searching, retrieving, transferring, using, and reporting all information pertinent to the condition, status, or care of patients.

coinsurance The proportional amount that an enrollee in an insurance program must pay for each unit of service provided.

competence The capacity to perform certain tasks, act in certain ways, or meet specific criteria. In health care, the capacity to understand and process information, and to make choices, regarding one's condition and treatment options. There are legal, ethical, and psychological definitions of competence, each of which employs different criteria.

computer A man-made assemblage of wires and integrated circuits with enormous potential, when properly used, to assist in the collection, analysis, and retrieval of information.

computer-stored medical record The use of computers to store, arrange, retrieve, and analyze the comprehensive patient record. The combination of many such records together constitutes a major part of a computerized **clinical information system** (see above).

conditions of participation Those standards established under federal regulations which must be met by any facility which receives federal funds for providing care or services to Medicare or Medicaid recipients.

consent An ongoing process of information exchange and shared decision making, with the intended result of a patient authorizing some medical procedure, plan of care, test, or treatment.

continuity of care Coordination of assessment and treatment offered by many LTC professionals, programs, and sites to a single elderly individual, to minimize duplication, cost, confusion and frustration of patients, families, and professionals.

copayment See **coinsurance**.

criteria In Quality Assurance, the measures or specific items which elaborate upon standards and clarify the explicit behaviors expected, and of whom they are required.

data base An organized collection of information, analyzed or not, most often about a specific topic or individual, or a collection of either.

data In information systems, the uninterpreted items which, when interpreted according to certain rules of **knowledge**, become **information**.

day hospital A program of intensive goal-directed medical, rehabilitation, or psychiatric services, which would otherwise be provided in a hospital setting, aimed at providing the services without the hotel costs and other attendant problems of hospitalization.

decision-making capacity A proposed alternate term for **competence**, which avoids the confusion associated with a primarily judicial process of competence determination.

deductible An amount of money that an enrollee in an insurance program must spend prior to the program paying anything for those specified benefits.

delegated review status In utilization management, this refers to a facility that conducts its own utilization review activities.

departmental staffing A medical staff arrangement wherein physicians are assigned to various departments, or are members of a single medical department, within the organizational structure.

diagnosis related group (DRG) A case-mix classification system upon which **prospective payment** to acute hospitals for Medicare-eligible patients is based, according to how each individual's diagnosis fits into certain predetermined diagnostic categories.

domiciliary care (DC) A hybrid of institutional and community-based care, referring to arrangements for providing food, shelter, and limited supervision in a group home setting, but at less than a **skilled** or **intermediate** care level.

ethics An attempt to provide a systematic review, analysis, and approach to making choices about moral issues.

ethics committee A committee within a health care facility intended to review and advise staff on cases presenting difficult ethical issues, such as patient choice or terminal care. Also known by such other names as "human values committees," "medical-morals committees," "bioethics committees," and "ethics advisory committees."

formal care Care provided for money by public or private agencies and organizations (e.g., nursing homes, home health agencies, adult day care centers).

geriatric evaluation units Usually hospital-based units, both inpatient and outpatient, intended to provide a thorough evaluation of a patient's problems with the goal of identifying remediable conditions, simplifying treatment regimens, assessing function, and developing treatment programs to maximize function.

geriatric specialty hospitals Sometimes referred to as "subacute" or "chronic" hospitals, these are licensed in some states as non-acute hospitals that provide acute, postacute, chronic medical and nursing services, plus patient assessments and such specialty services as care for incontinence and severe decubitus ulcers.

geriatrics The medical specialty of providing care for the elderly; especially, those elderly with multiple complex medical and social problems, requiring a comprehensive evaluation and management plan.

geriatrics service An organized, coordinated collection of programs for the assessment, treatment, and care of the elderly, either at an institutional, community, or governmental level.

gerontology The study of the social, biological, and psychological aspects of aging, and the provision of nonphysician services to the elderly.

geropsychiatric day hospital (GDH) A **day hospital** program offering intensive short-term psychiatric treatment to an older person whose problems are severe enough to otherwise require an inpatient stay plus continued supervised medical management.

governing body See **board**.

HCFA The Health Care Financing Administration, an agency of the US Department of **Health and Human Services**, responsible for the administration and monitoring of payments to physicians and institutions providing care to individuals covered under government-funded health programs.

Health and Human Services (HHS) The federal government cabinet-level department responsible for regulating health care and administrating most federal health programs in the U.S.

health maintenance organization (HMO) A community health organization which provides facilities, professional services, and supplies for a prepaid fee.

home health services A collection of home-based services, including any or all of the following: part-time or intermittent nursing care provided under the supervision of a registered nurse; physician; occupational or speech therapy; medical social services under a physician's direction; part-time or intermittent services of a home health aide; and medical supplies other than drugs.

hospice Formal multidisciplinary services which provide comfort and care to both a terminally ill individual and to the family. They may be hospital-based, LTC-based, home-based, or a mixture; the services include medicine, nursing, social, clergy, and psychological counseling.

hospital insurance Part A of Medicare, which may cover inpatient acute hospital and skilled nursing facility care, home health care, and hospice care.

infection control A program to prevent, control, and monitor the potential for, and actual occurrence of, infectious diseases in an institution.

informal care Care provided without charge by family, friends, and neighbors.

information management The orderly collection, storage, arrangement, retrieval, and analysis of information to facilitate its use, especially for decision-making.

information and referral A community-based nonmedical program serving one or several functions, including: providing lists of aging-related agencies, programs, and practitioners; providing information on self-care, prevention, illnesses, or medications; or providing triage and channeling of individuals into and within the system.

information In the **clinical information system,** the end result of interpreting clinical **data** according to certain rules or criteria.

inspection of care Monitoring by state Medicaid health facility licensing and regulatory agencies, or by a **peer review** organization, focusing on quality of care and utilization review.

instrumental activities of daily living Complex activities, associated with independent life (e.g., cooking, cleaning, using telephone, shopping, laundry, walking outdoors, managing money), which are frequently measured during the assessment of elderly persons.

intermediaries Organizations which handle claims from doctors and other suppliers of services covered under the medical insurance part of Medicare.

intermediate care facilities (ICFs) Nursing facilities licensed to provide care at less than **skilled,** but more than **domiciliary,** level .

Joint Commission on Accreditation of Hospitals (JCAH) The main accrediting organization for acute hospitals and long-term care facilities, based on request for review and voluntary acceptance of a set of standards.

key indicators In **quality assurance** or regulatory reviews, specific items, such as urinary tract infections or decubitus ulcers, which reviewers or surveyors look for to indicate positive or negative care, and which can help them decide whether additional more detailed investigation is indicated.

knowledge In **clinical information systems**, the rules, relationships, and experience by which data become information.

level of care The level of services and programs appropriate for an elderly individual's prognosis and needs, usually authorized after review by a **utilization review** individual or organization.

liability Accountability under the law for an act or error, regardless of whether the liable individual actually performed the act or made the error.

life care A hybrid of inpatient, home, and community-based services and benefits, ranging from housing through medical care, usually arranged as a package for an up-front entry fee plus additional monthly fees.

life expectancy The most likely length of life for an individual.

lifespan The maximum possible length of life for a given species.

living will A document especially relating to the eventuality of terminal illness, in which a person can express his wishes and issue directions for his care, prior to the time he reaches a state where this is no longer possible.

long-term care insurance Pooled risk approach which intends to cover (primarily) the costs of long-term care either at home or in a nursing home.

long-term care (LTC) A spectrum of health care programs and services outside the acute hospital, ranging from home-based to community-based to institutional.

long-term care medicine The application of knowledge and skills about the problems of the elderly, coupled with knowledge and skills about choosing and applying the many possible people, services, therapies, programs, options, and plans that might help deal with those problems.

Medicaid Title XIX of the Social Security Act, which provides medical care for certain low-income individuals and families.

medical executive committee (MEC) In formal medical staff organizations, the governing body, whose responsibilities include major policy-making decisions and review and renewal of privilege requests.

medical bylaws A document which defines the responsibilities, prerogatives, criteria for membership, leadership, and circumstances of monitoring and discipline, for all those providing medical care in an institution. They are effectively a contract between individual practitioners and the facility, in that the individual must agree to abide by them as a condition of membership or privileges, and failure to keep that agreement has enforceable consequences.

medical director The most often used title for a physician administrator, especially in the **nursing home**. **Principal physician** has been used to describe the primary physician in proprietary facilities.

medical staff The collection of individuals, including physicians, dentists, podiatrists, or other associated health care professionals, providing medical care to patients in a hospital or long-term care facility.

Medicare Title XVIII of the Social Security Act, which covers hospital, physicians', and other medical services for most persons 65 and over, disabled persons, and persons with end-stage renal disease.

negligence A legal term referring to conduct performed without due care or in violation of commonly accepted standards of practice.

no-code orders Physician orders specifically referring to whether and to what extent attempts at resuscitation should be made in the event a person suffers cardiopulmonary arrest.

nondelegated status A **utilization review** term for an institution whose reviews are conducted by an outside review organization or third-party payor.

nondepartmental A type of medical staff arrangement in which physicians are simply all grouped together as staff members, rather than further assigned to specific departments or division.

nursing home (NH) The primary long-term institution, and a central force in the long-term care continuum, maintaining at least three inpatient beds and providing a minimum of one personal care service (e.g., help with eating, walking, correspondence, dressing, bathing, or using the toilet). Such facilities commonly offer around-the-clock medical and nursing care, as well as other social and activities services, at a higher level than residential care facilities, which emphasize protected living arrangements and minimal assistance with psychosocial, activity, and personal care needs. Commonly covers the **intermediate** and **skilled** levels of care.

old-old The term often used to describe those elderly over the age of 75, as opposed to the **young-old**, between the ages of 65 and 75.

organized medical staff Formal medical staff arrangements, including a structure, by-laws, a governing body, officers, and certain committees. Medical staffs may be organized to varying degrees, depending on size, goals, and commitment of physician members.

outcome In **quality assurance**, the observed results of care and related activities upon the health, status, and well-being of patients.

overutilization In **utilization review**, the placement of patients in beds or programs for which they are receiving more medical, nursing, and ancillary services than they need for their given functional levels, prognosis, and psychosocial status.

patient care plan In long-term care, a coordinated multidisciplinary approach to management of an individual, incorporating goals, objectives, correlation of assessments, and some objective means of measuring progress in relation to those goals.

patient data base A collection of information about a patient, based on the measurements, observations, and analyses of health care professionals, including physicians. Both a patient medical history and medications list, and the list of books about geriatrics in a medical library, are considered data bases; but, whereas the latter is provided *to* or *for* the physician by others, the patient data base is created *by* the physician along with other health professionals.

Patient Care and Services (PaCS) A long-term care survey instrument and program mandated by the Department of Health and Human Services, intended to examine actual outcomes of care as well as facility paper compliance with standards and regulations.

peer review An analysis of care delivered within a program or facility, based on an examination of care rendered to individuals, especially as reflected in documentation and outcome of treatment.

Peer Review Organizations (PROs) Organizations under contract to the federal government to perform utilization reviews on patients receiving health care paid for by federal programs. The review focuses on the appropriateness and adequacy of those services and the approval or denial of payment based on such reviews.

physician extenders Nonphysician professionals, such as the nurse practitioner and physician assistant, who assist physicians in their assessment and follow-up of elderly patients in private practice, NHs, or other outpatient and inpatient settings.

physician administrator A physician assuming a managerial role in a health care facility or program. The **medical director** is one major subgroup of physician administrators.

policies Broad goals, objectives, and directions for any group or organization, including why things are to be done in certain ways, and what is to be achieved. These are in turn further clarified and implemented by **procedures** or protocols.

president Commonly used term for the **chief executive officer** of organizations, governments, or businesses.

principal physician The primary administrative or advisory physician in many for-profit (**proprietary**) nursing homes.

procedures Formal descriptions of how to do things, and who is responsible for doing them; a way of implementing **policies**.

process In **quality assurance**, the activities and procedures which characterize a service or program.

proprietary The term to describe those nursing homes which are operated primarily for profit, as contrasted to the nonprofit **voluntary** or governmental facilities.

prospective reimbursement Payment for service which is determined before the accounting period begins; any surplus or deficit accrues to the provider.

protective services A collection of social, legal, and medical services to assist those elderly who are unable to manage for themselves, because of psychological, medical, or financial problems or limitations.

proxy consent Consent offered by one person on behalf of another, which may be: 1. specific authorization, 2. general authorization with instructions, 3. general authorization without instructions, 4. substitute judgment, or 5. deputy judgment.

quality assurance (QA) The defined and organized program by which health care professionals, administrators, owners, or boards strive to assure quality patient care in a program or facility.

quality assurance tools Orderly methods of data collection and analysis to facilitate complete, accurate, and time-efficient collection of information. Such tools may be: patient-oriented (measurements or examinations of patient feelings, attitudes, responses, or characteristics), facility-oriented (measurements or examinations of facility setup, organization, staffing, policies, procedures, etc.), or professional-oriented (measurements or examinations of the activities, decisions, prescriptions, conduct, or documentation of those caring for the patient or operating the facility).

quality of life The relative extent to which a person is able to enjoy life, understand or acknowledge surroundings and other persons, and be free of extremes of pain and discomfort. A frequently used criterion for making medical and ethical decisions about subsequent management of older patients.

quality assurance plan A set of policies and goals which defines the organization, function, process, standards, criteria, tools, and information sources used in any **quality assurance** program.

quality of care The most appropriate care and management of individuals, considering their needs, desires, and prognosis, as well as limits of time, cost, and staffing.

respite care A program of supervised short-term institutional placement of individuals usually cared for at home or in the community, often to allow caretakers to take vacations, enjoy a break from responsibilities, or deal with emergencies.

respondeat superior The legal doctrine under which a superior of a facility is held responsible for the actions or errors of a subordinate or an employee, regardless of whether the superior or facility was directly responsible for those actions or contributed to those errors.

retrospective reimbursement Payment for service which is determined at the end of the accounting period and usually based upon actual costs.

skilled nursing facilities (SNFs) Nursing facilities offering medical and nursing services at a more intense level than **intermediate care**, but not as intense as **acute** or **chronic hospital** levels.

standards In **quality assurance**, broad statements describing expected degrees of performance or accomplishment. Standards not only establish acceptable norms, but also specify acceptable deviations from those norms.

structure In **quality assurance**, how things are established and organized, and their constituent personnel or parts.

supplementary medical insurance Part B of Medicare, which may cover doctors' services, outpatient hospital care, outpatient physician and speech therapy, home health care, and other health services and supplies.

underutilization In **utilization review**, refers to placement of a patient at a level of care less than optimal for his functional impairments, or his need for diagnosis, assessment, treatment, and follow-up.

utilization management (UM) The planning, organizing, directing, and controlling of the health care product in a cost-effective manner while maintaining high quality care and contributing to the overall goals of the institution. This is accomplished through the judicious use of resources to control inappropriate inpatient admissions, lengths of stay, and use of ancillary services.

utilization review (UR) The monitoring arm of utilization management, referring to the process of evaluating the use of medical care, services, and resources according to certain criteria.

voluntary Term used to describe nonprofit, long-term-care facilities; usually, those owned and operated by governments or religious or community organizations.

young-old The term often used to describe those elderly under age 75, as opposed to the **old-old**, over the age of 75.

Strategy Worksheets

The LTC physician—especially, the medical director—has certain specific tasks to accomplish. These worksheets represent a concise summary of the ideas and recommendations throughout this book, encompassing the major tasks a medical director might need to manage, in a form usable for planning or strategy sessions.

Task: Find Proper Placement and Services for LTC Patient (Chapters 2 and 8)

What is the individual's medical diagnosis, current condition, and prognosis?

_____

_____

_____

What was done for the individual in the acute care setting?

_____

_____

_____

What is the individual's current functional status and overall functional capabilities?

_____

_____

_____

What are the individual's personal goals and objectives, and understanding of his situation?

_____

_____

_____

What are the goals and objectives of family or other responsible parties?

_____

_____

_____

What are realistic goals and objectives, based on the above considerations?

_____

_____

_____

What resources are already available for the individual?

_____

_____

_____

What additional community programs and resources are available?

_____

_____

_____

Does the individual need case management or referral?

_____

_____

_____

What is the individual's financial and insurance status?

_____

_____

_____

From what agencies or individuals do I need additional information, and to whom should I send reports or requests?

_____

_____

_____

What forms or certification must I complete to validate eligibility or need for certain programs or agencies?

_____

_____

_____

Which programs and resources would best meet the individual's condition and goals?

_____

_____

_____

Which other health care professionals and agencies can assist in the management of this case?

_____

_____

_____

Task: Establish a Geriatrics Service (Chapters 2 and 13)

What is the target population?

_____

_____

_____

What are the needs and desires of the community?

_____

_____

_____

What programs and services are already available?

_____

_____

_____

Which programs are to be included?

_____

_____

_____

Where will these programs be based?

_____

_____

_____

Who will be responsible for managing the individual programs?

_____

_____

_____

Who will be responsible for coordinating the overall service?

_____

_____

_____

What costs are involved in setting up the service?

_____

_____

_____

What reimbursements are available for the services provided?

_____

_____

_____

Who will staff the programs and services?

_____

_____

_____

What equipment and supplies will be needed?

_____

_____

_____

What are the current and future trends for the population to be served?

_____

_____

_____

What operational policies and goals are needed?

_____

_____

_____

How will the services and programs be monitored and evaluated?

_____

_____

_____

Which existing facilities and programs will be involved?

_____

_____

_____

How will the services and programs be arranged and operated?

_____

_____

_____

Task: Choose a Medical Staff for a Nursing Home (Chapter 3)

What are the goals and objectives of the ownership, board, community, and administrator?

_____

_____

_____

What are the needs of the facility's residents?

_____

_____

_____

What are the facility's programmatic goals?

_____

_____

_____

What is the extent of the interest and participation of community practitioners?

_____

_____

_____

Who else is available to provide medical care, consultation, and services?

_____

_____

_____

Will there be any academic participation or teaching programs?

_____

_____

_____

Will there be other medical responsibilities besides nursing home care?

_____

_____

_____

What will be the specific duties and expectations of attending physicians?

_____

_____

_____

What are the pertinent laws, regulations, and accreditation requirements regarding physician coverage and services?

_____

_____

_____

What reimbursement exists, or could be sought, for physician services?

_____

_____

_____

Will the staff be organized or informal?

_____

_____

_____

Will the staff be open or closed?

_____

_____

_____

Will any physicians be employees of the facility?

_____

_____

_____

Will there be multiple medical departments, or a single department with several divisions?

_____

_____

_____

Will there be a separate medical executive committee, or will these functions be performed by the staff as a whole?

_____

_____

_____

Will bylaws be needed, and if so, who will be responsible for writing them?

_____

_____

_____

What should be included in the bylaws?

_____

_____

_____

What will the criteria and qualifications be for medical staff membership?

_____

_____

_____

What medical procedures should be allowed at the facility?

_____

_____

_____

What will the procedures be for corrective and disciplinary actions against privileges, including hearings and appeals?

_____

_____

_____

Task: Organize a Long-Term Care Medical Department (Chapter 4)

What are the goals and objectives of the institution or program to be served by physicians?

_____

_____

_____

What is the governing structure of the institution?

_____

_____

_____

What is the governing structure of the medical staff?

_____

_____

_____

What are departmental goals and objectives?

_____

_____

_____

Will there be some full- or part-time salaried staff?

_____

_____

_____

What contractual arrangements must be made for departmental staff?

_____

_____

_____

What policies and procedures need to be created or revised?

_____

_____

_____

How should policies and procedures be organized into specific categories?

_____

_____

_____

What standards are needed for physician performance?

_____

_____

_____

Which criteria and tools will I use to measure performance against these standards?

_____

_____

_____

How will I collect and analyze information about physician performance?

_____

_____

_____

How will this department interact with others?

_____

_____

_____

What medical privileges and practices are permissible in this setting?

_____

_____

_____

What committees should there be, and how should they be used?

_____

_____

_____

Task: Establish a Role as a Medical Director (Chapters 3 and 4)

Is my role as a program manager, staff administrator, or both?

_____

_____

_____

What are my job responsibilities?

_____

_____

_____

To whom am I answerable and responsible?

_____

_____

_____

Who is answerable to me?

_____

_____

_____

Is the staff closed or open?

_____

_____

_____

What authority do I have to require certain performance, and to enforce those requirements?

_____

_____

_____

Can I do the job that needs to be done, given these current expectations of authority and responsibility?

_____

_____

_____

What changes are needed in expectations or support to provide me with the means to accomplish necessary goals?

_____

_____

_____

What are the standards for medical practice and other physician responsibilities for this setting?

_____

_____

_____

What should be included in my medical director's agreement?

_____

_____

_____

What should be included in agreements between me and other medical staff?

_____

_____

_____

What should be the structure, function, and frequency of medical meetings?

_____

_____

_____

What education and training do I need, now and in the future?

_____

_____

_____

What is my time commitment?

_____

_____

_____

How, and how much, will I be compensated?

_____

_____

_____

What are my legal and professional liabilities?

_____

_____

_____

What are my interactions with the ownership or board?

_____

_____

_____

What are my interactions with the administration?

_____

_____

_____

How can I enhance my working relationships with administration, ownership, and board?

_____

_____

_____

Task: Provide Quality Care for the LTC Patient (Chapters 5, 6, and 10)

What are the patient's diagnoses, and how have they been determined?

_____

_____

_____

Has an adequate medical workup of signs and symptoms been done to rule out treatable problems?

_____

_____

_____

What is the patient's level of function?

_____

_____

_____

What information do I need to know about the patient, and what can I provide?

_____

_____

_____

What are the patient's medications, and can any of them be reduced or changed?

_____

_____

_____

What are the patient's wishes, objectives, and goals?

_____

_____

_____

How well does the patient understand what is going on?

_____

_____

_____

Who are the other professionals working with the patient, and what can they contribute to the care?

_____

_____

_____

What are reasonable goals and prognosis for the patient?

_____

_____

_____

How can I best communicate information to patient, family, and other staff?

_____

_____

_____

What can I add to the overall patient care plan?

_____

_____

_____

Task: Manage Ethical Dilemmas Posed by the LTC Patient (Chapter 12)

What is the individual's medical condition and prognosis?

_____

_____

_____

What other pertinent social, psychological, ethical, functional, and legal information about this person exists or is needed?

_____

_____

_____

What is the patient's understanding of this information?

_____

_____

_____

What is the patient's capacity to understand and process this information?

_____

_____

_____

Which criteria and tools have I used to determine the patient's decision-making capacity?

_____

_____

_____

Are there any correctable physical factors affecting the patient's decision-making capacity?

_____

_____

_____

Are any judicial proceedings, such as guardianship, necessary?

_____

_____

_____

What do family or other potential decision makers know or understand?

_____

_____

_____

What additional information do I need to provide to help this understanding?

_____

_____

_____

What does the patient want, or what did he say previously that he would want now?

_____

_____

_____

Does the patient have a living will, or other identifiable statements of wishes or intent?

_____

_____

_____

What do family or other potential decision makers wish for the patient?

_____

_____

_____

What are my personal feelings about appropriate goals and actions for this person?

_____

_____

_____

What do other staff think and feel about appropriate goals and actions for this person?

_____

_____

_____

Which other staff should provide information and opinions in the ethical decision-making process?

_____

_____

_____

Are any professionals available to assist in the ethical decision-making process?

_____

_____

_____

Is there an ethics advisory committee that I can call on for assistance?

_____

_____

_____

What are the options for action regarding this person?

_____

_____

_____

What are the likely risks and benefits of these various options?

_____

_____

_____

What decision is most likely to accomplish the goals and objectives for this person?

_____

_____

_____

Task: Devise a Medical Quality Assurance and Utilization Review Program for a Nursing Home Setting (Chapter 6)

What are the goals and objectives of the community and the facility?

_____

_____

_____

What are the regulations, laws, and voluntary accrediting standards pertinent to this setting?

_____

_____

_____

What are the appropriate geriatric medical facts and standards which serve as the source of principles of accepted practice?

_____

_____

_____

What are the standards and criteria for appropriate utilization of resources and services?

_____

_____

_____

How can these utilization criteria be made a part of the overall QA program?

_____

_____

_____

How will patient goals and prognosis, laws and regulations, resources and costs, and staffing be incorporated into the QA and UR program?

_____

_____

_____

Who are the key participants in the QA and UR program, and are all necessary disciplines represented?

_____

_____

_____

Who will draft the standards and criteria for this particular program or facility?

_____

_____

_____

What elements of structure, process, and outcome should be incorporated into our standards and criteria?

_____

_____

_____

How can we measure outcome reliably among our patients?

_____

_____

_____

What tools will be used to collect and analyze information?

_____

_____

_____

What subjects and sites will be covered by our QA program?

_____

_____

_____

How will the collected data be analyzed, and by whom?

_____

_____

_____

How will the results of our QA and UR analyses be reported to the physicians, both individually and collectively?

_____

_____

_____

What corrective actions will be used to improve compliance?

_____

_____

_____

How will we use QA and UR as an educational tool?

_____

_____

_____

How will the institution's QA and UR activities be broadly overseen?

_____

_____

_____

How often should we review and revise our QA and UR plans?

_____

_____

_____

Who will act as physician advisor for UR issues?

_____

_____

_____

What activities or programs can improve medical decision making on utilization?

_____

_____

_____

Task: Implement a LTC Clinical Information System (Chapter 9)

What are the institutions and who are the persons involved in my program who would be involved in the gathering, interpretation, and reporting of information?

_____

_____

_____

How will the accuracy of the data collection be assured?

_____

_____

_____

How will terminology and definitions be standardized, so that different observers will come up with consistent results?

_____

_____

_____

How and where will information be stored, so that it can be readily retrieved?

_____

_____

_____

What methods will be used for accurate and rapid information retrieval, and report generation?

_____

_____

_____

How can diagnoses be validated?

_____

_____

_____

How can we improve the accuracy of clinical observations, and the description of those observations in the medical record?

_____

_____

_____

How can the flow of information be enhanced among the many persons and institutions involved in care of the LTC patient?

_____

_____

_____

How can we improve the accurate interpretation of raw data, to turn it into useful information?

_____

_____

_____

How can the rules of clinical decision making be made readily available in a form useful for interpreting raw data?

_____

_____

_____

Who wants which reports from our data, and what do they want those reports to contain?

_____

_____

_____

What information about geriatrics do the professionals need to manage patient care, and how can they best access and retrieve that information?

_____

_____

_____

What basic elements of information about each patient should be contained in the medical record?

_____

_____

_____

What conclusions or opinions does the physician need to place in the medical record, based on that information?

_____

_____

_____

What are some tactics to improve physician compliance with documentation requirements?

_____

_____

_____

How can the information from our system be transferred to other users, institutions, or systems?

_____

_____

_____

Task: Employ Computers for a Nursing Home Clinical Information System (Chapter 9)

What information-related tasks or goals need to be accomplished?

_____

_____

_____

What current information system, if any, is used, and what are its strengths and weaknesses?

_____

_____

_____

What hardware and peripherals (mass storage, printers, etc.) will be needed?

_____

_____

_____

Who is assigned to manage or oversee the maintenance and operations of the system?

_____

_____

_____

How will physicians have input into the design and implementation of the system?

_____

_____

_____

What must be done to prepare the current clinical information system for computerization?

_____

_____

_____

What resources, and who, is the facility willing to commit to the design and management of the system?

_____

_____

_____

What safeguards will be used to protect data and patient and staff privacy?

_____

_____

_____

How will computerized information be stored and retrieved?

_____

_____

_____

How easily can reports be designed and redesigned?

_____

_____

_____

How readily can the format for information storage be modified?

_____

_____

_____

How easily can new information be added?

_____

_____

_____

Who will use the computer, and what will they be permitted to put into it?

_____

_____

_____

What software is available, and which will best meet our needs?

_____

_____

_____

How can we access the outside data bases?

_____

_____

_____

How can we link physicians with patient information in the nursing home, offices, hospital, and other outpatient sites?

_____

_____

_____

How will we test the system for accuracy and reliability before we use it?

_____

_____

_____

What user instructions need to be designed before we begin use?

_____

_____

_____

Who will provide technical support and maintenance of the system?

_____

_____

_____

Task: Set Up a Teaching Nursing Home (TNH) Program (Chapter 13)

What preliminary work needs to be done to organize the program and the participants?

_____

_____

_____

What is the organizational structure of the TNH program, and how does it fit into the overall academic and nursing home organization?

_____

_____

_____

What are the components of the program?

_____

_____

_____

Who are the key personnel, both medical and nonmedical, clinical and administrative?

_____

_____

_____

Which professional schools will be involved, and how will these interact with the medical school?

_____

_____

_____

Who will be responsible for supervision of trainees?

_____

_____

_____

What will be the managerial, supervisory, clinical, teaching, and research roles of involved physicians?

_____

_____

_____

What are the lines of accountability of both faculty and trainees?

_____

_____

_____

What are the time commitments of faculty and trainees?

_____

_____

_____

What are the overt and hidden costs of the program?

_____

_____

_____

How will initial and ongoing funding be arranged?

_____

_____

_____

How will performance of faculty and trainees be monitored?

_____

_____

_____

How will the program affect facility staffing, and will additional staff be needed?

_____

_____

_____

How will program management decisions be made?

_____

_____

_____

How will the community practitioner be accommodated by, and participate in, the teaching program?

_____

_____

_____

What are outside and internal sources of funds for beginning and continuing such programs?

_____

_____

_____

What will be the affiliations and relationships of facilities with one another, and with outside agencies or programs?

_____

_____

_____

How will the program affect the overall care of the elderly in the facility and the community?

_____

_____

_____

How can the results, cost, benefits, and drawbacks of the program be measured and assessed?

_____

_____

_____

To whom will progress and evaluation reports need to be sent?

_____

_____

_____

Task: Meet LTC Professional Geriatric Education Needs (Chapter 10)

Which professionals and other staff are to be involved in education programs?

_____

_____

_____

What topics need to be covered?

_____

_____

_____

What educational tools and resources are available?

_____

_____

_____

What are the community educational interests and needs?

_____

_____

_____

What are the educational needs of individual patients?

_____

_____

_____

What are some forums for educational presentations appropriate to a given setting?

_____

_____

_____

How can quality assurance evaluations be used as an educational tool?

_____

_____

_____

What sources of reference and geriatric information are available?

_____

_____

_____

Index